Fundamentals of Sensory Physiology

Edited by Robert F. Schmidt

With Contributions by
Helmut Altner Josef Dudel Otto-Joachim Grüsser
Ursula Grüsser-Cornehls Rainer Klinke
Robert F. Schmidt Manfred Zimmermann

Translated by Marguerite A. Biederman-Thorson

Third, Revised and Expanded Edition

With 143 Figures, Most in Color

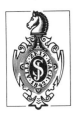

Springer-Verlag
Berlin Heidelberg New York Tokyo 1986

Robert F. Schmidt
Physiologisches Institut der Universität
Röntgenring 9, D-8700 Würzburg

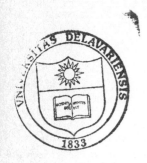

QP
431
.G8713
1986

Translation of „Grundriß der Sinnesphysiologie", 5. Auflage,
Heidelberger Taschenbücher, Band 136, 1985

ISBN 3-540-13225-2 5. Auflage Springer-Verlag Berlin Heidelberg New York Tokyo
ISBN 0-387-13225-2 5th Edition Springer-Verlag New York Heidelberg Berlin Tokyo

ISBN 3-540-15870-7 Springer-Verlag Berlin Heidelberg New York Tokyo
ISBN 0-387-15870-7 Springer-Verlag New York Heidelberg Berlin Tokyo

ISBN 3-540-10349-X 2. Auflage Springer-Verlag Berlin Heidelberg New York
ISBN 0-387-10349-X 2nd Edition Springer-Verlag New York Heidelberg Berlin

Library of Congress Cataloging-in-Publication Data
Grundriß der Sinnesphysiologie. English. Fundamentals of sensory physiology. Translation of: Grundriß
der Sinnesphysiologie. 5th ed. "Springer study edition." Bibliography: p. Includes index. 1. Senses and
sensation. I. Schmidt, Robert F. II. Altner, Helmut. III. Title.
QP431.G8713 1986 612'.8 85-30321
ISBN 0-387-15870-7 U.S.)

The use of general descriptive names, trade marks, etc. in this publication, even if the former are not
especially identified, is not be taken as a sign that such names, as understood by the Trade Marks and
Merchandise Marks Act, may accordingly be used freely by anyone.

Typesetting, printing and binding: Beltz, Hemsbach
2124/3140-543210

Preface to the Third Edition

Since 1978 this textbook, to the gratification of its authors and publisher, has found an undiminished readership. Recent research in sensory physiology has progressed so rapidly that this third edition, like the second, has required thorough revision. The understanding of pain, in particular, has increased to a remarkable degree. This development is reflected here in the appearance, for the first time, of a chapter devoted entirely to the subject "Nociception and Pain". In view of the great clinical significance of pain, it seemed necessary to broaden the scope of the discussion, so that in addition to the aspects directly related to sensory physiology consideration is given to the pathophysiology, pharmacology and psychology of pain.

The chapters present in earlier editions have also been carefully reexamined and, where necessary, revised and extended. Most of the illustrations provided for the first edition by the Stuttgart studio Gay & Benz have been retained. Some required alteration or replacement, and a number of new illustrations have been added. For the meticulous skill with which she transformed our ideas into graphs and drawings, we are most grateful to Mrs. Regine Gattung-Petith.

Our basic aim is unchanged – to give students with physiology as either a major or a minor subject an introduction, based on neurophysiology, to the fundamental physiological mechanisms underlying human sensations. We have taken care to keep the organization clear and the style of the text readable, despite the revision and expansion necessary to keep up with current developments. All the readers who, in surprisingly numerous letters, have conveyed their comments and suggestions have helped us greatly. We hope that we shall continue to receive assistance from this valuable source.

The test questions at the end of each section have also been reexamined and in part revised. Their purpose is not to familiarize the reader with this form of examination, which unfortunately is so popular today, but rather to provide an incentive for thinking over the material that has just been read. This active involvement in the learning process should not only assist memory but also raise ideas for further consideration.

On behalf of all the authors, I express sincere thanks for the help and support we have received from so many, above all our secretarial collaborators in the work of revision. Special thanks are due to Dr. M. A. Biederman-Thorson for her excellent translation, as well as to the production department of Springer-Verlag, Heidelberg, for efficient and congenial collaboration and to all the other members of the staff who, once again, have expertly guided the manuscript through the process of publication.

Würzburg, January 1986   Robert F. Schmidt

Preface to the First Edition

In the field of sensory physiology we are concerned with what our sense organs – and the associated central nervous structures – can do and how that performance is achieved. Research here is not limited to description of the physicochemical reactions taking place in these structures; the conditions under which sensations and perceptions arise and the rules that govern them are also of fundamental interest. Sensory physiology thus demands the attention of everyone who wishes to – or must – delve into the potentialities and limitations of human experience.

Our aim has been to guide the student with minimal prior training in biology and the other natural sciences into the realm of sensory physiology. Where other areas of neurophysiology are involved, reference is made to the companion volume produced by the same publisher, **Fundamentals of Neurophysiology** (2nd edition in English, 1978); the two together present an integrated introduction to the fascinating world of the neurosciences, with emphasis on its neurophysiologic and sensory physiologic aspects.

The first edition in English was translated from the third edition in German, which appeared in 1977. The two earlier editions in German, published in 1973 and 1976, were particularly well received by students of physiology, medicine, biology, and psychology. In preparing the third edition, we have carefully revised the text, expanded it in some places, and provided new illustrations throughout thanks to the help of Mr. Wolf-Rüdiger Gay and Mrs. Barbara Gay of Stuttgart, Germany. The book has thus been both brought up to date and made more readable. On behalf of all the authors, I express sincere thanks for the help and support that has been extended to us from all sides, especially by our secretarial co-workers.

Regarding this edition in English, I owe many thanks to Dr. Marguerite Biederman-Thorson of Oxford, England, for her excellent translation. Finally, I am most grateful to the publishers, Springer-Verlag, and their staff for their close collaboration and for the care they have taken in preparing the book.

Kiel, Germany, June 1978   Robert F. Schmidt

Table of Contents

List of Contributors

HELMUT ALTNER
Fachbereich Biologie
der Universität
Universitätsstraße 31
D-8400 Regensburg

JOSEF DUDEL
Physiologisches Institut der
Technischen Universität
Biedersteiner Straße 29
D-8000 München 40

OTTO-JOACHIM GRÜSSER
Physiologisches Institut
der Freien Universität
Arnimallee 22
D-1000 Berlin 33

URSULA GRÜSSER-CORNEHLS
Physiologisches Institut
der Freien Universität
Arnimallee 22
D-1000 Berlin 33

RAINER KLINKE
Zentrum der Physiologie
der Universität
Theodor-Stern-Kai 7
D-6000 Frankfurt 70

MANFRED ZIMMERMANN
II. Physiologisches Institut
der Universität
Im Neuenheimer Feld 326
D-6900 Heidelberg

1 General Sensory Physiology, Psychophysics

J. Dudel

As an introduction to the particular aspects of sensory physiology treated in this book, we shall consider the subject of "general sensory physiology" – the principles underlying all sensory perceptions. Such generalization is both possible and useful, not least because the different sense organs very much resemble one another, both in their organization and operation and in their connections to the central nervous system (CNS). On the other hand, in studying human sensory perception one encounters the *problem of subjectivity.* That is, environmental stimuli and the respective responses of our sense organs correspond to statements by the subject about his sensations and perceptions. Even muscle physiology, for example, has a subjective, "psychological" side. The subject identifies himself with certain movements of his limbs; he "wills" them or "expresses himself" with them. But by comparison, the high-level mental aspects of sensory physiology appear far richer and more fascinating. We experience our sensations as highly personal events, on which our moods depend; in surroundings from which sensory stimuli have been excluded – in a state of "sensory deprivation" – we become mentally unstable and ill. A human being, then, is "nothing other than the sum of his experiences" (D. Hume). Indeed, certain philosophical schools have been so impressed by the strong subjective component in all sensory experience as to maintain that only the subject exists – that the "environment" is a product of the mind. The general *psychophysical problem,* which so forcibly confronts us in sensory physiology, cannot be solved by the natural scientist, at least not yet. Psychophysical questions arise in very similar forms for all sense organs. Therefore a chapter on general sensory physiology should provide, along with a discussion of the basic organic mechanisms underlying sense-organ function, an introduction to the difficult questions of subjective sensory experience.

1.1 Basic Concepts in General Sensory Physiology

Sense organs. We experience our environment and the events taking place within our bodies not directly, and not in their entirety, but rather by way of specialized *sense organs.* The best known of these organs are the eye, the ear, the skin as an organ of touch, the tongue as an organ of taste, and the nose as an organ of smell. Each such organ is so constructed that it responds to a particular range of environmental influences and passes on corresponding information to the CNS.

The ranges of stimuli to which the sense organs are specialized can be explained in phylogenetic terms. Only those environmental events are detected that were *relevant to survival in the environment* of the primates from which we are descended. Consider, for instance, the electromagnetic waves striking the surface of the body. We experience no sensation of γ rays, X rays, or ultraviolet light. We can see, with our eyes, only light of wavelengths between 350 and 800 nm, to which the earth's atmosphere is relatively transparent. By contrast, we do not see infrared light; but we do sense long-wave heat rays by way of the heat sensors in the skin. Over the entire spectrum, radio waves elicit no sensations in humans. But other animals have adapted to habitats very different from ours by evolving other sense organs. For example, certain fish that live in very turbid water have a sense organ extremely sensitive to changes in electric field strength. With these they detect alterations in the electric field associated with pulses of current they themselves discharge. This information is used in orientation; the mechanism is like that of an echo-sounder or a radar installation.

Modality, quality, specific sensory stimuli. Each sense organ mediates sensory impressions that can vary in intensity but resemble one another in quality. A group of similar sensory impressions mediated by a particular organ is called a sense or, in a technically more precise term, a *modality.* Such modalities include the classic "five senses": sight, hearing, touch, taste, and smell. But it is easy to list other modalities. The skin itself senses not only pressure and touch, but also cold and warmth, vibration and pain. In addition to these modalities, comprising sensory impressions arising from the *external environment* and acting at the surface of the body, there are others mediated by sense organs within the body which reflect *its own state.* Examples of these are the sense of equilibrium and our knowledge of the relative positions of our limbs or the load on our muscles. Moreover, there are modalities associated with information about the state of our bodies of which we are not, or are only indirectly, aware. These include, among others, the osmotic pressure of the blood (thirst) or the blood's CO_2 tension (shortness of breath), as well as the amount of stretching of lungs and stomach. The definition of "modality" also holds for these interoceptive "senses". In each case they comprise a group of sensory impressions that resemble one another and are mediated by a particular kind of sense organ. The number of modalities, then, is far greater than five.

Within each individual modality, it is usually possible to draw further distinctions with regard to the kind of sensory impression, the *quality.* For example, the modality "vision" can be subdivided into the qualities lightness (position on the gray scale), red, green, and blue. Corresponding qualities in the sense of hearing are the different pitches of tones; the qualities of taste are sweet, sour, salty, and bitter.

A sensory impression of a certain quality is elicited when the appropriate environmental factors influence the sense organ. The quality "sour" is sensed when acids contact the tongue. The factors that elicit sensory impressions of a certain quality are called *specific sensory stimuli,* or simply *stimuli.* The stimulus acquires its quality by virtue of the reaction with the stimulus-detecting cells of the sense organs, the ***receptors.*** These cells are adapted to respond as strongly and specifically as possible to stimuli of their particular quality, both because of their positions and because of the presence of specialized cell organelles. The sense organs are located at sites exposed to their specific stimuli — the taste receptors on the tongue, and the light receptors in the retina of the eye, in the focal plane of a lens. The different kinds of receptor have special properties that guarantee the greatest possible effect of the specific stimulus quality. Again, take the visual cells of the retina as examples. Each contains a pigment that absorbs light of "its" particular quality. The details of this specialization of receptors for specific qualities are described in the next chapter. In general, the specific stimuli produce potential changes in the receptor cells, the receptor potentials (see Fig. 1–1); these in turn generate action potentials (cf. ***Fundamentals of Neurophysiology,*** Sec. 2.4) that are conducted to the centers via afferent nerve fibers. These action potentials are the same for all sensory qualities. The quality of the information they contain is determined entirely by the receptor type from which the relevant nerve fiber arises. Even when such receptors are stimulated by a strong "unspecific stimulus" it is interpreted as specific: when struck on the eye we see light — "stars." As long ago as the last century Johannes Müller formulated the "law of specific nerve energies" to describe this phenomenon.

Quantity, threshold. Whereas the kind of sensory impression is given by its modality and quality, its intensity can be termed ***quantity.*** The quantity of a sensory impression corresponds to the strength of the stimulus. Figure 1–1 shows the general nature of the response of a receptor to stimuli of increasing intensity. The receptor potential becomes larger, and the frequency of the triggered action potentials increases. Figure 1–1 B shows the relationship between stimulus intensity and the response elicited from a receptor. Such relations can be determined at various levels of the nervous system, as well as for subjective impressions and perceptions. The point of origin of the intensity/response curve is always an important characteristic; this is the smallest stimulus that just produces a response, the ***threshold stimulus*** S_0. In the case of the receptor cell, this may be determined as the smallest stimulus that just elicits an action potential (Fig. 1–1); it can also be measured, for example, in the auditory organ as the lowest intensity of a tone that is just perceived by a subject. The form of the intensity/response curve is characteristic of different receptors as well as of different sensory impressions; this aspect of the relationship will be discussed further in later sections.

We have now become acquainted with a number of the basic concepts of sensory physiology: modality, quality, quantity, and threshold. Figure 1–2 illustrates the correspondence between these concepts and their organic substrate, again using the example of the organ of sight.

Sensory impressions are characterized not only by modality, quality, and quantity; they also have the property of occurring at a ***particular time and place*** in the environment or in the body. Our eyes do not simply see light, but rather "pictures" of the space surrounding us. These pictures succeed one another in time, and they can also be recalled as having been associated with a particular point

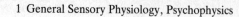

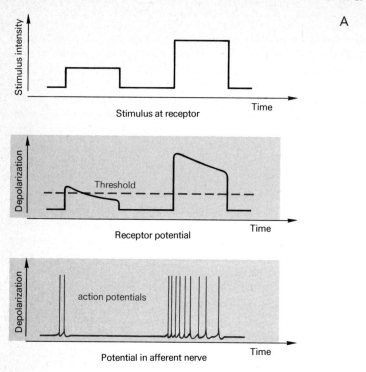

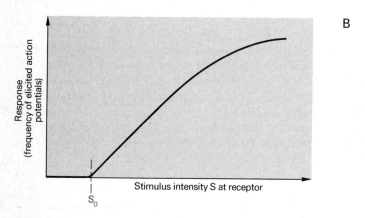

Fig. 1–1 A, B. Relationships between stimulus intensity and frequency of action potentials. **A** Time course of the receptor potentials and action potentials elicited by two stimuli of different intensity. **B** Dependence of the frequency F of action potentials in a receptor upon stimulus strength S. S_0 indicates the absolute threshold intensity of the stimulus

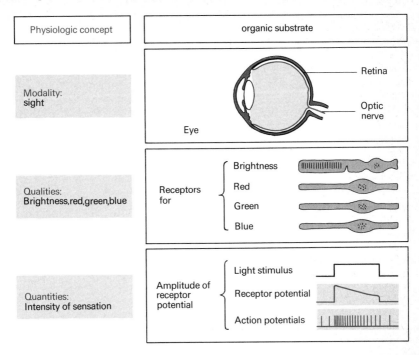

Fig. 1–2. Modality, quantity, quality, and their organic substrates; here the organ of vision is taken as an example

in time. The spatial and temporal aspects of sensory perceptions naturally correspond to the spatial and temporal properties of the stimuli.

Sensory impression, perception. The term *sensory impression,* which we have been using casually thus far, must now be explained more precisely. It is used to designate the simplest units, the elements of sensory experience. For instance, the perceived color "blue" and the taste "sweet" would be sensory impressions. It rarely happens that we receive such impressions in isolation; a combination of such sensory impressions is called a sensation. As a rule the pure sensation is accompanied by an interpretation, with reference to what has been experienced and learned, and the result is called *perception.* We express a perception when we say, "There is a chair".

Mapping between phenomenon and perception; objective and subjective sensory physiology. The chain of correspondences between the phenomena of the environment and their perception, indicated in the last paragraphs, is summarized in Figure 1–3. The boxes enclose basic phenomena of sensory physiology at successive levels; they are joined by arrows which indicate correspondence, not causality. The arrows stand for a relation that is called "mapping". That is, the excitation in a nerve can be regarded as a mapping of a sensory stimulus, and

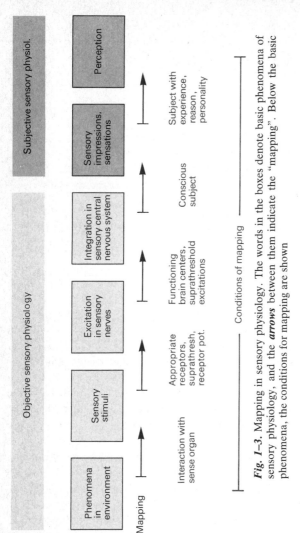

Fig. 1–3. Mapping in sensory physiology. The words in the boxes denote basic phenomena of sensory physiology, and the **arrows** between them indicate the "mapping". Below the basic phenomena, the conditions for mapping are shown

perception as a mapping of sensory impressions. The concept "mapping" denotes that there is a defined and unique representation by which points on an object are associated with (or "mapped onto") points on another, or more generally in mathematical terms, a unique association between members of two sets ($x \varepsilon A \mapsto y \varepsilon B$). The object itself is not the cause of its representation; the mapping may occur by means of a suitable device, for example, an aerial camera which projects an image of the object onto photographic paper. The mapping therefore is not only characterized by the object, but also by the special mapping conditions, the surveyor's instruments, the scale, the kind of projection, or the symbols of representation for specific details.

Thus under the boxes that denote the different levels in Figure 1–3 are listed the conditions that hold for mapping in each case. Environmental phenomena (at the *left* in Fig. 1–3) are sensory stimuli only if they interact with a suitable sense organ. Similarly, Figure 1–3 indicates that the excitation sent from a sense organ to the CNS and processed there becomes a sensory impression or sensation only if the CNS is associated with a subject capable of consciousness. The mapping relationship indicated by the arrows in Figure 1–3, from environmental phenomena to the integrative processes in the sensory CNS, can in principle be described as physical and chemical processes in the structures of the body. This realm of sensory physiology is therefore called *objective sensory physiology.* By contrast, the mapping between these objective phenomena — a sensory stimulus and the subsequent responses of the nervous system — and a conscious sensation cannot be described in terms of physical and chemical processes. The realm of sensations and perceptions, as it is related to sensory stimuli, is therefore termed *subjective sensory physiology.*

The proposition that subjective sensation and perceptions are not accessible to description in physicochemical terms must be qualified. From the point of view of the natural sciences, such an assertion is simply a statement of the present state of knowledge. The natural scientist will attempt to apply his methods to subjective phenomena as well, and there are impressive examples of success, as the discussion of *psychophysics* in Sections 1.3 and 1.4 shows. However, many professionals in other academic areas think that the response of the subject, the realm of the psyche, is fundamentally inexplicable in the framework of the natural sciences.

Sensory physiology, then, is divided into two parts: the description of the responses of the nervous system to a stimulus — objective sensory physiology, and analysis of the statements the subject makes about his sensations and perceptions — subjective sensory physiology. The terms *objective* and *subjective* in this context ought *by no means to be taken as value judgments* with regard to the correctness of a statement. The sentence "red is a warm color" can be just as "correct" as the sentence "the frequency of discharge in the sensory nerve fiber rises with the intensity of a sensory stimulus." As biologists, and especially as scientists who study humans, we must treat subjective statements about sensations and perceptions in just as unprejudiced a way as we do recordings of cell potentials. Section 1.3 will show that it is possible to make very precise statements, using the appropriate terms, about the objects of subjective sensory physiology; quantitative mathematical relationships can be established in this field as well. Even though the relation between stimulus and sensation can only be described by the term "mapping", and the qualitative distinction between physical stimulus and subjective sensory impression seems unbridgeable, the study of sensory physiology can employ the *methods of behavioral physiology,* briefly treated in the next section, to serve a certain *mediatory function* between physics and subjectivity.

By answering the following questions (designated by "Q" here and throughout the book) you can test your knowledge of the subject matter of the section. In deciding upon your answer, you should wherever possible not refer back to the text. Jot down your answers on a sheet of paper and then compare them with the Answer Key beginning on p. 277

Q 1.1. A group of sensory impressions that resemble one another and are mediated by a particular sense organ is called... When sensory impressions of different kinds can be distinguished within a modality, they are termed...

Q 1.2. Identify the words in the following list that designate modalities with M, those that designate qualities with Q, and those that represent quantities with I.
a) Hearing (   )
b) Intensity of sound (   )
c) Red (   )
d) Taste (   )
e) Stretching of the lungs (   )
f) Sour (   )
g) Pitch (   )
h) Intensity of the color red (   )
i) Cutaneous cold sense (   )

Q 1.3. Choose the term that best describes the relationship between a sensory stimulus and the sensation:
a) Cause and effect
b) Objectivity
c) Mapping
d) Increase in specificity
e) Quality

1.2 Relation Between Stimulus and Behavior; Conditioned Reflex

The central nervous reactions elicited by a sensory stimulus may lead to responses of the whole organism, which may be directed outward or inward. If one hears an unexpected noise on one side, one turns the head in that direction; a deer in the woods behaves in just the same way. When monkeys in a zoo see their keeper at feeding time, they become restless and noisy. The appearance of some obstruction when we are driving causes us not only to brake and swerve aside; muscle tonus is also increased, and the heart beats faster. In all these examples, specific sensory stimuli have given rise to more or less complex changes in the activity of the animal or man. Such activities, usually *interpretable as goal-directed,* are in general termed *behavior.* Changes in behavior resulting from a sensory stimulus can be described by an observer, and they can also be recorded by appropriate measuring devices. We regard such behavioral changes as explicable, in principle, by the responses of the animal's nervous system to the stimulus, even though we may not yet understand these responses in detail. Studies of behavior from the point of view of sensory physiology are thus a part of objective sensory physiology. Certain basic concepts and methods in this area, an area also in the domain of animal psychology and the psychology of learning, will be surveyed here.

Stimulus, behavior, reflex. If the hindpaw of a cat is stimulated painfully (for example, by pinching), it will pull the paw away by bending the joints of the leg. This behavior of the cat is called the flexor reflex in neurophysiology (cf. *Fundamentals of Neurophysiology,* p. 168). Part of an animals's behavior, then, consists of stereotyped reactions to certain stimuli, the *reflexes* (*Fundamentals of Neurophysiology,* p. 106). Among the reflexes some (for instance, the flexor reflex) are *innate* or *unconditioned,* being based on fixed neuronal connections between receptors and effectors. But in the context of sensory physiology, the *acquired reflexes* are of particular interest. In these reflexes, the functional connection between receptors and effectors is formed by *learning processes.* The animal learns to respond regularly to a certain stimulus with a certain activity. Such reflexes are also called *conditioned,* because they are found only under the condition of previous learning. An example is the "automatic" braking by an automobile driver confronted with an obstacle.

Conditioning. The acquisition of conditioned reflexes by many animals can easily be examined in the laboratory. The first procedure for doing this was developed by PAVLOV, and is called the *classic conditioning procedure.* In this method an unconditioned reflex is first triggered — for example, a dog is offered food, and the flow of saliva is thereby excited. Then the stimulus for the unconditioned reflex (the presentation of food in this example) is repeatedly accompanied by an arbitrarily selected second stimulus; for example, a bell may be rung at the same time the food appears. If this combination is repeated frequently, the dog will eventually respond by salivating when the ringing of the bell occurs by itself; at that stage, a *conditioned reflex* has been formed. That is, in the classic conditioning procedure the association between the adequate stimulus for an unconditioned reflex and an arbitrarily chosen test stimulus makes the latter a stimulus for a conditioned reflex.

This method of classic conditioning has the disadvantage that the experimental animal acquires the conditioned reflex passively by association. Conditioned reflexes can more easily be developed by the process of *operant conditioning.* In operant conditioning the desired response to a stimulus (i. e., the conditioned reflex that is the goal of the training) is rewarded – for instance, by a small amount of food. The reward *reinforces* the behavior, and the animal quickly learns to respond to the test stimulus with the correct conditioned reflex. The procedure of operant conditioning resembles that in other types of training, in which suitable rewards (or punishments) are used in connection with certain patterns of behavior. But *in contrast to the training* of horses or dogs, in operant conditioning the role of a human "trainer" is eliminated as far as possible. Conditioning is done by apparatus that automatically gives the stimulus, records the response, and presents the reward in accordance with the set criteria. A well-known example of such an apparatus was developed by SKINNER and is called the "Skinner box"; this can be used to condition various kinds of small animals (Fig. 1–4). It consists of a cage for the experimental animal, with a stimulus display on the front wall. In the example shown this is a light. On the same wall a lever is mounted, and the animal is supposed to learn to press this lever when the stimulus is presented. A further attachment to this wall, in the cage of Figure 1–4, is a food container. An automatic device places a portion of food into the container as a reward, whenever the correct response, pressing on the lever, follows the selected stimulus.

Another element of the Skinner box in Figure 1–4 is a recording instrument that keeps track of the rate of correct responses to the test stimuli given repeatedly in a program over a certain time. From the record one can see how rapidly and to what extent the conditioned reflex has been learned; the *learning curve* from such an experiment is shown at the top of the figure. On every day of the experiment (abscissa) the test stimulus was given 100 times, and the percentage of correct responses (ordinate) was recorded. The diagram shows that the curve rises during the first days, then flattens out and after about 10 days reaches a plateau of nearly 100% correct responses.

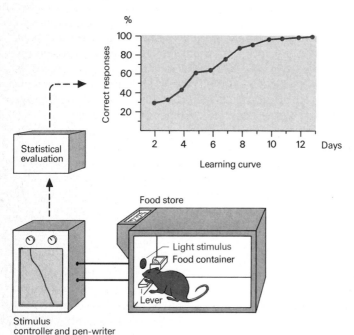

Fig. 1–4. Operant conditioning in a Skinner box. The experimental animal can respond to a stimulus presented via the controlling apparatus by pushing the lever, and is then automatically rewarded with food. The stimuli and their consequences are recorded on the pen-writer. Above the Skinner box is a learning curve derived from such records, with days since the start of conditioning on the abscissa and the percentage of correct responses to the test stimulus on the ordinate

An advantage of devices like the Skinner box is that large numbers of them can be set up in parallel and that the experimental program – the test stimuli and the criteria for the correct response — for such an array can be automatically controlled. Today such experiments are usually controlled by computers, which also perform the statistical evaluation of the results. The test stimuli used in such programs can be varied over a wide range, which is particularly important in the experiments in sensory physiology that will now be discussed. The procedure of *operant conditioning* of reflexes, however, has also been used very successfully in *other fields.* Experimental psychologists study learning behavior, pharmacologists determine the effects of drugs on learning and on the performance of the conditioned reflexes, biochemists block enzyme systems, and neurophysiologists measure changes in the pattern of neural discharge during the learning process.

Measurement of dark adaptation by operant conditioning. As an example of the relation between behavior and sensory stimulus, we shall now consider in detail the way the method of operant conditioning can be used to determine the increase in sensitivity of the visual sense of a pigeon as it adjusts to darkness — the process of *dark adaptation.* As you know from personal experience, we see "nothing" when we suddenly move from bright sunlight into a dimly lit room. But once we have spent some time in the room, we can gradually detect more and more objects in our surroundings; the sensitivity of our vision increases. We have *adapted* to the lower light level (for further discussion see Sec. 1.4). The experiment to be described now is designed to determine whether a similar dark-adaptation process occurs in the pigeon.

Before the experiment itself is begun, two conditioned reflexes are established: The pigeon pecks key A (in the arrangement of Fig. 1–5 A) when it sees a stimulus light, and key B when it sees no stimulus light. Control of the stimuli in the apparatus is set up in such a way that closing of a contact by depression of key A reduces the intensity of the stimulus light somewhat, while closing of the contact at key B has the reverse effect. Now, when the stimulus light shines brightly at the beginning of the experiment the pigeon will peck key A, and it continues to do so until the intensity of the light becomes so low that it is no longer visible to the bird. When the pigeon sees no stimulus light, according to its previous training, it will peck key B. The stimulus-controlling arrangement then increases the light intensity, and key B will be pecked until the pigeon again sees the stimulus light. Operating both keys in this way, the pigeon will set the light at an intensity that fluctuates about the threshold intensity. Figure 1–5 A, then, shows a method for the *measurement of the absolute visual threshold* of the pigeon, by means of two quite complex learned behavior patterns.

The same apparatus can be used to measure the *dark-adaptation curve.* Before the experiment of Figure 1–5 B, the pigeon is kept in brightly lit surroundings; when the experiment is begun, the experimental chamber is darkened. By pecking the two keys, A and B, the pigeon continually resets the light intensity to correspond to its absolute visual threshold; the change in this threshold as the experiment progresses is shown in Figure 1–5 B. Shortly after the room is darkened

A

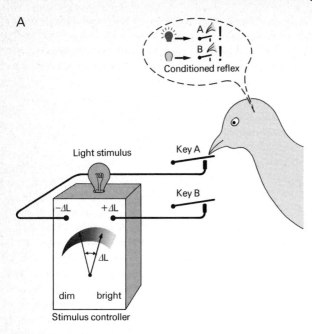

B

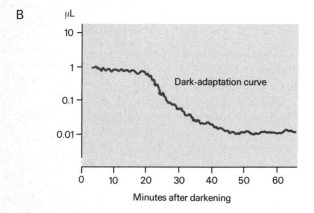

Minutes after darkening

Fig. 1–5 A, B. Determination of the visual threshold in a behavioral experiment on a pigeon. *A* Diagram of the experimental arrangement. The pigeon pecks key *A* when it sees light, and as a result the next light stimulus is reduced. Pecking of key *B*, when no light is visible, increases the next light stimulus. *B* Gradual change in the threshold stimulus intensity set by the pigeon, after the bright background illumination is switched off. Modified from BLOUGH: J. Comp. Physiol. Psychol. *49,* 425 (1967)

the threshold is about 1 microlumen (μL; note the logarithmic scale on the ordinate). The threshold does not remain constant; in the first 20 min it declines slowly, but then a more rapid decline sets in, until after 50–60 min a constant level of 0.02 μL is reached. During *dark adaptation*, then, in 1 h the *absolute threshold* has fallen to about 1/100 of the value in the light-adapted pigeon. This *dark-adaptation curve* measured by means of conditioned reflexes in the pigeon closely resembles, in form and time course, the corresponding curve measured in humans by methods of subjective sensory physiology(cf. Fig. 5–17).

Similar behavioral experiments can be used to determine other threshold values, by establishment of the appropriate conditioned reflexes. For example, the technique has been used to measure visual thresholds at different wavelengths of light in mammals, frogs, fish, birds, and even octopus, so that the absorption curves of the *visual pigments* used by these animals could be characterized. Correspondingly, after suitable conditioning *auditory thresholds* or *tone-discrimination thresholds* can be determined. The threshold for tone discrimination is the smallest difference in pitch (frequency) of two tones for which the tones can just be determined to be different. That is, it characterizes the ability to distinguish tones. A procedure for the measurement of a *tone-discrimination threshold,* in analogy with the dark-adaptation curve in Figure 1–5 B, would be roughly as follows: The animal is trained to perform behavior A when two identical tones are heard in succession, and behavior B when the two successive tones are different. The stimulus consists of a reference tone and a subsequent, variable comparison tone. The stimulus control operates so that following behavior A the difference in pitch is increased, and after behavior B it is decreased. Thus the tone-discrimination threshold associated with the reference tone will automatically be set.

By establishing appropriate conditioned reflexes, then, very detailed *studies of the sensory physiology* of animals can be made. Many of the rules governing sensory physiology to be presented in the next section as pertaining to human "subjective sensory physiology" can also be demonstrated in this way in animals as a *relation between stimulus and behavior*, though we cannot mention further examples here. In the area of subjective sensory physiology it is usually verbal statements about sensations and perceptions that are related to the sensory stimuli (Fig. 1–3). But *speaking* is nothing other than a *form of behavior.* The method for determining tone-discrimination thresholds described in the preceding paragraph could thus be applied in the same way to a behavioral experiment on an animal and to the subjective sensory physiology of a human. Behavior A would simply amount to the subject's statement "I hear one tone," and behavior B would be the statement "I hear two tones." Formally, then, the natural scientist could regard subjective sensory physiology as a special chapter of the sensory physiology of animal behavior.

Our sensations and perceptions are accompanied by the consciousness of our *subjectivity* and our *identity,* and many believe that this constitutes the specifically human aspect of our responses to phenomena in our environment and to sensory stimuli (see Fig. 1–3). To me, as a natural scientist, it seems very difficult to ascertain whether animals also have some consciousness of subjectivity and identity. But if this should be the case, the difference between the subject of this section and that of the next would be a quantitative rather than a qualitative one.

Q 1.4. Give a definition, in your own words, of the conditioned reflex.

Q 1.5. Which of the following statements apply to the procedure of operant conditioning?
a) The conditioned reflex is reinforced by rewarding the correct response.
b) The test stimulus is paired with the adequate stimulus for an innate (unconditioned) reflex and by repetition of the procedure becomes the stimulus for a conditioned reflex.
c) A conditioned reflex becomes an unconditioned reflex by frequent repetition.
d) The conditioned reflex is established by active collaboration of the animal.

Q 1.6. The learning curve of a conditioned reflex:
a) Describes the frequency of mistakes as a function of the difficulty of the task
b) Describes the frequency of correct responses as a function of the time spent in practice
c) Is flat at first and later rises rapidly
d) Is steep at first and eventually reaches a plateau
e) Can be determined only for higher animals

Q 1.7. Which of the following procedures is (are) suitable for determining the point visual acuity (the smallest distance between two dots at which they can be detected as separate) of a cat?
The cat has learned to press lever A when it sees *one* dot, and lever B when it sees *two* dots.
a) The stimulus-control apparatus is programmed so that pairs of dots varying in separation from 0 to 5mm are presented in random sequence. The dot separation at which the cat presses lever A exactly as often as lever B ist point visual acuity.
b) The stimulus-control apparatus is arranged in such a way that when the cat presses lever A the distance between the two dots is increased, and when it presses lever B, the distance is reduced. After a large number of trials the separation is set at a value corresponding to the point visual acuity.

1.3 Measurement of the Intensity of Sensations; Psychophysics

In *subjective sensory physiology* we are concerned with the statements a human being makes about external phenomena. As experiments, we present him with specific sensory stimuli and record what he says. As long as the hypotheses proposed on the basis of these statements are testable by the results of further experiments — that is, as long as the hypotheses can possibly be ruled out experimentally (cf. K. R. Popper's doctrine of falsifiability) — subjective sensory physiology is an area of natural science; as such, it is often termed *"psychophysics"*. It is also possible to treat sensory experience in a way oriented more toward the humanities, as may be done in Gestalt psychology, esthetics, or epistemology. Here we shall consider only the psychophysical side of subjective sensory physiology.

As far as the methodologic approach to subjective sensory physiology is concerned, we can in principle ignore all that we know about sense organs, receptors, and centers in the brain — our interest is directed entirely toward the response of the human subject to a sensory stimulus. Nevertheless, subjective and objective sensory physiology cross-fertilize one another to an extraordinary degree. Most of the questions asked in objective sensory physiology were originally formulated on the basis of discoveries in the subjective branch of the field; in many areas the two approaches give results that can be correlated, and often new findings from objective experiments can be verified in the form of subjective experiences.

The remainder of this chapter can give but a brief *introduction* to general subjective sensory physiology. In the chapters concerned with the individual sense organs special results of subjective sensory physiology are presented. Here we shall cite only a few principles and illustrate them by examples. We shall pay particular attention to the measurement of the intensity of sensations in this section, and in the next turn to the spatial and temporal aspects.

Subjective measures. In objective sensory physiology, both the strength of the stimulus and the amplitude of the response can be measured by physical or chemical means. The intensity of a taste stimulus, for instance, can be given in terms of the concentration of a stimulus substance in a solution, in millimoles per liter, and the response to the stimulus can be determined as the frequency of action potentials in a nerve from the tongue. By contrast, subjective experiments cannot use the physical/chemical measurement system to establish the intensity of the sensation resulting from a stimulus. Therefore a new *subjective measurement system* must be introduced.

A system of measurement must have a defined elementary unit and a fixed procedure by which a particular number of such units can be assigned to the quantity to be measured. Therefore appropriate units must be established for the various sensations. One such subjective *unit*, frequently selected, is the *absolute threshold for sensation;* this is taken as the reference intensity of sensation, and other degrees of sensation are expressed as multiples of that threshold sensation. But one can also establish a standard sensation by using as a unit of sensation that level elicited by a unit stimulus. Three important methods used to quantify the intensity of sensations will now be described.

Estimation of the multiple of a sensation intensity. One possible way of determining the intensity of a sensation is in terms of the subject's *estimate* of how much

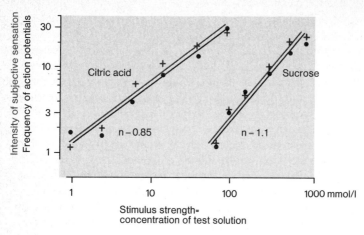

Fig. 1–6. Dependence of the subjective intensity of the sensation of taste *(red, crosses)* and of the frequency of the action potentials in fibers of the nerve mediating taste *(black, circles)* upon the concentration of citric acid and of sucrose solution. The scales of both ordinate and abscissa are logarithmic. The slopes of the lines correspond to the exponents n of power functions with $n = 0.85$ and 1.1. Modified from Borg et al.: J. Physiol. *192*, 13–20 (1967)

stronger a given sensation to be measured is, as compared with a standard sensation unit. Since this procedure involves the ratio between the sensation and a unit sensation, it is also termed the establishment of a **ratio scale.** Figure 1–6 illustrates an example of the procedure. The subjects were told to taste solutions of citric acid or sugar, in the concentrations indicated on the abscissa. They then said how many times stronger the test solution tasted than a standard solution offered for comparison. The subjective intensity of sensation thus obtained is indicated (on the ordinate) by the red crosses. The data points can be quite well approximated by straight lines. Ordinate and abscissa are both logarithmic, so that the straight lines correspond to power functions; the sensation intensity I is proportional to the nth power of the suprathreshold stimulus $(S - S_0)$:

$$I = k \cdot (S - S_0)^n \qquad (1\text{--}1)$$

where k is a constant and S_0 the threshold of the stimulus. To see why this represents a straight line, note that if one takes logarithms of both sides of Eq. (1–1),

$$\log I = n \cdot \log (S - S_0) + k' \qquad (1\text{--}2)$$

where k' (equal to $\log k$) is another constant; thus $\log I$ is a linear function of $\log (S - S_0)$. The slope of the straight line obtained by plotting the intensities of both stimulus and sensation on logarithmic scales (as in Fig. 1–6) is given by the exponent n. In the case of citric acid n is 0.85, and for sugar solutions it is 1.1; this difference is found routinely even in different subjects.

Power functions like those of Eq. (1–1) can describe the relations between stimulus and intensity of sensation over wide ranges; they are called *Stevens' power functions* after their discoverer. In the area of objective sensory physiology, too, the relationship between the intensities of a stimulus and a response can often be described by Eq. (1–1). For comparison, Figure 1–6 includes an example of such a result.

That is, Figure 1–6 shows not only the dependence of *intensity of sensation* upon *stimulus intensity,* but also the *neural response* to the stimulus. It was possible to obtain these data because the subjects were patients who required an operation on the middle ear (stapes mobilization) to treat a hearing difficulty. As part of the surgical procedure, the nerve (chorda tympani) in which taste fibers pass from tongue to brain is exposed. During the operation action potentials could be recorded from this nerve, as a quantitative measure of the neural response to taste stimuli. The *action-potential frequencies* thus determined are plotted as the black circles in Figure 1–6. These data can also be approximated by straight lines, with the same exponent n that was found in subjective measurement. That is, in the *mathematical description* there is a very extensive *agreement* between the *subjectively estimated* intensity of sensation and the *objectively determined* intensity of response of the sensory neurons.

Cross-modality comparison of intensity. In the experiment of Figure 1–6, the intensity of sensation was estimated as a multiple of the sensation elicited by a standard stimulus. Many subjects find it difficult to make numerical statements about such relations. This difficulty can be circumvented by using a procedure in which the intensities of two modalities are compared, an example of which is given in Figure 1–7. In this experiment the subject is required to press his hand against a force meter (a hand dynamometer) with such a strength that the pressure corresponds (subjectively) to the intensity of sensation elicited by a test stimulus — for instance, a tone. The loudness of the tone as sensed by the subject is measured in terms of the amount of pressure exerted by the hand — that is, intensities are compared intermodally. Figure 1–7 shows the sensation intensities thus measured for many different modalities, represented as "hand pressure" on the ordinate as a function of the various stimulus intensities on the abscissa. The data for each modality, plotted in this double-logarithmic coordinate system, lie on a straight line; that is, they can be described by power functions. The steepest slope is obtained in the case of pain produced by the application of electric currents to the skin. This slope corresponds to an exponent n (of the power function) greater than 1. The other extreme is represented by the sensation of light; here the exponent is much less than 1.

The magnitudes of the exponents for the various *modalities* are considered in the chapters on the individual sense organs. Here we shall simply point out that these relationships are open to functional interpretation. For example, when a pain or heat stimulus increases, the intensity of the sensation rises markedly (n

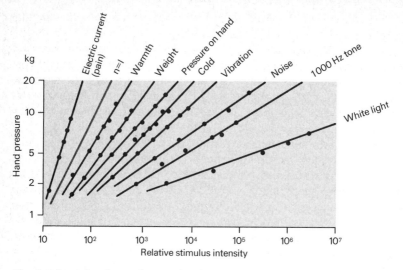

Fig. 1–7. Intensity of sensation as a function of stimulus intensity. The sensation intensity was measured by cross-modality intensity comparison, using the force exerted upon a hand dynamometer (ordinate). On the abscissa, the intensity of stimuli of the various forms is given in arbitrary units. The scales of both ordinate and abscissa are logarithmic, so that the straight lines correspond to power functions. Modified from STEVENS: Am. Sci. **48,** 226–253 (1960)

greater than or equal to 1); such sensations have the character of a **warning** against more severe damage. On the other hand, it is plausible in terms of function that in the case of light stimuli, which range in amplitude over 5–6 decades, the intensity of sensation increases relatively gradually and thus enables a given range of sensations to correspond to a wider range of stimuli.

Cross-modality intensity comparisons, then, permit precise and extensive measurements of the intensity of sensation for different modalities. As Figure 1–7 shows, this procedure gives exponents n of the power function which agree very well with those obtained in the procedure described above — the estimation of the relation to a standard stimulus. Another notable property is that the relationship between the neural response and the stimuli — measured by the techniques of objective sensory physiology –reveals exponents very like those resulting from the subjective procedures in both Figure 1–6 and Figure 1–7.

Measurement by means of difference-threshold steps. A third procedure used in subjective sensory physiology is that in which intensity of sensation is expressed as the number of **difference-threshold steps** needed to go from the absolute threshold (or another standard) to the intensity to be measured. The difference threshold (or difference limen) is the smallest change in the stimulus parameter that can just be detected. It is often called the "just noticeable difference" (j. n. d.). Intensity measurements on this basis are made as follows: First the threshold stimulus intensity for the form of stimulus to be measured is determined for the individual subject. This absolute threshold is assigned the value "1." Then the stimulus intensity is increased until the subject detects a change. This difference threshold is assigned the value "2". This procedure is repeated until the sensation has reached the intensity to be measured; the sensation at this stimulus intensity is given the value N_i. If N_i is thus determined for various sensation intensities, the *dependence of sensation intensity N_i upon stimulus intensity* can be plotted. Here again one obtains a power function, with exponents like those determined by the two other psychophysical procedures and by objective measurements.

Psychophysical measurements made by means of the number of difference-threshold steps, then, give results equivalent to those of the above procedures with respect to intensity determinations. But the procedure can also be applied to other stimulus parameters — to dimensions of sensation other than intensity. *Difference thresholds* can be determined not only for intensity but for *temporal duration, spatial displacement, extent of area,* and so on. For each of these dimensions the difference threshold is to be regarded as a *unit* specific to the individual subject, so that quantitative relationships between magnitudes in different dimensions can be given.

Thus, by determining the number of difference thresholds, *combinations* of change in various stimulus parameters or dimensions of perception can be studied quantitatively. Such an experiment is presented in Figure 1–8. The graph gives the results obtained with two subjects (shown in black and red); both the area a and the intensity i of a stimulus (consisting of pressure on the ball of the thumb) were varied, and these were plotted in arbitrary units on the ordinate and abscissa,

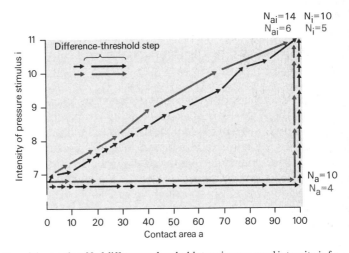

Fig. 1–8. Determination of the number N of difference-threshold steps in area a and intensity i of a pressure stimulus experienced by two subjects (*black* and *red*). On the ordinate is the intensity of the pressure stimulus, and on the abscissa the contact area over which the stimulus was presented, both in arbitrary units. The length of the *arrows* in each case signifies the size of one difference-threshold step. Further explanation in text. Modified from BERGSTRÖM, LINDFORS: Acta Physiol. Scand. *44,* 170–183 (1958)

respectively. Starting with a pressure of 6.7 and an area of 1, the contact area was enlarged and the difference-threshold steps of the stimulus area reached during the increase plotted as horizontal arrows. The subject "black" required $N_a = 10$ such steps to reach stimulus area 97. Then, with the stimulus area held constant at 97, the intensity i was increased and the difference thresholds plotted as vertical arrows. Subject "black" again required $N_i = 10$ threshold steps to reach pressure 10.5.

Now comes the interesting part of the experiment: Pressure and area of the stimulus can also be increased at the same time, so that the **simultaneous difference thresholds** for change of intensity and area can be determined. Such simultaneous increases, in the experiment of Figure 1–8, started from the values (contact area = 1, pressure intensity = 6.7). The successive difference thresholds are plotted as diagonal arrows. Eventually, as a result of the simultaneous change of pressure and area, the curve arrives at the final value reached in the first part of the experiment — pressure 10.5 and area 97. To reach this point, $N_{ai} = 14$ simultaneous difference-threshold steps were required.

Thus in this experiment we have obtained the results $N_a = 10$, $N_i = 10$, and $N_{ai} = 14$. We can see that these numbers approximately satisfy the following relation:

$$N_{ai} = \sqrt{N_{ai} + N_i} = \sqrt{100 + 100} = 14.1 \tag{1–3}$$

But this is the equation for the **hypotenuse of the right triangle** having sides N_a and N_i. The numbers of difference thresholds correspond mathematically to the lenghts of the side of the triangle enclosed by the curves of Figure 1–8.

Subject "red" was less sensitive than the subject "black", so that the same increase in stimulus area and intensity was achieved with only four or five difference threshold steps in each case. Accordingly, the value $N_{ai} = 6$ for this subject was smaller than that for the first subject. But $N_{ai} = 6$ again corresponds quite well $\left(\sqrt{4^2 + 5^2} = \left(\sqrt{41} = 6.4\right)\right)$ to the length of the hypotenuse of a right triangle with short sides of lengths 4 and 5.

It is therefore possible to describe simultaneous changes in different dimensions of a sensation by a **rectangular system of coordinates.** One can say, then, that these dimensions are **orthogonal** to one another, and that a Pythagorean relationship holds. The validity of an orthogonal relationship of this kind has been demonstrated for the dimensions of the modalities light sense, pressure sensation, and hearing, over certain ranges of intensity. The fact that simultaneous changes in different dimensions of a sensation can be described by an orthogonal relationship makes it possible to apply **subjective** sensory physiology to the study of relations between **sensations and complicated forms of stimuli** approaching the natural stimulus forms in our surroundings. For instance, when we feel an object the pressure and the contact area change simultaneously and continuously.

Examination of the difference thresholds in Figure 1–8 reveals yet another aspect of great significance in general sensory physiology. The lengths of the individual arrows indicate the size of the change ΔS of the stimulus that corresponds to a difference threshold. Now, as the stimulus amplitude S increases, the arrows become longer; on the average they are about proportional to the stimulus amplitude. On the basis of similar observations in the last century, Weber formulated **Weber's rule:**

$$\frac{\Delta S}{S} = \text{const.} \tag{1-4}$$

As applied to pressure stimuli on the skin, this rule means that whenever the magnitude of the stimulus is changed, the difference threshold is about 3% of the starting pressure.

If Weber's rule is taken to be generally valid, it can be concluded that the reaction to a stimulus is proportional to the logarithm of the stimulus amplitude. This relationship is called the **Weber-Fechner law**, and often referred to as the "fundamental law of psychophysics." However, this "law" holds only in limited ranges of intensity, and is not valid for all modalities. Another relationship, the abovementioned Stevens' power function $F = k \cdot (S - S_0)^n$, has a far greater range of applicability.

Let us illustrate this difference with an example from the area of vision. The responses of cells in the visual cortex can be described by the Stevens function over a range of brightness of at least 1:10,000 (cf. Fig 1–7), whereas the Weber-Fechner law holds, to a good approximation, only in an intermediate range of brightness corresponding to an intensity ratio 1:100.

Q 1.8. List the basic dimensions of perception.

Q 1.9. Which of the following procedures can be used to measure the intensity of sensation?
a) Special psychophysical determination of the subjective intensity
b) Measurement of the time taken for the sensation to fade away
c) Determination of the number of difference-threshold steps taken as the stimulus is increased from the absolute threshold to the sensation intensity to be measured
d) Estimation of the ratio of the intensities of a standard sensation and the sensation to be measured.

Q 1.10. Measurements of a particular light sensation, in response to a bright area, could be achieved by the following procedure: First the intensity of a point light source was increased in $N_i = 3$ difference-threshold steps, and then the area of the light source was enlarged in $N_a = 4$ difference-threshold steps. If brightness and area are increased simultaneously, starting from the absolute threshold, how many difference-threshold steps will be required to reach the same intensity of sensation?

1.4 Spatial, Temporal, and Affective Aspects of Sensation

Spatial dimension of sensation. Sensations have not only the dimensions of quality and quantity thus far discussed, but also those of space and time. First let us consider the spatial dimension. Our sensations are referred to the space surrounding us; we perceive stimuli coming from a certain place as being of varying extent and at varying distances from us. These parameters of sensation can be specified by measurement. For example, *spatial resolution thresholds* are measured as the smallest distance between two stimulus sources at which they can just be detected as separate. Figure 2–4 (p. 35) shows the result of such an experiment, in which two needle tips were placed on the skin. As another instance, the size or extent of a stimulus was measured in the experiment of Figure 1–8 (abscissa; here the variable is the area over which pressure is applied) by counting the difference-threshold steps.

That experiment has already made it clear that the impression of intensity of a sensory stimulus is enhanced by enlargement of the area over which the stimulus acts. This implies that the sensations elicited by the various elements within the stimulated area at least partially *summate.* This summation follows the Pythagorean theorem [Eq. (1–3)] over certain ranges of some modalities, and is thus not a linear summation for suprathreshold stimuli — doubling of the stimulus area does not increase sensation to twice the original intensity. In the case of *threshold stimuli,* on the other hand, the *combination can be linear.* When the stimulus is a light source, the product of threshold light intensity I_0 and luminous area A is constant:

$$I_0 \cdot A = \text{const.} \tag{1–5}$$

Thus if the threshold light intensity is 20 with a luminous surface of area 1 (arbitrary units), an increase in area to 10 would be accompanied by a decrease of the threshold light intensity to 2. Note that Eq. (1–5) holds only for small parts of the visual field; once a critical area is exceeded, the threshold light intensity becomes independent of the stimulus area. Relations like that of Eq. (1–5) hold for other modalities as well. The nearly linear spatial summation of threshold stimuli is the basis for the detection of large signals in poor lighting. In a nearly dark room an alarm clock with a large dial can still be read, but not a wrist watch.

So far we have been concerned with the dependence of quantity of sensation upon the spatial extent of the stimulus. A more interesting aspect is the way perception is influenced by a second stimulus spatially distinct from the first. Under such conditions facilitatory and inhibitory effects appear, which can best be described in the case of contrast phenomena.

Contrast. Contrast, as applied to visual perception, denotes the ratio of the brightnesses of adjacent parts of the viewed pattern — for example, the ratio of the brightness of a dark cupboard to that of the bright wall against which it stands. Contrast can be similarly defined for other sensations (e.g., the loudness of a speaker as compared with a background noise). Only if there is sufficient contrast do objects become so distinct from the background as to be detectable. When the brightness differences between the various parts of a visual pattern are too small, the picture becomes vague and unclear, and if it is on a television screen we use the electronic facilities provided to increase the contrast.

It is a general property of sensory perceptions that the contrasts involved are increased — that **contrast enhancement** occurs. When you look at any fairly large dark area against a light background, the edge of the dark area looks darker than the middle, and around the dark object there is a small strip of background that appears brighter (cf. also Fig. 5–11). Contrast enhancement of this sort can also be demonstrated quantitatively. In the experiment of Figure 1–9, the subject looked at a surface on which a dark area at the left adjoined a light area on the right; the objective brightness distribution, measured with a physical device, is shown by the black curve. The red curve shows the **subjectively sensed** brightness distribution. This is determined by instructing the subject to set a comparison brightness at a level felt subjectively to be just as bright as the different portions of the transition region of the viewed pattern. The subjective brightness change is much sharper than the objectively measured transition. Moreover, subjectively the edge of the dark area is darkened, with a minimum in the subjective brightness at −10 min of

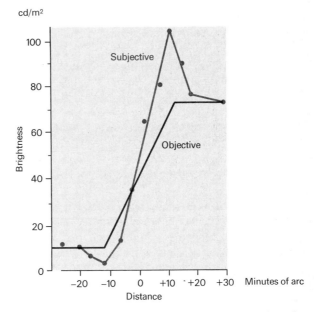

Fig. 1–9. Contrast enhancement. Transition from a dark area on the *left* to a light area on the *right;* the curves represent values along a line perpendicular to the edge (position 0 on the abscissa). On the ordinate is the brightness of the viewed surface. The **black curve** shows the objective brightness distribution measured with a photometer and the **red curve,** the subjective distribution. The latter was obtained by having the subject set a comparison area to a brightness perceived as equal to that at each position on the test pattern. Modified from LOWRY, DE PALMA: J. Opt. Soc. Am. *51,* 740 (1961)

arc, and there is a subjective brightening at the edge of the bright surface, with a subjective brightness maximum at + 10 min of arc. Subjective contrast enhancement, then, can readily be measured.

The fact that just on the left of the edge in Figure 1–9 (between −20 and 0 min of arc) the sensed brightness is much less than that within the dark area indicates *inhibition;* the light area on the right reduces the subjectively sensed brightness in the adjacent dark area. Thus the intense light stimulus not only leads to a sensation of high intensity, but diminishes or inhibits the sensation of light in the neighboring parts of the pattern. The enhanced brightness just to the right of the edge in Figure 1–9 (between 0 and + 15 min of arc) also depends upon this mechanism of inhibition in adjacent areas. Within the uniformly bright area (to the right of + 10 min of arc) neighboring bright parts of the pattern inhibit one another reciprocally, whereas at the margin of the bright area some of the inhibition by adjacent (darker) parts of the pattern is eliminated; the sensation is thereby relatively "disinhibited." The marked inhibitory function of the bright areas can be illustrated with the example of a black-and-white television set. When the set is turned off, the screen is a light gray. Once it has been turned on the electrons striking the screen produce light — that is, the only change the screen can actually undergo is to become brighter than light gray. But parts of the picture we see are definitely a deep black. They are black only because very bright parts of the picture are next to them, and these inhibit the sensation of brightness in the adjacent black parts of the picture. The significance of this inhibition can be characterized by the paradoxial formulation *"black is white with a brighter surround."* The black pile of coal in the summer sun is objectively much brighter than white snow in the evening twilight.

Phenomena similar to contrast enhancement and inhibition by adjacent stimulus sources are to be found in other modalities. In fact, corresponding inhibitory mechanisms are found to operate during stimulus processing in the sense organs and in the sensory nervous system; cells excited by strong stimuli reduce the sensitivity of neighboring cells by "surround inhibition" (cf. "receptive field," Chaps. 3 and 4; "surround inhibition," *Fundamentals of Neurophysiology,* Chap. 4).

Figure 1–9 showed that at an objective brightness transition, contrast is enhanced in the elicited sensation. Another elegant way of revealing the influence of the spatial surroundings on the intensity of sensation is shown in Figure 1–10. The experiment is based on estimation of the sensed brightness of a circular light source as the luminance of the stimulus (plotted on the abscissa) is changed. The relationship between intensity of stimulus and sensation is shown by the red line in the diagram. It has a very shallow slope; when the luminance is increased by 30 dB — that is, by a factor of 1000 — the intensity of sensation increases only a little more than tenfold. The low rate of rise of sensation intensity with increasing intensity of white light was also shown in Figure 1–7. The exponent of Stevens' power function for light stimuli is about 1/3 [cf. Eq. (1–1)]. Once the response to a circular source was established, this source was surrounded by a luminous ring of variable intensity, and the estimation of brightness of the central spot was

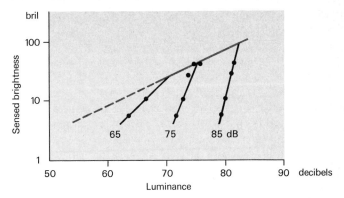

Fig. 1-10. Inhibition of the sensation of brightness by a bright surround. The **red line** shows the perceived brightness of a target area fixated by the eye, as a function of the objective luminance; double logarithmic plot. The **black lines** indicate the brightness sensed when the target area is surrounded by a ring with luminance 65, 75 or 85 d B. Modified from STEVENS: Psychophysics. New York — London — Sydney — Toronto: John Wiley 1975

repeated. If the surrounding ring was relatively dim, with luminance 65 dB, the left black curve resulted. At low stimulus light intensities it rose rather more steeply than the red control curve, and joined the latter at about 70 dB. When the luminance of the surrounding ring was increased, the curves became progessively steeper until at a surround intensity of 85 dB the slope of the curve relating sensed brightness to stimulus-light intensity was quite large. At this surround illumination the light sensation increased by a factor of 10 when the stimulus intensity was only tripled. The bright light surrounding the stimulus light source, then, increased the exponent of Stevens' power function from 1/3 to 3. This means that the **high surround luminance greatly increases contrast** — that is, it increases the brightness difference sensed for a particular difference in stimulus intensity.

The deflection of the red curve of Figure 1-10 into the black segments when the surround illumination is switched on also makes it quite obvious that the surround illumination decreases or **inhibits** the intensity of sensation. For instance, whereas without surround illumination a stimulus light luminance of 80 dB elicits a sensed brightness of 70 units, at a surround illumination of 85 dB the same stimulus gives rise to a sensation of brightness amounting to only 10 units. The inhibition is well known in the form of the **blinding effect** of the headlights of oncoming cars. Near the dazzling headlights the dimly lit street disappears, and of the cars ahead only the taillights and no other details are visible. The contrast enhancement with bright lighting of the surround is reproduced by artists when they paint beaches or snowy landscapes in bright sunlight; the brightness gradations become hard, with sharp transitions. Pictures of evening twilight, on the other hand, are characterized by soft shadings.

The time dimension of sensation. The last of the dimensions of sensation to be discussed is time. Time itself is sensed as present, remembered as past, and anticipated as future. A good deal could be said in this regard, for instance, about the span of time that we perceive as the immediate present, the "psychological moment." Difference thresholds can be determined for time intervals; the smallest discernible durations of periodic stimuli, for example, are measured as the flicker-fusion frequency. The sense organs turn out to be sluggish, and unsuitable for precise time measurements.

The aspect we shall consider in greater detail is the influence of *stimulus duration* upon the *intensity of sensation.* Stimulus durations summate as do stimulus areas. This *summation is linear* for short stimuli in the vicinity of the threshold; there, a doubling of the stimulus duration doubles the intensity of sensation. This effect is shown in Figure 1–11 for the visual sense. With durations

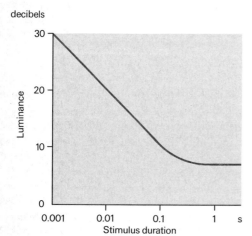

Fig. 1–11. Temporal summation at the absolute visual threshold. The ***red curve*** indicates the minimal luminance (ordinate) a light stimulus of the duration given on the abscissa must have to be just perceptible. Double logarithmic plot. For stimulus durations shorter than 0.1 s the curve has a slope of –1; in this range, duration and threshold intensity of the stimulus are inversely proportional. Modified from MARKS: Sensory Processes, New York — London: Academic Press 1974

less than 0.1 s, the threshold light intensity decreases in inverse proportion to the stimulus duration; in this range it holds that

$$I_0 \cdot t = \text{const.} \tag{1–6}$$

The product of threshold stimulus I_0 and stimulus duration t is constant. This relationship, "Ricco's law", is entirely analogous to that governing the spatial summation of threshold stimuli [Eq. (1–5)]. If a critical stimulus time is exceeded, summation no longer occurs; the threshold in Figure 1–11 is independent of duration for stimulus durations above 1 s. Relationships like that of Eq. (1–6) also hold for other modalities. For instance, Eq. (1–6) reflects the common experience that we can see very rapid movements only in bright light. The acrobat, whose quickness we are meant to admire, is centered in the spotlight, while the magician prefers dim illumination.

Very brief stimuli thus summate in our sensations. Long stimuli, by contrast, lead to inhibition — and to *adaptation.* A uniformly maintained stimulus is sensed as progressively weaker with time. A good example of this adaptation is given by the sensation of warmth: A bath can seem to be unpleasantly warm when one first gets in, but after a short time the sensation of heat fades away. The result of a measurement of subjective adaptation is shown in Figure 1–12. In this experiment,

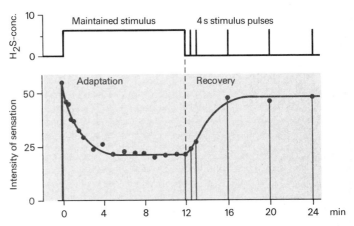

Fig. 1–12. Adaptation of an odor sensation. Above *(black),* stimulus amplitude (hydrogen sulfide, concentration $6.5 \cdot 10^{-6}$ by volume); below *(red),* intensity of sensation, estimated by four subjects in ten trials each, as multiples of a standard intensity. Modified from ECKMANN et al.: Scand. J. Psychol. *1,* 177 (1967)

a *constant odor stimulus* consisting of a certain concentration of hydrogen sulfide was presented. During the stimulus the subject was asked to estimate the intensity of the smell as a multiple of a standard odor intensity (ratio scale; cf. Fig. 1–6). Immediately after the odor stimulus was turned on, the subjects estimated a sensation intensity of 56. Then the *subjective intensity fell* sharply within a few minutes, levelling off after about 5 min at a constant intensity of about 20. This fall-off in sensation intensity, from 56 to 20 with a constant stimulus, is typical adaptation. Figure 1–12 also shows the recovery from adaptation, the return of full sensitivity after the end of the maintained stimulus. Following the termination of the prolonged stimulus, brief test stimuli are given, and estimates of the associated sensation intensity are made each time. The subjective sensitivity returns with a time course resembling that of adaptation — first rapidly, and then more slowly.

Adaptation, and recovery from it, can be demonstrated for most of the qualities of perception; the particular cases are treated in the chapters on special sense organs (cf. also Fig. 5–17). The most important exception to this rule is the sensation of pain, which does not adapt (cf. Fig. 4–2). The consequence of **adaptation,** like that of **contrast enhancement,** is that we can perceive changes in stimuli very much better than we can perceive a constant situation. Both mechanisms serve to select and emphasize only the essential stimuli among the great number to which the body is exposed. We also actively generate such contrast-enhancing temporal changes in stimuli; when we want to feel a fine tactile pattern in relief, we stroke it lightly with our fingertips. Our eyes carry out continual small jerky movements so as to shift the image of the environment on the retina and thus increase appreciably the acuity of vision (cf. the comment on stabilized retinal images, p. 146.

Affective and intentional aspects of sensory perception. In addition to the dimensions discussed, sensory perception frequently involves affective shadings, which can be expressed by the word pairs pleasant/unpleasant, comfort/discomfort, beautiful/ugly, and so on. This factor is particularly marked in the case of odors,

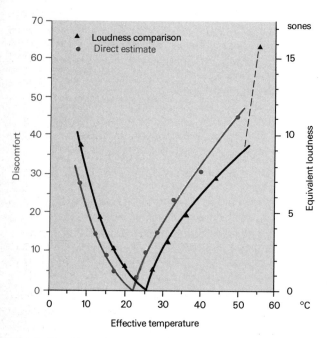

Fig. 1–13. "Discomfort" as a function of temperature. On the abscissa the "effective skin temperature" produced by irradiating the subject (in air at +4°C) by an infrared lamp set at different intensities. The degree of discomfort at each temperature was estimated by the subjects (*circles, red curve and ordinate*) or indicated by setting a sound source to the equivalent loudness (*triangles, black curve and ordinate*). Effective temperatures of 22°–24°C were felt to be "neutral". Modified from Stevens: Psychophysics. New York — London — Sydney — Toronto: John Wiley 1975

which we often can describe with no better terms than "refreshing" or "disgust-ing". The intensity of the affects produced can be measured and compared with the stimulus, in an experiment like that of Figure 1–13. Subjects in a room with air temperature 4 °C were exposed to infrared radiation so that the effective temperature at their body surfaces had the values shown on the abscissa of the diagram. The subjects were then told to state the *degree of their discomfort* at the various temperatures. They did this either by estimating its intensity (red curve, procedure of Fig. 1–6), or by cross-modality intensity comparison (black curve, procedure of Fig. 1–7). The two curves nearly coincide. Discomfort was minimal between 22° and 26°C, a range corresponding approximately to the normal skin temperature. Warming and cooling beyond this range caused a sharp rise in discomfort; with cooling, the exponent of the curve was actually 1.7 — about as large as the exponent measured for pain (Fig. 1–7). Pain could, after all, be regarded as an extreme form of discomfort. Discomfort and comfort, as a rule, have an effect on behavior. We avoid extremes of both cold and heat, and seek out pleasant warmth. The very sharp rise of discomfort during cooling perhaps protects us from the dangers of hypothermia.

To conclude this incomplete outline of subjective sensory physiology, we should recall once again that we usually do not simply submit passively to sensations; rather, on the one hand they incite us to act, and on the other we often induce them actively by directed movements. It is this *willing of sensation* that makes it my personal experience, causes it to occupy my personal time, makes it an event pertaining to myself; and because this experience is repeatable — and thus predictable — it can become a basis for my actions.

Q 1.11. Which of the following statements about threshold light intensity is false?
   a) It decreases with enlargement of the light-source area.
   b) It increases with intensified illumination of the surroundings.
   c) It rises as the square root of stimulus duration.
   d) It decreases during a long period in the dark.
   e) It can be lowered by spatial summation.

Q 1.12. Adaptation to a sensory stimulus is the term describing the observation that:
   a) Maintained stimuli are perceived as weaker than short stimuli of equal intensity.
   b) A weak stimulus is sensed as more intense if it is repeated frequently.
   c) After a long intense stimulus the sensitivity to brief test stimuli slowly increases.
   e) During a long stimulus the intensity of sensation associated with additional small test stimuli of the same quality decreases.

2 Somatovisceral Sensibility

R.F. Schmidt

In addition to the special sense organs (such as the eye and ear) treated in later chapters of this book, in practically all its tissues the body has receptors (sensors) that detect signals from the surroundings or from the body itself and convey them to the central nervous system. All these sensory systems together constitute the *somatovisceral sensibility.* As illustrated in Figure 2–1, the receptors in the skin, the joints and the skeletal muscles with their tendons are customarily termed the somatosensory system, to distinguish them from the visceral sensory system.

Within the somatic system, superficial sensibility is mediated by receptors located in the skin, and deep sensibility by those in the underlying muscles, tendons and joints. The modalities associated with the skin, with superficial sensibility, are the senses of touch (mechanoreception) and of temperature (thermoreception). These, together with deep sensibility and visceral sensibility, are treated in this chapter. The sense of pain, common to all tissues, is considered separately in Chapter 4.

The *receptors* (sensors) for somatovisceral sensibility can be assigned to four basic types, as illustrated in the lower part of Figure 2–1. In one category are those responsive to mechanical, thermal or chemical stimuli — the mechanoreceptors, thermoreceptors and chemoreceptors. In another are the nociceptors, which respond only to stimuli that are harming or threaten to harm the body. Such stimuli are called "noxious" stimuli (the Latin "noxa" means "damage"). Mechanoreceptors are involved chiefly in the skin's sense of touch and in deep sensibility, thermoreceptors mainly mediate the sense of temperature, and chemoreceptors are most often associated with visceral sensibility.

The signals received by the receptors for somatovisceral sensibility are transmitted to, and processed in, diverse parts of the peripheral and central nervous systems. These aspects are described in Chapter 3. The following four sections of this chapter are concerned mainly with the psychophysical aspects of somatovisceral sensibility, on one hand, and on the other with correlations between the discharge of somatovisceral receptors and the sensation this activity produces.

2.1 Mechanoreception

This section is concerned with the detection of mechanical stimuli at the skin and the central processing of such signals — that is, with *mechanoreception* (sometimes

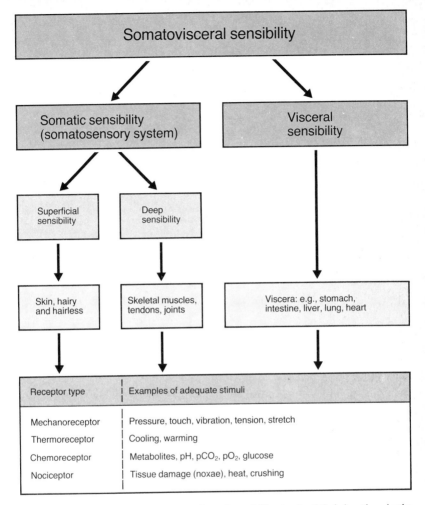

Fig. 2–1. Survey of the components of somatovisceral sensibility *(top)*, of their locations in the body *(middle)*, and of the four basic types of somatovisceral receptors with their adequate stimuli

called the sense of touch). This modality comprises four qualities: the sensations of ***pressure, touch, vibration, and tickle.*** In the following, after a discussion of the subjective perception of mechanical stimuli, it will be shown that the skin contains a number of mechanoreceptors with properties (adequate stimuli, threshold, forms of discharge and of adaptation) that appear to make them particularly suitable to serve in mediating one or another of these qualities.

Sensation threshold and intensity function of mechanical stimulation of the skin. In experiments designed to determine the threshold for sensation of a mechanical stimulus to the skin, the results depend strongly on the stimulation method used.

With the oldest procedure, in which threshold and distribution of mechanosensitivity are tested by means of hairs or bristles, it turned out that with light pressure stimuli (in the 0.1–0.5 g range; for method of calibration see Fig. 2–2 A) sensations of pressure or touch (i. e., tactile sensations) could be elicited only at certain points on the skin. These points were called **touch points.** The results of such an experiment are shown in Figure 4–3 (p. 124). Regions of the skin with many touch points are the fingertips and lips, in particular, whereas on the upper arms, upper thighs and back the touch points are especially sparse.

Such experiments, to determine the touch points of a skin area and their thresholds to pressure stimuli, are informative but difficult and tedious. Moreover,

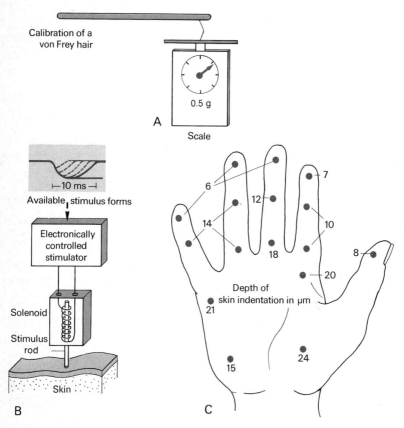

Fig. 2–2 A–C. Threshold and distribution of mechanical sensitivity on the skin. *A* Calibration of a "von Frey hair"; the force (in milligrams) at which the hair or the (nylon) bristle just bends is measured. A graded set of such stimulus hairs can be used to determine the thresholds and distribution of the touch points, and the thresholds and receptive fields of mechanoreceptors. *B* Example of mechanical stimulation of the skin with an electronically driven rod. *C* Distribution of the sensation thresholds to stimuli of the form shown in *B,* expressed in microns of indentation. Modified from LINDBLOM, LINDSTRÖM. In: ZOTTERMAN, Y. (ed.): Sensory Functions of the Skin in Primates. Oxford: Pergamon Press 1976

they have the disadvantage that because of the punctate nature of the stimulus it is not easy to make a direct comparison with the stimuli ordinarily encountered, which tend to cover an appreciable area. Modern stimulating devices, with which the form, duration, and intensity of the stimuli can be varied over a wide range, make use of exchangeable rods, the ends of which contact the skin over different areas. With such an apparatus, using the stimulus form shown in Figure 2–2B, a measure of the tactile sensation threshold of the inner surface of the right hand was obtained, as shown in Figure 2–2C. Here the threshold is expressed in terms of the minimal depth of skin impression (in micrometers) necessary to produce a just detectable sensation of touch.

Indentations of the skin of the order of magnitude of 0.01 mm (10 μm) thus suffice to produce tactile sensations when they occur on the inner surface of the hand. The thresholds of the fingertips are distinctly lower than those of the rest of the hand surface. This result agrees with everyday experience. It is, however, surprising to find that the thresholds of the tips of index and middle fingers are not

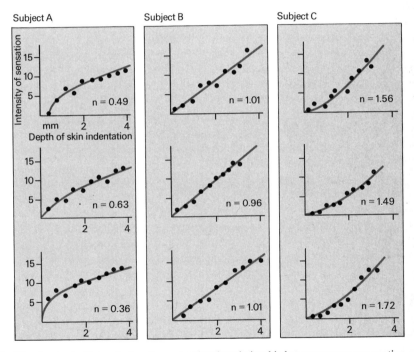

Fig. 2–3. Psychophysical intensity functions, showing the relationship between pressure sensation and stimulus intensity. Pressure pulses 1 s in duration are applied to the inner surface of the hand with the apparatus shown in Figure 2–2 B, and the depth to which the skin is indented is measured. The three subjects *A, B* and *C* assigned to the stimuli numerical values reflecting the intensity of their sensations. Each experiment was repeated three times (the three curves in each column). The *solid curves* are power functions fitted to the data points; the exponent of the function is shown on the *right* in each diagram. Modified from KNIEBESTÖL, VALLBO. In: ZOTTERMAN, Y. (ed.): Sensory Functions of the Skin in Primates. Oxford: Pergamon Press 1976

appreciably different from those of the other fingers. In the same study — again rather unexpectedly — it was found that the tactile sensation thresholds of the blind do not differ distinctly from those of normal subjects.

With suprathreshold mechanical skin stimulation, one can measure the dependence of sensation intensity upon stimulus intensity, using the psychophysical methods described on pp. 15–21. Figure 2–3 serves as an example of such an investigation. It shows the results for three subjects (A, B and C) in a graph relating the amplitude of a pressure stimulus (abscissae) to the subjectively experienced stimulus intensity (ordinates). This *intensity function* was obtained three times for each subject; the results showed clearly that the function is remarkably reproducible for a given individual, but varies widely among different individuals. This finding is clearly expressed in the exponents of the power function fitted to the data. In evaluating intensity functions of this kind (for further examples see Figs. 1–6 and 1–7) it is therefore necessary to take account not only of the conditions of the experiment but also of the interindividual differences in subjective sensation.

Spatial resolution. The skin's spatial resolution capacity for tactile stimuli has traditionally been measured by finding the smallest distance between two tactile stimuli at which the two are just discerned as separate. This "spatial discrimination threshold" can easily be studied with a pair of pointed compasses (with blunt tips, so that pain stimuli are avoided). If the two tips are set on the skin at the same time, so that the *simultaneous spatial threshold* is tested, results like those shown in Figure 2–4 are obtained for adults. These are *measures of the spatial resolution* of tactile stimuli in the regions of the body tested. It is consistent with everyday experience, as well as with the distribution of the touch points mentioned above, that the simultaneous spatial thresholds of the tip of the tongue and of the fingers, as well as the lips, are particularly low (order of magnitude 1–3 mm), whereas on the back and the upper arms and thighs they are of the order of 50–100 mm. Moreover, they are distinctly higher along the long axis of the limbs than on a circumferential line (try it for yourself).

In blind people, other conditions being the same, the spatial discrimination threshold is no better than in normal subjects. This finding agrees with the absence of a difference in sensation of light touch stimuli (see above); the same thing is found in the case of vibration stimuli.

If the spatial resolution of an area of skin is tested by applying the tips of the compasses in sequence, one has a test not of simultaneous but of *successive spatial thresholds.* If you try both of these experiments on a subject you will see that the successive spatial threshold is *clearly lower than the simultaneous threshold,* often amounting to only a quarter of the simultaneous threshold (e. g., 1 mm rather than 4 mm). The reasons for this difference lie partly in the mechanical properties of the skin, but mostly in the way it is innervated and the central connections of the afferent nerve fibers (cf. Sec. 3.3).

The skin's spatial resolution of mechanical stimuli can also be tested in other ways than by measuring the simultaneous and successive spatial thresholds. For

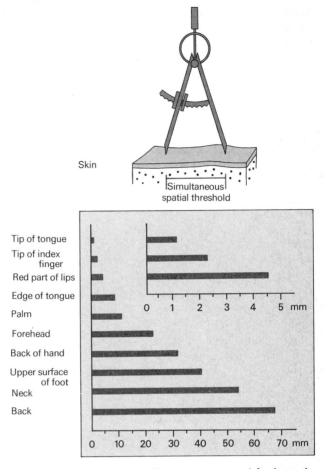

Fig. 2–4. Simultaneous spatial thresholds in the adult. The *inset* at *upper right* shows the simultaneous spatial threshold of the three skin areas just to their left, with the abscissa expanded by a factor of 10. The length of the *bars* indicates, for each region of the body, the smallest distance between two simultaneously applied point stimuli for which the two points are still detected as separate. Modified from WEBER and LANDOIS

example, one can measure the smallest detectable difference in length of two edges placed on the skin, or how long a single edge must be for the subject to detect whether it is oriented lengthwise or crosswise. On the forearm, for instance, where the simultaneous spatial threshold is 30–40 mm, the smallest detectable difference in length of two edge stimuli is 5–10 mm and, on average, a minimal edge length of 17 mm is needed to distinguish the medio-lateral from the proximo-distal orientation.

Tests of mechanoreception. In clinical examinations, sensitivity to touch is usually tested by stimulating the skin with a wisp of cotton or the like and asking the patient what he feels, and where he thinks the stimulus is located. Discrimination between sharp and dull is tested by applying the tip and head of a glass-headed pin, in irregular sequence. Such examinations also routinely involve asking the patient if he can recognize numbers written on his skin with a rounded object such as the fingertip or the head of a pin. The numbers are first written large, and then progressively smaller.

The **sense of vibration** is examined clinically by putting a tuning fork in contact with a bony place (e. g., on the elbow or shin bone). In an experiment, or when a more detailed examination is desired, it is better to use an electrical vibrator or loudspeaker system driven by a sine-wave generator. The object as a rule is to find

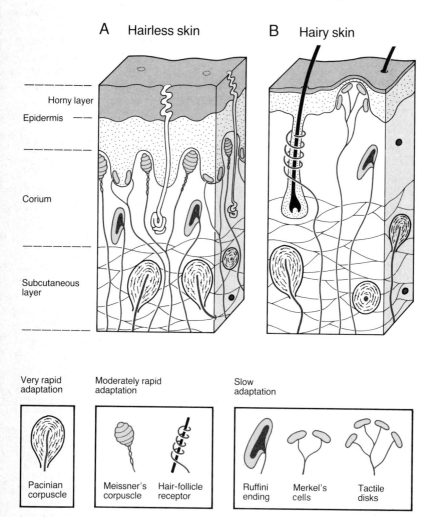

Fig. 2–5. Schematic representation of the structure and position of mechanoreceptors in the hairless (**A**) and hairy (**B**) skin. For details see text (cf. also Table 2–1)

the absolute threshold for the conscious sensation of vibration. Its minimum lies at frequencies near 150–300 Hz. The minimal amplitudes of vibration required at these frequencies are on the order of 1 μm (cf. Fig. 2–9 E, p. 40).

Clinical measurements, wherever possible, should include **bilateral comparison** — a test of the same parameter at the corresponding place on the other side of the body — and even slight differences should be noted. The routine examinations in a doctor's office are relatively crude as compared with what mechanoperception can in fact achieve; slight, but diagnostically important disturbances of mechanosensibility are not always detected.

Survey of histologic structure, afferent innervation, and adaptation in cutaneous mechanoreceptors. Figure 2–5 illustrates the kinds of mechanoreceptors to be found in hairless (A) and hairy (B) skin regions of humans and other mammals (e. g., monkeys and cats). All of these receptors are innervated by myelinated, rapidly conducting afferent nerve fibers of group II (diameter 5–12 μm, conduction velocity 30–70 m/s; cf. Table 1–1, p. 10 and Table 2–2, p. 67 in **Fundamentals of Neurophysiology,** 3rd Ed.). At these high conduction velocities, an impulse elicited peripherally arrives at the spinal cord within a few milliseconds.

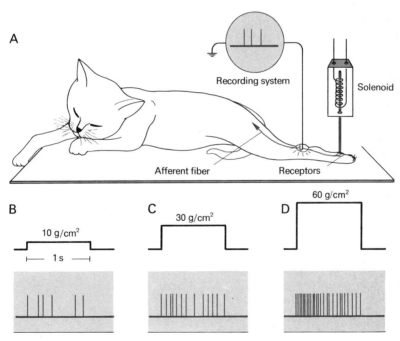

Fig. 2–6. **A** Diagram of an experimental arrangement for study of the stimulus/response behavior of receptors in the skin. **B, C, D:** impulses (action potentials) discharged by a pressure receptor in the hairless sole of the cat's paw (lower, red records) during stimulation with various stimuli of constant force (upper records). The forces are given in grams/square centimeter. The receptor was not spontaneously active

In experiments on animals, the ***stimulus/response behavior of cutaneous receptors*** is determined by recording the action potentials in a single afferent nerve fiber (Fig. 2–6A). Similar recordings can be obtained in humans by inserting metal microelectrodes through the skin into the nerve to be examined, until the activity of single afferent nerve fibers is picked up. By stimulating with suitable devices (cf. Fig. 2–2 A, B) or applying weights the experimenter attempts to excite the receptor associated with the fiber and thus derive the relationships between stimulus and response.

When the responses to constant pressure stimuli are studied in the various receptors shown in Figure 2–5, it becomes apparent that the receptors can be divided into three types on the basis of the measured differences in ***adaptation:*** those that adapt ***very rapidly,*** sending out only one or two impulses per pressure stimulus (Pacinian corpuscles; cf. Fig. 2–9), ***moderately rapidly,*** with discharges that cease about 50–500 ms after the onset of the pressure stimulus (Meissner corpuscles, hair-follicle receptors; cf. Fig 2–8) and ***slowly,*** continuing to discharge stimulus-induced action potentials even when the pressure is maintained for a long time (Merkel's cells, tactile disks, Ruffini endings; Figs. 2–6 B, D and 2–7).

Table 2–1 shows the classification based on this criterion (adaptation to a constant pressure stimulus; headings above the columns). This grouping dates from a time when it was easy to fix the intensity and duration of a tactile stimulus (using von Frey hairs, for example), whereas other parameters of the stimulus, such as the velocity or acceleration of skin indentation, were not readily variable. When the characteristics of the response with respect to these parameters are

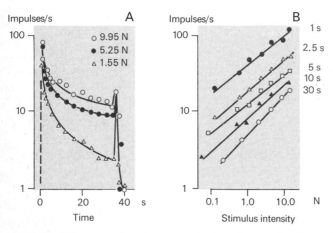

Fig. 2–7 A, B. Response of a pressure receptor to various constant-force stimuli. ***A*** Time course of the receptor discharge (ordinate in impulses per second, logarithmic scale) during three stimuli 40 s in duration (abscissa) at intensities indicated by the symbols in the graph. ***B*** The relationship between stimulus intensity (abscissa) and receptor discharge (ordinate) at various times after the onset of the stimulus. Both axes are logarithmic. The threshold stimuli at each time during the maintained stimulus were subtracted from the applied intensities. Each point in ***A*** and ***B*** is the average of ten individual measurements

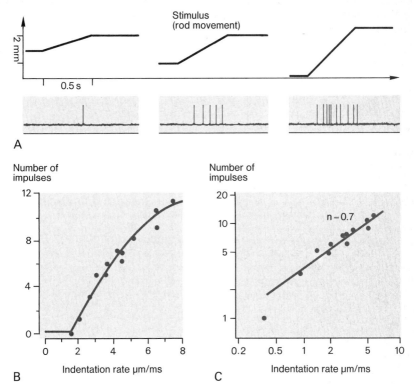

Fig. 2–8 A–C. Response behavior of a mechanoreceptor with intermediate adaptation rate (velocity detector). In *A* are original records *(red)* of the responses to three mechanical stimuli in which the skin was indented by a rod at different rates *(black ramps)* for the same period of time. **B, C** The relationship between rate of indentation (abscissa in micrometers/millisecond) and magnitude of receptor response (ordinate, number of impulses per stimulus), in linear *(B)* and double logarithmic *(C)* plots. The threshold stimulus 1.6 μm/ms has been subtracted from the values in *(C)*. Modified from ZIMMERMANN

considered, it turns out (as will be shown below) that the receptors adapting rapidly or very rapidly to pressure stimuli can be interpreted differently. That is, they do not code primarily the intensity of the tactile stimulus (as the slowly adapting receptors do), but rather can be said to provide information about its velocity or acceleration. The labels at the bottom of the columns in Table 2–1 take account of this finding.

Pressure receptors (intensity detectors). In slowly adapting receptors the instantaneous discharge rate continues to reflect stimulus intensity throughout even very long pressure stimuli (Figs. 2–6 B, C, D, and 2–7 A). When the relationship between stimulus intensity and impulse frequency is plotted on double logarithmic coordinates (Fig. 2–7 B), it is evident that the data points can be joined by straight lines. This means that the relationship is a power function of the form (impulse frequency) = (stimulus intensity)^n (cf. Sec. 3.1, p. 71). From a functional

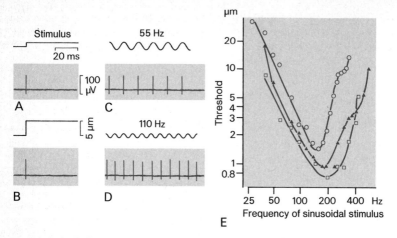

Fig. 2–9 A–E. Response of Pacinian corpuscles (acceleration detectors). *A–D* Responses to mechanical square-wave stimuli of different intensities *(A, B)* and mechanical sinusoidal stimuli at 55 and 110 Hz *(C, D)*. The amplitudes of the sinusoidal stimuli are just above the threshold for a one-spike-per-cycle response of the receptor. The calibrations apply to all records. *E* Amplitude threshold (ordinate) of three Pacinian corpuscles as a function of the frequency (abscissa) of mechanical sinusoidal stimuli. The stimuli were applied at the site of maximal sensitivity of each receptor (sole of cat's paw). Both scales are logarithmic

viewpoint, such receptors serve as ***intensity detectors;*** that is, they measure the strength or depth of impression of a mechanical stimulus to the skin. Because they do not adapt completely even after a considerable time (Fig. 2–7 A), they also signal the ***duration*** of a pressure stimulus.

The slowly adapting intensity detectors in hairless skin (e. g., the inner surface of the hand) are called ***Merkel's cells*** (Fig. 2–5, Table 2–1). These lie in small groups

Table 2–1. Classification of cutaneous mechanoreceptors according to rate of adaption (headings above the columns) and adequate stimulus (at the bases of the columns)

	ADAPTATION TO CONSTANT PRESSURE STIMULUS		
	Slow	Moderately rapid	Very rapid
Hairless skin:	Merkel's cells, Ruffini endings	Meissner corpuscle	Pacinian corpuscle
Hairy skin:	Tactile disks, Ruffini endings	Hair-follicle receptor	Pacinian corpuscle
	Intensity detector	Velocity detector	Acceleration detector
	CLASSIFICATION BY ADEQUATE STIMULUS		

in the lowest layers of the epidermis, where it sends peglike projections into the papillae of the corium. Merkel's cells can also be found in hairy skin, but there they are located in special *tactile disks* — small regions raised above the surface of the skin (Fig. 2–5 B).

In the corium of both hairless and hairy skin is another slowly adapting receptor, the *Ruffini ending* (see Fig. 2–5). Many of these (unlike the Merkel's cells) have a "resting" discharge, when no stimulus is present. Furthermore, they respond not only to pressure stimuli perpendicular to the skin surface, but also to stretching of the skin. Some of the Ruffini endings on the inner surface of the human hand are direction-sensitive; that is, when the skin is stretched in one direction their discharge rate increases, whereas stretching in the perpendicular direction reduces the resting activity (cf. Fig. 2–10). Therefore the Ruffini endings transmit information about the direction and intensity of shear forces within the skin and between skin and underlying tissues. Such forces are produced during joint movements, for instance, or when one uses tools.

Touch receptors (velocity detectors). If one moves a few hairs on the back of the hand without touching the skin itself, and keeps them bent into the new position, a sensation is felt only while the hairs are moving. As soon as they are held motionless in the new position the sensation ceases. This indicates that the receptors in the hair follicles record not so much the extent of hair displacement as the movement itself — or, perhaps, the velocity of the hair movement.

In hairless skin, too, there are receptors that respond in a comparable way. An example is shown in Figure 2–8. Only during the steady (ramp) movement of the stimulus rod does the receptor respond; there is no discharge after movement has stopped, although the stimulus (indentation) continues. The frequency of the impulses is clearly dependent on the velocity with which the rod presses into the skin, as shown both by the original records in A and by the diagram in B. When the data are plotted on double logarithmic coordinates (C) it becomes apparent that the curve relating discharge rate and stimulus velocity (the first time derivative) is nearly a straight line; the relationship is described by a power function. These receptors, then, can be called *velocity detectors* (Table 2–1).

The velocity detectors with intermediate rates of adaptation found in hairless skin are the *Meissner corpuscles,* receptors in the papillae of the corium (Fig. 2–5 A). Their counterparts in hairy skin are the *hair-follicle receptors,* located on the intracutaneous parts of the hairs (Fig. 2–5 B).

"Tonic" receptors such as pressure receptors, so called because of their maintained responses, signal primarily the intensity of a stimulus. Correspondingly, *"phasic"* receptors respond as velocity detectors, and there are also intermediate (phasic-tonic) forms. Sometimes, in analogy with the terms used for technical sensing devices, these are called proportional (P), differential (D), and PD receptors, respectively.

Vibration receptors (acceleration detectors). Figure 2–9 A, B shows the response behavior of the third receptor type, when stimulated with square-wave stimuli.

Regardless of stimulus strength (stimulus *A* is just above threshold, stimulus *B* several times the threshold intensity), the receptor discharges only one impulse for each square-wave stimulus. That is, it adapts very rapidly (Table 2–1). This receptor can transmit no information about the depth of skin indentation, nor about the rate of indentation.

During sinusoidal stimulation (Fig. 2–9 C, D), however, each cycle of the sine wave elicits action potentials. If the amplitude of the sinusoidal oscillation is set at a level such that each cycle elicits precisely one action potential, it becomes evident that the minimal amplitude required depends on the frequency of oscillation in a characteristic way. At 110 Hz (D) it is smaller than at 55 Hz (C). Figure 2–9 E shows the relationship between the minimal oscillation amplitude required to produce one action potential per cycle (ordinate) and the frequency of oscillation (abscissa). A rise in stimulus frequency from 30 Hz to 200 Hz is accompanied by a sharp decrease in threshold; in the double logarithmic plot shown here the slope of the curve in the range 30–200 Hz is about -2. The relationship between threshold amplitude S_0 and frequency f can thus be written as $S_0 = \text{const.} \cdot f^{-2}$, which indicates that the adequate stimulus for these receptors is the second time derivative of indentation depth, the acceleration of skin displacement. We can therefore call these receptors *acceleration detectors* (Table 2–1). At frequencies above 200 Hz the threshold of the receptor rises, and at considerably higher frequencies (400–1000 Hz) a 1:1 response is no longer obtainable. Acceleration detectors can be excited by stimuli to both hairy and hairless skin.

As was shown in Table 2–1, the *Pacinian corpuscles* in the fatty tissue of the subcutaneous layers of both hairless (Fig. 2–5 A) and hairy (B) skin act as acceleration detectors. These are relatively large neuronal end structures, enclosed by connective tissue arranged in layers as in an onion. Apart from the subcutaneous fat, they are also found in varying numbers on the tendons and fascia of muscles, on the periosteum and in the joint capsules.

Mechanosensitive free nerve endings in the skin. Each skin nerve, in addition to its myelinated afferents, contains a large number (50% or more of its fibers) of unmyelinated (group IV or C) axons. Some of these are efferent postganglionic sympathetic fibers, supplying structures such as the smooth musculature of the cutaneous vessels and the hair follicles. But this category includes afferent fibers as well; these terminate in free nerve endings, not in corpuscular structures. The receptor functions of these free nerve endings of group-IV fibers are in certain cases still unknown. Some of them, however, are *thermoreceptors,* and many are *nociceptors* (cf. pp. 123–126). A few are sensitive to low-intensity touch stimuli. Such *mechanoreceptors* with unmyelinated afferent fibers have been found in hairy and — rarely — in hairless skin.

Because of the low conduction velocity of group-IV fibers (on the order of 1 m/s), a considerable time elapses between stimulation of the free nerve endings and the arrival of the afferent impulses in the CNS. For example, an impulse in a group-IV fiber from the toe of an adult takes about 1 s to reach the spinal cord (a distance of about 1 m), whereas an impulse in a group-II fiber (conduction velocity 50 m/s) requires only about 20 ms to cover the same distance. Many reflexes induced by mechanical stimuli, and most of our subjective sensations, have shorter latencies than the conduction times in group-IV fibers would allow. For this reason alone, such fibers cannot be involved in these fast reflexes, at least not in their early stages.

Examination of the *response behavior* of mechanosensitive group-IV receptors reveals another important difference from the corpuscular mechanodetectors discussed above: Skin stimuli of identical intensity give rise to very different responses. This implies that receptors of this type cannot signal changes in stimulus intensity accurately. That is, with respect to measurement of stimulus intensity, the precision of single mechanoreceptors innervated by unmyelinated nerve fibers is very poor. No more than two intensity levels can be discriminated. This imprecision suggests that these receptors are *threshold detectors* — sensors that signal only the presence of a stimulus at a particular place on the skin. In addition, they may participate in transmitting weak mechanical *stimuli moving over the skin* (for instance, a crawling insect). The possibility has also been discussed that their activation, alone or with other receptors, induces the *sensation of tickle.*

Receptive fields of mechanoreceptors. The receptive field of a mechanoreceptor is the area within which an applied stimulus of specified intensity can elicit a response of the receptor. The intensity ordinarily used is some small multiple of the threshold intensity — for example, a factor of four or five. Receptive-field extent on the inside of the human hand, as measured in this way, is diagrammed for the four types of mechanoreceptors in hairless skin in Figure 2–10. In A are the receptive fields of 15 *Merkel-cell units.* They are small; their area is ordinarily 3 to 50 mm², which corresponds approximately to diameters of 2 to 8 mm. The receptive fields of the *Ruffini endings,* which also adapt slowly, are relatively large (B). As has been mentioned, these receptors are characterized by direction-sensitivity. The differences in size of the receptive fields of the rapidly adapting receptors are still more pronounced. The receptive fields of the *Meissner corpuscles* (C) are just as small as those of the Merkel's cells, whereas those of the *Pacinian corpuscles* (D) cover a broad area — a whole finger, for instance, or half of the entire palmar surface.

In hairy skin the receptive fields of the Ruffini endings and Pacinian corpuscles are of the same size as in hairless skin, and the receptive fields of the tactile disks are small, like those of the Merkels's cells. As a rule, however, one nerve fiber supplies two to three tactile disks, so that a single afferent unit has two or three separate small receptive fields. The hair-follicle receptors are organized differently; here one afferent nerve fiber supplies as many as a few hundred neighboring hair follicles, so that these fibers have large receptive fields. Conversely, each hair follicle is innervated by many afferent fibers. That is, the afferent innervation of the hair follicles is characterized by marked divergence and convergence.

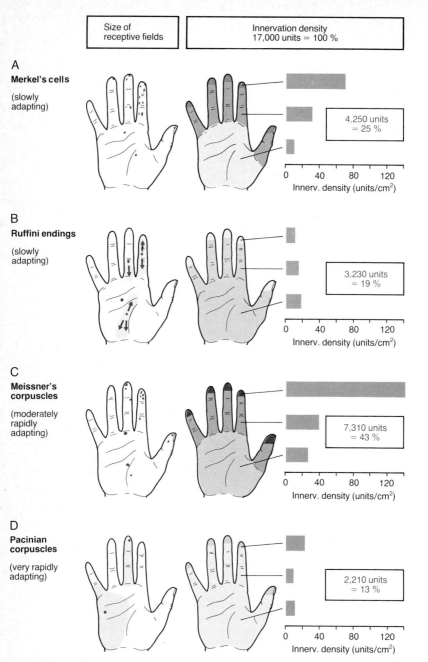

Fig. 2–10. Receptive fields and innervation densities of mechanoreceptors with corpuscular end structures and group-II afferent fibers, on the palmar surface of the human hand. From VALLBO and JOHANSSON 1984

Innervation density of mechanoreceptors. The inner surface of the human hand is supplied by about 17,000 mechanoreceptive nerve fibers of group II. The proportions of the different types of mechanoreceptors and their distribution density over the fingertips, proximal finger surfaces and palms are shown in Figure 2–10. The Meissner corpuscles are relatively numerous (43%); their remarkable density (ca. 140 per cm^2) at the fingertips certainly bears the main responsibility for the fine spatial resolution in this region. It is likely that the innervation density in the lips and the tip of the tongue is similarly high, but as yet no detailed data are available for these or any other skin areas apart from the palm. On the whole, it appears that the rapidly adapting receptors are clearly in the majority in the hand (both hairy and hairless parts) of humans, apes and other mammals. This makes sense from a functional viewpoint, because changes in stimulus phenomena as a rule are more important to the organism than the absolute magnitudes of intensity, duration or frequency of a stimulus.

Receptor function and mechanoperception. At the end of the 1960's a technique was introduced by which the activity of single afferent nerve fibers could be recorded in humans, with metal microelectrodes inserted through the intact skin (i.e., transcutaneously). Such experiments not only provided the results cited above (see Fig. 2–10 and associated text) but also made it possible to carry out neurophysiological and psychophysical measurements at the same time. For example, one could test whether the threshold for conscious sensation of a tactile stimulus to the skin coincides with the threshold for response of one or more of the various mechanoreceptor types, or whether the sensation threshold is clearly above the receptor threshold, so that sensation occurs only when mechanoreceptors are excited by stimuli well above threshold.

In the case of the human hand, it turned out that the *excitation of a single Meissner corpuscle* in the skin of the inner surface of a finger produces a tactile sensation, even if the receptor discharges only one impulse (with an impression depth of 5–10 μm). For vibration stimuli above 60 Hz, again, excitation of one or a few Pacinian corpuscles suffices to produce a sensation of vibration. The Merkel's cells and Ruffini endings are not involved in the perception of such small stimuli, because their thresholds are several times higher than those of the two other receptor types.

For stimuli to the palm, however, the sensation threshold is distinctly higher than that of the rapidly adapting mechanoreceptors. That is, on the inner surface of the fingers the threshold of the mechanoreceptors determines the sensation threshold, whereas in other skin areas the sensation threshold is higher due to central mechanisms. Evidently the central nervous system pays more attention to impulses from skin areas of tactile importance than to those from less important areas.

When suprathreshold tactile stimuli are presented, both the psychophysical intensity curves (Figs. 1–7, 2–3) and the discharge-vs.-intensity curves of pressure receptors (Fig. 2–6) are described by power functions, the exponents of which may have similar values. However, it remained an open question whether the form of the psychophysical intensity function is mainly a reflection of the receptor discharge or is also fundamentally affected by central nervous processes. Simultaneous measurement of pressure-receptor discharge and the intensity of subjective sensation in response to pressure stimuli to the human skin have largely resolved the question, in favor of the second alternative. That is, the exponents for the discharge function of single receptors and for the intensity function of the associated sensations are usually so far apart as to imply a fundamental involvement of the central nervous system in shaping the psychophysical intensity functions.

Q 2.1. Arrange the following skin regions according to the magnitude of the simultaneous spatial threshold. Begin with the area that has the lowest threshold.
a) Edge of the tongue
b) Red part of the lips
c) Tip of the index finger
d) Palm of the hand
e) Back
f) Back of the hand

Q 2.2. Which of the following terms applies to the Pacinian corpuscle?
a) Intensity detector
b) Acceleration detector
c) Threshold detector
d) Velocity detector
e) Pressure detector

Q 2.3. Which of the following histologic structures has/have the characteristic of an intensity detector?
a) Pacinian corpuscle
b) Meissner corpuscle
c) Merkel's cell
d) Hair-follicle receptor
e) Ruffini ending

Q 2.4. Which type of afferent nerve fiber supplies the hair-follicle receptors?
a) Group Ia
b) Group Ib
c) Group II
d) Group III
e) Group IV

Q 2.5. Which of the receptors in the following list are velocity detectors?
a) Pacinian corpuscles
b) Tactile disks

c) Hair-follicle receptors
d) Meissner corpuscles
e) Merkel's cells

Q 2.6. Which of the following statements applies to the mechanosensitive units with unmyelinated afferent fibers (group-IV fibers)?
a) These units display a very constant stimulus/response behavior.
b) The conduction velocity of the afferent fibers is over 2 m/s.
c) The number of discriminable intensity steps is more than three.
d) Only statements b and c are correct.
e) All the statements (a–d) are false.

Q 2.7. The receptors in the human fingertip with the highest innervation densities are
a) the Meissner corpuscles
b) the Merkel's cells
c) the Pacinian corpuscles
d) the Ruffini endings
e) It is not possible to say anything about the innervation densities of the various receptor types.

Q 2.8. Two of the receptor types listed in Question 2.7 have small, sharply delimited receptive fields. These are the
a) Ruffini endings and Pacinian corpuscles
b) Ruffini endings and Meissner corpuscles
c) Meissner and Pacinian corpuscles
d) Merkel's cells and Ruffini endings
e) Merkel's cells and Meissner corpuscles

2.2 Proprioception

In the waking state we are aware of the orientation of our limbs with respect to one another. We also perceive the movements of our joints, and we are able to state fairly accurately the amount of resistance opposing any movement we make. These abilities together constitute the *deep sensibility* mentioned at the beginning of this chapter. The three qualities of this modality are the senses of position, of movement, and of force; these will be discussed below. Then we shall turn to the receptors involved, which are located primarily in the muscles, tendons, and joints. Finally it will be shown that the structure of the tactile world — like our total subjective impression of the position of the body in space — is an integrative achievement of the nervous system, in which sensory modalities other than deep sensibility, and the motor system as well, play crucial roles.

According to Figure 2–1 (p. 31), the main receptors for deep sensibility are those in the joints, muscles and tendons. Because these receptors receive stimuli from the body itself and not the surroundings, they are called *proprioceptors,* and deep sensibility is usually termed *proprioception.* It should be kept in mind, however, that cutaneous receptors can also be excited during joint movements (by stretching and compression of the skin; see Fig. 2–9) and in this way may make a contribution to deep sensibility (see below).

Qualities of proprioception. In the dark, or with eyes closed, one is aware of the position of one's own limbs and the orientation of their parts with respect to one another. This proprioceptive quality is called the *sense of position.* Strictly speaking, the sense of position informs us of the angles at each of our joints, and thus of the relative positions of the limbs. When we have not moved our limbs for a long time, or when we awaken from a long sleep, our sense of their positions is usually well preserved. Apparently, then, the sense of position displays little or no adaptation.

The amount of bending at the joints cannot be described with any degree of accuracy without special practice, either in degrees of angle or in any other verbal form. But we can easily demonstrate the precision with which we are informed of the relative positions of the different parts of our limbs by the following two experiments. First, any position taken by one limb, whether adopted actively or imposed passively (by an experimenter), can be imitated without visual control by the corresponding limb on the other side. Second, we can find very accurately any point on one limb (whether specified by ourselves or by an experimenter) with the fingers of the contralateral hand, again with no visual control.

When we change the angle at a joint without visual control — for example, when we pull in or extend the lower arm at the elbow — we perceive both the direction and the velocity of the movement. This quality of proprioception is called the *sense of movement.* Here the threshold for perception depends on the extent and the velocity of the change of angle. This threshold is distinctly lower at the proximal joints (e. g., the shoulders) than at those more distal (e. g., the finger joints).

Our ability to estimate the amount of muscular force that must be exerted in order to make a movement or to maintain the position of a joint against a resistance is also a quality of proprioception. We call it the *sense of force.* Because the force a muscle must exert depends on the resistance opposing the movement, we could use the expression "resistance sense" as a synonym for the sense of force, but this term has not come into common use.

In determining experimentally the performance of this sense, one inevitably encounters difficulties in eliminating or controlling contributions from cutaneous mechanoreceptors. However, it can easily be shown that the discriminatory ability of the sense of force is distinctly better than that of the pressure sense of the skin. It is very much more difficult to estimate the weight of an object if it is set on the skin than if it is lifted — a fact that everyone turns to advantage in ordinary life.

Proprioceptors. As mentioned at the beginning of this section, these are receptors in subcutaneous structures (joints, muscles, tendons), which together with cutaneous mechanoreceptors can mediate deep sensibility. Their role with regard to the senses of position, movement and force will be considered in the following paragraphs. The joint receptors will be treated in somewhat more detail; properties of the muscle receptors (muscle spindles, GOLGI tendon organs) can be found in Sections 4.2 and 6.1 of *Fundamentals of Neurophysiology,* and those of the cutaneous receptors are discussed in the preceding Section 2.1, from page 30 on.

First we shall describe the *joint receptors.* Their afferent nerve fibers usually run together in special joint or articular nerves. Each joint nerve contains a number of thick myelinated (group II) and thin myelinated (group III) afferent nerve fibers as well as unmyelinated afferents (group-IV fibers). There are usually distinctly more fibers in the last category than the first two. The group-II fibers and a few of group III end in mechanosensitive *corpuscular receptor structures* (mainly GOLGI-MANZONI and paciniform corpuscles and Ruffini endings). The rest of the group-III fibers and all those of group IV terminate in *free nerve endings* that innervate the joint capsules and ligaments. For example, the afferent innervation of the knee consists of about 400 myelinated (groups II and III) and 800 unmyelinated afferents (in addition there are about 800 unmyelinated sympathetic efferents).

When a joint moves, the joint capsule is compressed and stretched. Therefore the mechanosensitive *corpuscular receptors* could provide information about the position of a joint as well as about the direction and velocity of its movement. That is, in principle they could mediate the sense of position and movement (but not of force). But in experiments on animals, at least, these receptors have been found to have mainly phasic (dynamic) responses, which moreover are elicited by movement in more than one direction — for example, by flexion as well as extension and rotation of the joint. The most that could be concluded by observing the discharge of a single joint receptor of this kind is whether a joint movement is occurring or not.

Little is known about the response characteristics of the free nerve endings with thin myelinated and unmyelinated nerve fibers (groups III and IV). Many of these afferents probably have nociceptive functions; that is, they do not respond until the joint movement threatens to go beyond the physiological working range of the joint, or when damage to the joint (by injury or inflammation) occurs. Apparently the *joint nociceptors,* like many other nociceptors (see p. 123), can be stimulated not only by strong mechanical stimuli but also by certain chemical stimuli (e. g., bradykinin, serotonin, prostaglandin, K^+ ions); that is, they are multimodal nociceptors. Excitation of these receptors produces joint pain.

The *non-nociceptive free nerve endings* seem to be mainly mechanosensitive receptors, activated both by local stimuli (pressure on the joint capsule) and by joint movements. Research on these has been scanty, and little information is available about either their receptive properties or their role in proprioception. It appears that the tonic (static) components of their responses are more pronounced than is the case with the corpuscular joint receptors. Nevertheless, it is still impossible to draw reliable conclusions about joint position from the discharge of a single receptor or even a number of receptors of this type.

On the whole, given the known properties of the mechanosensitive low-threshold joint receptors, it seems likely that these receptors contribute in mediating the sense of movement, though they may also play a role in the sense of position. Other findings also point in this direction. If transmission through the articular nerves is interrupted, either by illness or by local anesthesia, the sensations of position and movement are severely impaired.

But the *muscle-spindle receptors* are also involved in sensing position and movement; in humans, if these receptors are selectively stimulated with small-amplitude vibrations applied to the tendon (e. g., 100 Hz, amplitudes of a few micrometers), the subject's judgement of his actual joint position deteriorates to a remarkable degree. Such false impressions of position become evident when the subject is asked to set the corresponding joint on the other side into the same position as that set by the experimenter, without visual control.

The most likely detectors of force sensations are the stretch receptors in the musculature — the *muscle spindles and tendon organs.* But it should be remembered that the discharge rate of the muscle spindle afferents depends not only on the momentary length of the muscle, but equally on the activity of (and hence tension in) the intrafusal muscle fibers excited by the γ motor axons (cf. *Fundamentals of Neurophysiology,* Sec. 6.1). It has also been shown that animals cannot be conditioned to selective stimulation of the group-I fibers. Therefore it must be assumed that the sense of force is mediated also by *other receptors* than those just mentioned.

In addition to the articular, muscle and tendon receptors, *receptors in the skin* over the joints may possibly contribute to proprioception. The slowly adapting RUFFINI endings in particular, as described in the preceding section, are excited by stretching of the skin, in some cases in a clearly direction-specific manner (Fig. 2–10 B). The extremely sensitive PACINIAN corpuscles, with their large receptive fields, would also be expected to be activated by joint movements. Experiments on human skin have now supported this expectation. They have shown that joint movements can excite cutaneous mechanoreceptors of all four types, the PACINIAN corpuscles most frequently and the RUFFINI endings next most frequently. On the other hand, the role of the skin receptors in proprioception should not be overestimated, because proprioceptive ability deteriorates only slightly when the skin regions over the joints are locally anesthetized.

Central integration. Evidently, then, none of the receptor systems considered above is independently capable of mediating the information necessary for one or another quality of proprioception. It follows that perception in this modality must require the *simultaneous activation of various receptor systems* in particular combinations, and the central integration of such afferent inputs (Fig. 2–11, red-shaded elements). This *integrative processing,* as in the case of other sensory inputs, begins in the *subcortical sensory nuclei.* For example, in the thalamus neurons have been found with responses that accurately reflected joint position over more than 90 °. There must be remarkably precise and subtle convergence onto such a neuron of many proprioceptive signals, and it may be that only a small proportion of these come from the joint receptors themselves.

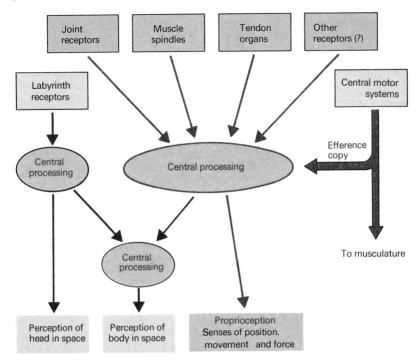

Fig. 2–11. The origin of proprioceptive sensations. The afferent inputs from proprioceptors are integrated with the motor efference copies (or "corollary discharges") in the nervous system, to allow perception of position, movement and force. The information coming from the receptors of the vestibular organ, together with proprioception, contributes to the perception of the body in space

This central integration also involves signals from nonsensory sources. One such input — which constitutes an important and still little-understood aspect of CNS processing — derives from the central motor systems. They appear to send a "memo" (*efference copy* or *corollary discharge;* on the right in Fig. 2–11) of their signals to the muscles, to interact centrally with the sensory input from proprioceptors. These efference copies give advance information about the intended muscle activity and the movements that will result. Thus they can be used to *eliminate ambiguity in afferent information.* In the muscle spindles, for example, ambiguity is introduced by the γ-fiber activity, and other receptors may be activated by external stimuli as well as by movement (e. g., cutaneous mechanoreceptors near joints).

Another aspect of proprioception that has so far received little attention is that the static position of a joint need not necessarily be communicated by the maintained discharge of tonic receptors. It is entirely conceivable that the central nervous system can *derive joint position from phasic proprioceptive signals* and store this information in memory so that it is available until the next change in joint position occurs. In this case the sense of position would not be dependent on special receptors with a prolonged tonic discharge.

Body scheme and body position. Signals from peripheral proprioceptors and central efference copies are thus the major variables that serve to keep one's internal picture or *scheme of the arrangement of the body* up to date, according to the movements of head, trunk, and limbs. Proprioception, along with inputs from the equilibrium organ (labyrinth receptors, see p. 224), which notify us of the position of the head in the earth's field of gravity, ultimately work together to keep us informed about the *position of the body in space* (left in Fig. 2–11).

Consciousness of the spatial disposition of our bodies is astonishingly firmly anchored in us, and appears to be separable from the afferent influx from the proprioceptors. Consider, for example, the fact that even after partial or complete amputation of a limb, the great majority of patients still feel the missing limb for a long time, often for the rest of their lives. The illusion is frequently so persuasive that the patient experiences his *phantom limb* more intimately than his remaining one. Sometimes the patient is able to "move" the phantom limb at will (an influence of efference copy?); in other cases he feels it to be in an unalterable, permanent position. It often happens that somatosensory sensations arise in the phantom limb. Unfortunately many of these are unpleasant — occasionally they are so painful that the *phantom-limb pain,* which is difficult to alleviate therapeutically, becomes a heavy or even unbearable burden on the patient.

The structure of the tactile world. Our concepts of space are formed largely by visual perceptions. But many properties of the environment can be better experienced by one's hand, as it touches and feels. For example, think of properties such as liquid, sticky, firm, yielding, soft, hard, smooth, rough, velvety — and the many others recognized by a combination of proprioception, mechanoreception, and cutaneous thermoreception. An important point here is that these properties are discerned poorly, if at all, by passive touching (laying the object on the hand, or simply putting the hand on the object and holding it still). However, by moving the hand one has little trouble in recognizing structure and form. The superiority of the "feeling" hand over the motionless one derives in part from the activation of many more cutaneous receptors, owing to the motion; adaptation is circumvented, so that detailed information about distortion of the skin is sent centrally. Moreover, when the hand moves proprioception contributes its share to the recognition of form and resilience of the objects touched.

Q 2.9. Name the three qualities of proprioception that you learned in this section.

Q 2.10. Which three of the following receptors count as proprioceptors?
a) Hair-follicle receptors
b) Joint receptors
c) Golgi tendon organs
d) Meissner corpuscles
e) Muscle-spindle receptors
f) Pacinian corpuscles
g) Tactile disks

Q 2.11. The joint receptors with free nerve endings and fine afferent nerve fibers of groups III and IV are not involved in proprioception *because* all of them are nociceptors.
a) Both statements as well as the conjunction are correct.
b) Both statements are correct, but the conjunction is wrong.
c) Only the first statement is correct.
d) Only the second statement is correct.
e) Both statements are incorrect.

Q 2.12. Which of the following properties of a body are only or primarily detectable by touching, and not by visual impressions?
a) Angular
b) Sticky
c) Round
d) Dark
e) Soft
f) Velvety
g) Fluid
h) Bright
i) Elastic

Q 2.13. Which of the following receptor types probably participate in producing the sensation of a resistive force? (Choose the two you think most important).
a) Merkel's cells
b) Hair-follicle receptors
c) Joint receptors
d) Pacinian corpuscles
e) Muscle-spindle receptors
f) Golgi tendon organs
g) Tactile disks

2.3 Thermoreception

In this section we shall discuss the *sense of temperature* (synonyms: thermoreception, thermoperception) of the skin. This sensory modality can be assigned two qualities, on the basis of both objective and subjective findings. These are the senses of *cold* and *warm*. Properties of this system in humans include the following: In the skin there are specific cold and warm points, at which only sensations of cold or warmth can be elicited. Reaction-time measurements have indicated higher conduction velocities for sensations of cold than for warmth. By selective blocking of nerves it is possible to prevent either the cold sensation alone or the warm sensation alone. Finally, there are specific cold and warm receptors in the skin. These serve not only as sensors for conscious sensations of temperature; they also participate in the thermoregulation of the body. In the latter task they are supplemented and reinforced by temperature sensors in the CNS (e. g., in hypothalamus and spinal cord). As a rule we are not conscious of the activity of these central thermoreceptors; they will not be discussed here.

In the analysis of thermoreception it has proved helpful to study those physiologic processes that can be recorded while the skin temperature is constant separately from recordings of those that appear during a change in skin temperature. Accordingly, in the following discussion of psychophysical results first the *static* and then the *dynamic* temperature sensations will be considered; the same sequence will be followed in the discussion of thermoreceptors per se.

Static temperature sensations (constant skin temperature). When you get into a warm (~ 33° centigrade [°C]) bath, you first experience a clear sensation of warmth. After some time this sensation fades away, even if the water temperature is kept constant. You are no doubt also familiar with the opposite phenomenon — when you jump into a pool with water at about 28°C on a hot summer day, you first feel that the water is cool. After some time, however, the sensation of cold tends to die away. At least in an intermediate temperature range, then, warming or cooling give rise only temporarily to the respective sensations of warmth or cold. In this range of temperatures there is an essentially complete adaptation of temperature sensation to the new skin temperature.

The temperature range within which complete adaptation of the temperature sensation occurs is thus a neutral zone (sometimes called the "comfort" zone). Above or below this neutral zone, permanent sensations of heat or cold are produced even when the skin temperature is kept constant for a long time (the best-known example is perhaps feeling that one's feet are cold for hours at a time). The upper and lower temperature limits of the neutral zone are 36°C and 30°C, respectively, for a skin area of 15 cm^2. When smaller areas of skin are studied, the zone expands, and with larger areas it becomes narrower (an indication of central summation of the impulses coming from the thermoreceptors). In experiments with naked humans in a climate-controlled room, the range narrows to only 33°–35°C.

The *maintained sensations of warmth* that persist at constant skin temperatures above 36°C are more intense, the higher the temperature of the skin. At temperatures of more than 43°–44°C the sensation of warmth gives way to a painful heat sensation (heat pain). Similarly, at temperatures below 30°C the *maintained cold sensation* increases in intensity, the colder the skin. Actual cold pain sets in at skin temperatures of 17°C and lower, but at skin temperatures as high as 25°C the sensation of cold has an unpleasant component, especially when large areas of skin are affected. (Man is a tropical creature, intolerant of skin temperatures much below 30°C.)

Measurements of the *time course of adaptation* after a stepwise change of skin temperature within the neutral zone have shown that it takes many minutes for the temperature sensation produced by the step to be replaced by a neutral sensation. Even outside the neutral zone there is (incomplete) adaption after a new skin temperature has been established, as we know well from ordinary experience. Dipping the hand into warm water (42°C) initially gives rise to a strong sensation of warmth; this falls off rapidly at first, then more slowly, until a maintained warmth sensation of low intensity is reached.

Studies of the *static temperature sensation on the inner surface of the hand* indicate that there, even with very long adaptation times (30 min or more) within the temperature range 27°–40°C, reproducible estimation of skin temperature is possible; that is, there is *no complete adaptation*. Figure 2–12 shows means of

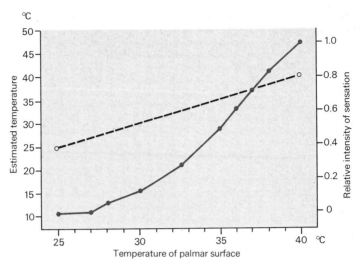

Fig. 2-12. Psychophysical intensity function (*solid red line*) for the perception of temperature of the palmar surface, as a function of the actual skin temperature after an adaptation time of 30 min. Left ordinate: estimates in degrees centigrade (Celsius). Right ordinate: estimates in relative units. The *dashed line* indicates the shape and position the curve would have if the actual and estimated skin temperatures agreed. Average for 18 subjects. Modified from HENSEL et al.: In ZOTTERMAN, Y. (ed.): Sensory Functions of the Skin in Primates. Oxford: Pergamon Press 1976

static temperature estimates by 18 subjects, as a function of the constant temperature at which the palmar surface was actually held. The subjects were asked both to give their skin temperature in centigrade (degrees Celsius, left ordinate) and to estimate its position on a relative scale between the highest (40°C) and the lowest (25°C) temperature. Their estimates, in centigrade, were most accurate when the actual temperature was near 37°C; at higher and lower temperatures the temperatures estimated were distinctly above or below the correct value. The skin temperatures 25°C and 27°C were estimated to be 10°! In these experiments temperatures around 34°C were felt to be neither cold nor warm, so that this region can be regarded as a (very narrow) neutral zone. At 37°C the subjects had a pleasant, maintained sensation of warmth.

Dynamic temperature sensations. The sensations appearing during changes in skin temperature can be considered to be determined by three parameters: the initial temperature of the skin, the rate of change of temperature, and the size of the area of skin affected by the stimulus.

The *influence of starting temperature* upon the threshold for a sensation of warmth or cold is shown in Figure 2-13. At low skin temperatures — for example, at 28°C — the threshold for a warmth sensation is high and that for a cold sensation low. If the starting temperature (abscissa) is shifted upward, the warmth thresholds decrease and those for cold increase. In other words, a cool skin (e. g., 28°C) has to be cooled further by less than 0.2°C in order for the maintained cold

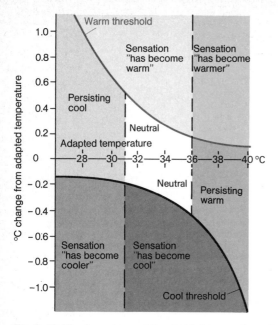

Fig. 2–13. The dependence of thresholds for sensations of warmth and cold upon the initial skin temperature. Starting at the temperatures shown on the abscissa, to which the skin had been adapted for some time, the skin temperature had to be changed by the number of degrees (centigrade or Celsius) shown on the ordinate in order to elicit a sensation of cold or warmth. The diagram is valid for all temperature changes at a rate of more than 6 °C/min. Modified from KENSHALO. In: ZOTTERMAN, Y. (ed.): Sensory Functions of the Skin in Primates. Oxford: Pergamon Press 1976

sensation to give way to the sensation "colder". The same skin must be warmed by almost 1°C before a sensation of warmth occurs. However, if the initial temperature is 38°C a slight warming (< 0.2°C) elicits the sensation "warmer", whereas the skin must be cooled by around 0.8°C if a "cooler" sensation is to be experienced.

We should also mention a peculiarity of this response that is not apparent in Figure 2–13. When the change is such that the temperature moves out of the neutral zone (31°–36°C in Fig. 2–13), cooling or warming cause a shift from a neutral sensation to a sensation of cold or warmth. On the other hand, if the skin is warmed up from a temperature of 28°C (for example), before reaching the warmth threshold shown in Figure 2–13, the subject says that the skin is "less cool" and then "neutral". Conversely, when the skin is cooled down from a high temperature, the first feelings are „less warm" and then "neutral", before a sensation of cold appears. These *sensations of decreasing intensity* of an existing cold or warmth sensation are distinctly different from those described as the occurrence of a sensation of warmth or cold.

A final conclusion to be drawn from Figure 2–13 is that at *a given skin temperature,* depending on the stimulus conditions, sensations of *either warmth or cold* can be produced. For example, when the starting temperature is 32°C warming by 0.5°C gives rise to a sensation of warmth, whereas cooling by 0.5°C from an initial 33°C produces a distinct sensation of cold. You can easily convince yourself of the phenomenon just described by repeating Weber's "three-bowl experiment"; fill one bowl with cold, one with lukewarm, and the last with warm water and then put one hand in the cold water and the other in the warm water. Now if you move both hands to the bowl with the lukewarm water, you will have a clear sensation of warmth in one hand and of cold in the other.

As Figure 2–14 shows, the *rate of temperature change* has little effect on the warmth and cold thresholds, as long as the change is more rapid than 0.1°C/s (6°C/min). With slower temperature changes both thresholds increase steadily. This is true even when the temperature changes at rates slower than those shown in Figure 2–14. For example, cooling of the skin by 0.4°C/min (0.0067°C/s) from a starting temperature of 33.5°C gives rise to a sensation of cold only after the temperature has fallen by 4.4°C, 11 min after the change was begun. When cooling is very slow, then, a person may not notice that large regions of his skin have become quite cold (with concomitant loss of heat from the body), especially if his attention is distracted by other things. It is conceivable that this factor is involved when one catches a cold.

With respect to the *size of the skin area* affected by a change in temperature, the thresholds to cooling or warming of small areas are higher than when large areas are stimulated; moreover, with a given suprathreshold change in skin temperature

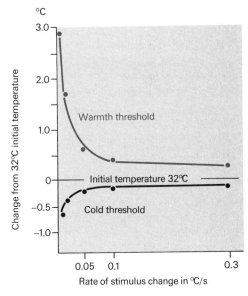

Fig. 2–14. The dependence of cold and warmth thresholds on the rate of temperature change. The starting temperature in all cases was 32 °C. Modified from KENSHALO. In: ZOTTERMAN, Y. (ed): Sensory Functions of the Skin in Primates. Oxford: Pergamon Press 1976

the intensity of the sensation increases with the stimulated area. That is, in both the threshold and the suprathreshold region there is a central nervous *spatial facilitation* of the impulses coming from the thermoreceptors. This is especially clear in experiments in which the stimulus is given bilaterally. For example, when heat stimuli are applied simultaneously to the backs of both hands, the threshold is lower than when either hand is stimulated alone.

Cold and warm points; spatial thresholds. The sensitivity of the human skin to cold and heat is localized at different points in the skin. That is, there are cold points and warm points. These are distributed over the skin in varying density, though on the whole they are less numerous than the touch points of the mechanoreceptor system. A comparison of the densities of cold and warm points on the skin has shown that there are clearly more of the former than the latter. For example, the hand surfaces have 1–5 cold points per square centimeter, but only 0.4 warm points per square centimeter. The greatest density of cold points is in the most temperature-sensitive region of the skin, the face. Here there are 16–19 cold points per square centimeter. Individual warm points cannot be resolved on the face, probably because deep in the skin the warm receptors are so close together that a thermode placed on the surface always excites several at once. The warmth sensitivity of the facial skin appears as a uniform sensory continuum.

The low density of cold, and especially of warm points as compared with the grain for mechanoreceptors makes it understandable that the simultaneous spatial thresholds to temperature stimuli are relatively large. The spatial thresholds for cold stimuli are lower than those for warmth. Moreover, there are considerable differences in the longitudinal and transverse directions. For example, on the thigh the simultaneous spatial threshold for warm stimuli in the longitudinal direction is 26 cm and in the transverse direction, 9 cm; the corresponding values for cold stimuli are 16.5 and 2.9 cm.

Cold and warm receptors. In primates (including man), and in many other animals as well, the presence of *specific thermoreceptors* has been established conclusively. They share the following characteristics:
- Maintained discharge at constant skin temperatures, with discharge rate proportional to skin temperature (static response, Fig. 2–15)
- A rise (or fall) in discharge rate during a change in skin temperature (dynamic response, Fig. 2–16)
- Insensitivity to nonthermal stimuli
- Threshold sensitivity comparable to the sensation thresholds to thermal stimulation of the skin
- Small receptive fields (1 mm^2 or less), each afferent fiber supplying only one or a few warm or cold points
- Conduction velocities of the afferent nerve fibers below 20 m/s, and in some species as low as 0.4 m/s.

An example of the discharge rates of thermoreceptors *at constant skin temperature* is shown in Figure 2–15. The mean static frequencies in the two

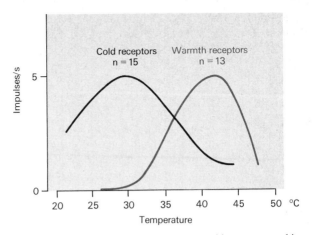

Fig. 2–15. Responses of cold *(left)* and warm *(right)* receptors in the monkey skin at constant skin temperature. The action potentials were recorded from thin filaments of the associated nerves, as in the sketch in Fig. 2–6. The data are means for the steady discharge frequencies of the populations of cold and warm receptors indicated in the figure. Modified from KENSHALO. In: ZOTTERMAN, Y. (ed.): Sensory Functions of the Skin in Primates. Oxford: Pergamon Press 1976

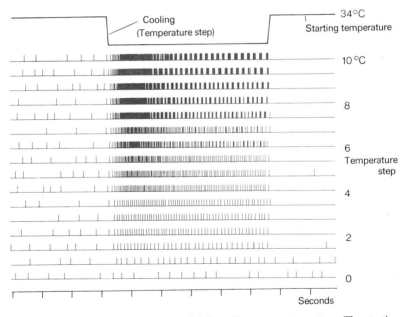

Fig. 2–16. Behavior of a cold receptor during brief, cooling temperature steps. The starting temperature was 34 °C for each record. The amplitude of each cooling step is given in degrees Celsius at the right. Particularly when the steps are large, the phasic-tonic behavior immediately after the cooling, as well as the occurrence of bursts of discharges during cooling, are clearly evident. Records from a filament of the median nerve to the skin of a monkey, made with the technique shown in Fig. 2–6. Modified from DARIAN-SMITH et al.: J. Neurophysiol. **36**, 325 (1973)

populations (cold and warm receptors) form "bell-shaped" curves, with the maximal activity of the cold receptors at about 30°C and that of the warm receptors at about 43°C. (The individual activity maxima of single cold receptors lie between 17 °C and 36°C; those of single warm receptors are between 41°C and 47°C).

The behavior of thermoreceptors during a *change in the skin temperature* is illustrated with the example of a cold receptor during cooling and rewarming (Fig. 2–16). Cooling elicits dynamic responses dependent on the size of the temperature step; within a few seconds, these give way to the new static response. When the skin is rewarmed to the original temperature there is a transient cessation of activity before the initial frequency of discharge (shown at the beginning of each record and in the bottom trace) is once again resumed. The behavior of warm receptors subjected to temperature change is the mirror image of the above. Warming causes them to discharge at a higher rate, and during cooling there is an undershoot in frequency, followed by return to a steady level.

The *histologic structure* of the thermoreceptors is not yet entirely clear. They are probably *free nerve endings* of thin nerve fibers of groups III and IV, with the cold receptors in human skin lying in and just below the epidermis, and the warm receptors more in the upper and middle layers of the corium. The cold receptors of humans are supplied mainly by thin myelinated nerve fibers (group III) and the warm receptors by unmyelinated fibers (group IV). (Hence the more rapid response to cold stimuli, mentioned above.)

Receptor function and thermoreception. There is no doubt that the activation of thermoreceptors by thermal stimuli is responsible for temperature sensations. However, as will be apparent in the following comparison of the receptive and subjective responses, receptor activity is reflected in consciousness only after considerable *central nervous integration* of the influx from the periphery. We have mentioned that spatial summation of temperature stimuli occurs; this is one aspect of such processing.

As Figure 2–15 shows, with skin temperature held constant in the subjective neutral zone (31°–36°C) both warm and cold receptors discharge impulses. Thus thermoreceptor activity per se, at least at low frequencies, does not necessarily give rise to subjective sensations. Sensations arise only if impulses reach the CNS at a sufficient rate. The *maintained sensations of warmth* above 36°C can be interpreted in similar terms, as the result of the steadily increasing discharge rates of the warm receptors as temperature rises; above 43°C, because of the additional excitation of heat receptors, the sensation of warmth gives way to a painful heat sensation. The *maintained cold sensations* below 31°C, on the other hand, cannot be so simply ascribed to the increase in static discharge of the cold receptors. That is, the lower limit of the neutral zone and the position of the maximal average discharge rate of the cold receptors are, for practical purposes, the same. Furthermore, the average discharge rates at 25°C and 33°C (for example) are about the same, but at the lower temperature there is a lasting sensation of cold and at the higher, a neutral sensation. In this case, therefore, additional information is required to decide on which side of the bell-shaped curve the actual skin temperature lies. One way in which this could be derived is from the presence or absence of simultaneous discharge of the warm receptors; alternatively, the CNS could make use of the fact that many cold receptors tend to discharge in short bursts in their intermediate frequency range (Fig. 2–16). As a final example of the central modifications the peripheral inputs undergo before they are reflected in consciousness, remember that the time course of *subjective adaptation* to a new skin temperature extends over *many minutes* (p. 54), whereas the *thermoreceptors* adapt to a new temperature within a *few seconds* (Fig. 2–16). Evidently the central nervous activity induced by the transient efferent influx dies out slowly.

Special forms of temperature sensation. One common feature of the sense of temperature is the occurrence of *after-sensations*. For instance, if you press a cold metal rod against your forehead for about 30 s and then remove it, a distinct feeling of cold persists even though the skin is warming up again, so that a feeling of warmth might be expected. WEBER, who studied this curious situation, believed that the persistent cold sensation came from a spread of the cooling into the surrounding skin. But direct recordings from thermoreceptors have shown that the cold receptors, having been greatly cooled, continue to discharge during rewarming — at first even at an increasing rate. The after-sensation is thus a "normal" cold sensation. Corresponding sensations of warmth have also been described. Very strong warm stimuli (too-hot bath water) often elicit a *paradoxical cold sensation*. This is presumably based on the fact that the cold receptors, normally silent above 40°C, discharge again transiently when rapidly warmed to more than 45°C.

The *heat sensation* that occurs regularly at skin temperatures above 45°C is not yet entirely understood in terms of neurophysiologic correlates. It appears, however, that there are special heat receptors (see p. 125). Because the heat sensation also has a painful character, and since heat stimuli are injurious, the heat sensation is more appropriately considered a quality of pain than one of thermoreception. A strong negative affective component also characterizes the sensations of "oppressive closeness" and of chill. Both are accompanied by autonomic reflexes — sweating and expansion of the blood vessels in the former, and shivering and vasoconstriction in the latter. These are ordinarily elicited either by external stimuli or by psychological causes, though more rarely pathologic processes in the CNS may be implicated.

Clinical examination of the sense of temperature is usually limited to testing of the cold and warm sensations with two test tubes, one containing hot water and the other ice water. Spatially delimited disturbances of the sense of temperature can be diagnostic of spinal-tract damage or blocking. Usually the sense of pain is also affected, because the nociceptive afferents pass centrally along the same paths (see p. 91). Under such conditions mechanoreception and proprioception may be unaltered.

Q 2.14   Which of the following statements is (are) correct?
  a) With the skin temperature kept constant at 10°C, after a short time no further sensation of temperature is detectable.
  b) With the skin temperature kept constant at 25°C there is a permanent sensation of warmth.
  c) With the skin temperature kept constant at 33°C there is a permanent sensation of warmth.
  d) With the skin temperature kept constant at 20°C there is a maintained sensation of cold.
  e) All the above statements are false.

Q 2.15   Which of the following statements is (are) false?
  a) The threshold for a temperature sensation in response to a constant change in temperature is independent of the starting temperature.
  b) With a constant starting temperature, the appearance of a temperature sensation is independent of the rate of temperature change.
  c) Depending on the starting level and direction of temperature change, at intermediate skin temperatures a sensation of either warmth or cold can appear.
  d) In the neutral zone the subjective adaptation to a new temperature lasts precisely as long as the dynamic response of the thermoreceptors elicited by the temperature change.

Q 2.16.   The following statements apply to the sense of temperature:
  a) There are no cold or warm points: temperature sensitivity is distributed uniformly over the skin.
  b) The ability to resolve warm stimuli (simultaneous spatial threshold) is poorer than that for cold stimuli.
  c) The relation of cold sensitivity to warm sensitivity is the same at all places on the human skin.
  d) The part of the face with the best temperature sensitivity is the tip of the nose.
  e) The ability to resolve thermal stimuli (simultaneous spatial threshold) is poorer than that for mechanical stimuli.

Q 2.17.   Which statement is correct? The warm receptors
  a) do not discharge when the skin is at a constant temperature of less than 25°C.
  b) behave as purely tonic sensors.
  c) are supplied predominantly by group-II fibers.
  d) mediate the heat sensation at high stimulus intensity.
  e) are identical with the histologically identifiable Merkel's cells.

Q 2.18.   Which statement is correct? The cold receptors
  a) are supplied predominantly by group-I and group-II fibers.

b) are identical with the histologically identifiable Meissner corpuscles.
c) are normally silent at temperatures above 45°C.
d) discharge exclusively in proportion to the momentary skin temperature.
e) have spinal conduction pathways in common with mechanoreceptors.

2.4 Visceral Sensibility

Like the somatic nerves to skin, muscles and joints, the visceral nerves to the internal organs in the chest and abdominal cavity contain a high percentage of afferent nerve fibers. In the parasympathetic vagus nerve 80–90% of the fibers are thought to be afferent, in the sympathetic splanchnic nerve 50%, and in the parasympathetic pelvic nerves at least 30%. Thus the visceral receptors, with their afferent nerve fibers, make a considerable contribution to somatovisceral sensibility (cf. Fig. 2–1, p. 31).

The afferent fibers in the visceral nerves differ from those in the somatic nerves in the subjective effect of their activity. That is, we are conscious of the centripetal activity of visceral afferents only to a very small extent, and often only under special circumstances. This in itself implies that the main function of the visceral component of somatovisceral sensibility is something other than mediating sensations from the viscera. This other function can best be described as the *homeostatic role of the visceral receptors.* The signals they transmit are used by the autonomic parts of the central nervous system to detect departures from the normal state of the "internal milieu" of the body so that they can be corrected. For example, when the blood pressure falls or the carbon dioxide concentration in the blood becomes too high, appropriate adjustments are made to preserve homeostasis (the constancy of the internal milieu, one of the most fundamental prerequisites for animal and human life).

Of course, many signals from somatic receptors are also used to monitor homeostasis, regardless of whether the same signals simultaneously generate conscious sensations or not. In the skeletal muscles, for instance, there are receptors that respond to the accumulation of metabolic products (metabolites) during muscular work; the activity of these "metaboreceptors" causes more blood to flow through the muscle, to carry away the metabolites. We are not conscious of the activity of these receptors. On the other hand, activation of warm receptors in the skin initiates an increase in blood flow through the skin, and at the same time a sensation of warmth occurs.

On the whole, the available information about the total number of somatovisceral receptors and about their responses to stimuli is still very incomplete. Nevertheless, the current state of knowledge justifies the speculative conclusion that the *homeostatic functions* of the somatovisceral receptors *far outweigh their role in our sensory experience.* To put it another way: only a minute fraction of the centripetal activity in somatovisceral nerve fibers gives rise to conscious sensations. The phenomena of somatovisceral sensibility can be arranged in order of the varying degree to which they can reach the level of consciousness. At one end are receptors such as the Meissner corpuscles of the fingertips, which can cause a sensation of touch by discharging only a single impulse (see p. 45). At the other are receptors such as the glucose receptors in the liver (see p. 266), which apparently have no access at all to the conscious level. Between these extremes is a large intermediate region; we can become conscious of the activity of receptors here, given the appropriate spatial and temporal facilitation and convergence.

Many somatovisceral receptors are involved in *synthetic sensations* such as deep sensibility and the perception of the position of head and body in space (cf. Fig. 2–11 and associated text). Typical synthetic sensations mediated by the visceral receptors are those of *thirst* and *hunger.* These *general sensations* are the subject of a separate chapter in this book (Chapter 10, beginning p. 256). The other sensations mediated by visceral receptors — except for pain, to which another separate chapter is devoted (Chapter 4, beginning p. 117) — are treated in the following paragraphs.

Cardiovascular system (circulatory system). The volume of blood propelled through the body by the heart in a given time is matched to the varying demands of the tissues. This adjustment, and the associated maintenance of a constant blood pressure, is achieved with the aid of special mechanoreceptors which continually measure the blood pressure in the large vessels and the filling of the atria of the heart (*pressure receptors* in the aortic arch and in the carotid bodies, *stretch receptors* in the atrial walls). To all appearances, we are unaware of the life-long activity of these receptors. But we can perceive the activity of the heart, especially in extreme situations (e. g., great physical effort or severe mental tension, such that one's heart "pounds"). What are the receptors that mediate these perceptions of the heartbeat?

In the course of a cardiac cycle the heart changes considerably in shape, volume and position. During a heartbeat the left and right ventricles each expel 70 ml of blood; the volume of the heart is therefore reduced by this amount. During this process, the pressure in the left ventricle rises from nearly 0 mm Hg to 120 mm Hg (systolic blood pressure), and that in the right ventricle rises to 25 mm Hg. The pressure waves are conducted as pulse waves into the periphery of the body (from the left heart) and into the lungs (right heart). The jerky systolic contraction of the heart can be felt as an "apex impulse" by placing the fingers on the left side of the chest (5th intercostal space), and often is actually visible. It also produces the first heart sound; the second sound is produced at the end of systole by the closing of the aortic and pulmonary valves.

The mechanical forces acting on the chest wall *probably excite many mechanoreceptors* in the muscles, tendons, joints and subcutaneous tissue of the chest and spine — especially when the heart begins to work harder, so that the pressures mentioned above rise considerably and increases in stroke volume and heart rate raise the cardiac output to several times the resting level (5 l/min). The pulse waves also excite a large number of mechanoreceptors in the periphery of the body, Pacinian corpuscles in particular. Ordinarily we are unaware of the activity of all these somatic receptors, perhaps because we have learned to prevent this unimportant information from reaching the level of consciousness. This **afferent inhibition** is apparently overcome by the increased influx of afferent signals when heart activity intensifies, and then we notice the heartbeat.

It is conceivable that this afferent inhibition can be reduced voluntarily — for instance, by biofeedback training. Success at such training could enable a person to perceive the heartbeat even under "normal conditions". However, no clear and consistent results have yet been obtained in this regard.

Pulmonary system (respiratory system). We are ordinarily not conscious of the rhythmic activity of breathing, although at each breath many *somatic* mechanoreceptors in the chest and diaphragm are activated, along with numerous *visceral* mechanoreceptors in the thoracic and abdominal cavities. Again, there is evidently afferent inhibition that prevents us from receiving this information, which as a rule is not important to us. But we can turn our attention to our breathing at any time, so as to perceive the respiratory movements and voluntarily modify them.

The reflex control of involuntary breathing movements by the central nervous system requires information from both the mechanoreceptors just discussed, which provide data on the duration and depth of inspiration and expiration, and chemoreceptors that signal the carbon dioxide and oxygen tensions of the blood and thus indicate whether the respiratory minute volume is appropriate to the ongoing metabolism. We are aware of the activity of these chemoreceptors only in extreme cases; we feel **starved for air,** as though we are suffocating, when the oxygen supply falls far behind the demand and the carbon dioxide content of the blood rises sharply.

In the mucosa of the airways — the nose, throat, trachea, bronchi and bronchioles — there are many receptors that respond to noxious mechanical (foreign bodies, mucus) and chemical stimuli and trigger coughing reflexes. The properties of these nociceptors are described on pp. 123 ff.

Gastrointenstinal system. The gastrointestinal canal is actually **part of the body surface,** although it is closed off from the outer surface by mouth and anus. Its surface is therefore much more exposed to stimuli of external origin — substances in food and drink, and the products of their decomposition — than are the other internal organs. In this situation it is not surprising that we are more aware of mechanical, thermal and chemical events in the gastrointestinal region than in the other viscera. Insofar as these events produce feelings of hunger and satiety, they are discussed beginning on p. 256. Here we consider certain other aspects of gastrointestinal sensibility.

From the esophagus to the rectum, **tactile stimuli** to the gastrointestinal canal elicit no sensation. Only at the opening of the rectum, the anal passage, is touch perceived. On the other hand, **stretching** of the organ wall (produced experimentally, for instance, by inflating a balloon) seems to be sensed throughout the gastrointestinal canal, though the sensations vary. When the stomach walls are stretched, one perceives a feeling of satiation or fullness (see p. 267), whereas stretching of the rectum reliably causes an urge to defecate. Stretching of the small or large intestine is also noticed and is often ascribed to intestinal gases; the site of stretching cannot be precisely localized. *Excessive stretching* anywhere in the gastrointestinal system appears to cause pain.

Warm and cold stimuli are perceived throughout the esophagus and in the anal passage, but not in the stomach or intestine. *Alcohol,* however, can give rise to a warming or burning feeling in the stomach as well as the mouth and esophagus.

It has long been claimed from surgical experience that an unanesthetized human feels no sensation at all when his stomach, small and large intestine, or appendix are touched with warm or cold instruments, cauterized (cut with a glowing wire), crushed with forceps or clamps or cut with a scalpel. Given the anesthesiological and surgical techniques generally in use today, it is no longer possible to test this claim.

Renal system (kidneys, urinary bladder, urinary ducts). The formation of urine in the kidneys and its transport into the bladder give rise to no sensations, even though both kidney and ureter are well supplied with afferent nerve fibers. But if the bladder becomes stretched by the accumulation of urine within it, this filling is perceived and one feels the *need to urinate.* Of course, it is an everyday experience that the threshold for perception can vary widely, depending on one's state of attentiveness and activity. That is, one may feel the need to urinate when the bladder is nearly empty or when it is almost maximally filled.

Q 2.19. In the course of a cardiac cycle excitation of visceral and somatic receptors in the thoracic cavity occurs. Perception of the heartbeat is probably ascribable to excitation
a) of pressure receptors in the aortic arch,
b) of stretch receptors in the atria,
c) of stretch receptors in the lungs,
d) of mechanoreceptors in chest wall and spine,
e) All of the above receptors participate equally in perception of the heartbeat.

Q 2.20. Which of the following statements is false?
a) In the entire gastrointestinal canal touch stimuli are clearly perceived,
b) Stretch of the rectum causes one to feel a need to defecate,
c) Cold stimuli to the esophageal wall are perceived as cold,
d) Highly concentrated alcohol causes a burning feeling in the stomach,
e) Warm stimuli in the small intestine are not perceived.

Q 2.21. The respiratory minute volume is adjusted mainly by way of activity of the following receptors:
a) Mechanoreceptors in the chest wall,
b) Stretch receptors in the lung,

c) Mechanoreceptors in the diaphragm,
d) Chemoreceptors for carbion dioxide and oxygen tension,
e) Mucosal receptors in the airways (nose, throat, trachea, bronchi, bronchioles).

3 Neurophysiology of Sensory Systems

M. Zimmermann

The term "sensory systems" is applied to those parts of the nervous system that receive signals from the environment and from the interior of the body, and conduct and process these signals. This chapter is a general introduction to the mode of operation of these sensory systems, relying chiefly upon examples taken from the somatosensory system (the cutaneous senses). The greatest emphasis is laid upon the objective, neurophysiologically measurable processes; the subjective perceptions and their psychophysical correlates have been discussed at some length in Chapter 1.

3.1 Transformations of Stimuli in Receptors

The adequate stimulus; classification of receptors. A receptor is a specialized nerve cell. It signals the states and/or changes of state in its vicinity to the CNS. The states of the surroundings, and their changes that affect the receptors, are called *stimuli.* Stimuli are objectively measurable quantities, such as mechanical deformation of the skin, temperature, and electromagnetic radiation (light).

Physiologic studies have revealed that each receptor responds especially readily to one stimulus type. This property is generally called the *specificity of receptors;* the stimulus that is effective in each case is sometimes called the *adequate stimulus* for the receptor. In the case of some receptors the adequate stimulus can be inferred from everyday experience. For example, we can easily determine that the adequate stimulus for the receptors in our eyes is light radiation, whereas we do not ordinarily detect thermal or mechanical stimuli with these receptors.

Each receptor, then, is capable of transducing for the CNS information about only one certain aspect or dimension of the environment. That is, the receptor has a *filter function.* Hence it appears useful to classify receptors on the basis of their adequate stimuli. The receptors of mammals fall into the following four groups: *mechano-, thermo-, chemo-, and photoreceptors.*

Within each of the four groups we can discern a certain degree of specialization. For example, there are distinguishable types of photoreceptors, each responding to light of a different wavelength; these receptors are said to be wavelength- or color-specific. Thermoreceptors can be subdivided into warm and cold receptors. Among the mechanoreceptors one can also observe specialization to various parameters of the stimuli: in the skin, for example, there are receptors for vibration and other receptors for pressure.

The receptor potential. In the following paragraphs we consider the processes in the receptor — when exposed to adequate stimulation — which result in an action potential in the afferent fiber. The example taken is the crustacean stretch receptor, a mechanoreceptor located between certain muscle fibers of the animal; it is sensitive to stretch (Fig. 3–1).

When a microelectrode penetrates the receptor cell the potential initially recorded, as in all nerve cells, is the resting potential (e. g., −80 mV in Fig. 3–1). Under adequate stimulation — when the surrounding muscle is stretched — the membrane potential changes in a depolarizing direction. This depolarization brought about by the stimulus, the departure from the resting potential, is called the *receptor potential.*

The receptor potential lasts as long as the stimulus (the length change ΔL in Fig. 3–1). But even though the square-wave stimulus is maintained, the receptor potential falls from its initial maximum value (a depolarization by about 40 mV from the resting potential in Fig. 3–1) to a lower level. The decline in the effect of a stimulus held for some time at a constant level can be observed in practically all receptors; it is called *adaptation* (for further discussion see p. 71).

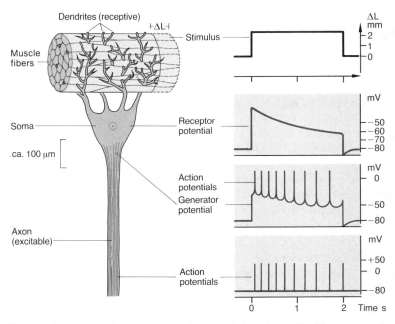

Fig. 3–1. Diagram of the electrophysiologic measurements that can be made with a crustacean stretch receptor. During stimulation (change in length of the associated muscle by ΔL) a microelectrode in the soma records the receptor potential, which arises in the receptive region (the dendrites). As a generator potential, it triggers conducted action potentials in the excitable axon

The receptor potential results from an *increase in membrane conductance* which is nonspecific, affecting *all kinds of small ions* (Na^+, K^+, Ca^{2+}, Cl^-). Under normal conditions the only one of these that can bring about depolarization is the Na^+ ion, for only this ion has an equilibrium potential in a depolarizing direction with respect to the resting potential. Consequently, Na^+ ions must be the chief causative agent in the production of the receptor potential. The increase in membrane conductance described for receptors is like that at the subsynaptic membrane of excitatory synapses — for instance, at the motor endplate.

The membrane conductance increase that leads to the receptor potential is localized in a specialized region of the receptor cell, the *receptive membrane* (the dendrites in Fig. 3–1). A receptor potential arises only when the stimulus affects this specialized region. The receptive membrane region, then, is spatially distinct from the other parts of the cell — for example, from the electrically excitable (impulse-conducting) membrane of the axon. It can be distinguished pharmacologically as well; the excitable membrane can, for example, be selectively poisoned by application of tetrodotoxin (TTX), so that action potentials can no longer be elicited there. The receptive membrane, and thus the receptor potential, by contrast, are largely unaffected by TTX.

Vertebrate photoreceptors are exceptional in that when stimulated by light they produce a hyperpolarizing receptor potential (see p. 174). However, during synaptic transmission to the higher-level neurons in the retina a depolarization is induced — an excitatory postsynaptic potential (EPSP) which triggers conducted action potentials in the ganglion cells.

The transduction process; primary and secondary sensory cells. The intermediate events between arrival of a stimulus and appearance of a receptor potential are still little understood; they are grouped under the heading *transduction processes.* This term comprises chiefly molecular-biological events occurring in the receptor membrane and/or in intracellular structures (in general called organelles). In the region of the receptor there are many of these organelles, such as the membrane disks of photoreceptors, which contain the light-sensitive visual pigment molecules (see Fig. 5–27) and the hairlike outgrowths (cilia) of the receptors of the inner ear (see Fig. 6–3). These are accessory structures that render the receptor especially sensitive to its particular adequate stimulus.

Many receptors consist of two linked elements, a nerve ending and a cell of nonneural origin such as a Merkel's cell in the skin (see Fig. 2–5) or a sensory cell in a taste bud (see Fig. 8–3). The transduction process is thought to take place in the nonneural cell. Such cells are called *secondary sensory cells.* In an electron micrograph, the contact region between the cells looks like a synapse. For this reason it is postulated that there is synaptic transmission from the secondary sensory cell to the nerve ending.

A *primary sensory cell*, on the other hand, is a receptor in which stimulus transduction occurs directly at the nerve cell or nerve ending. Examples of these are the stretch receptor (Fig. 3–1), the olfactory receptors (see Fig. 9–2) and the free nerve endings of the skin, which have various functional specializations.

The receptor potential as a generator of conducted action potentials. The receptor potential spreads electrotonically (cf. *Fundamentals of Neurophysiology,* Chap. 2) to the adjacent parts of the cell. As a result, the axon is depolarized (Fig. 3–1). When the depolarization reaches the threshold of the axon membrane, an action potential is triggered. The action potential is conducted along the axon to the CNS. The receptor potential, then, acts as an electrical stimulus to the axon; for this reason it is also called the *generator potential.*

If the duration of the generator potential exceeds that of the first action potential it can trigger further action potentials, until the stimulus and thus also the generator potential come to an end. That is, during a prolonged generator potential the afferent fiber discharges repetitively. The conversion of the stimulus into conducted action potentials may be called *transformation.* Transformation would thus comprise the following subevents: transduction, conductance increase in the receptor membrane, receptor potential, transcellular (e.g., synaptic) transmission (in the case of secondary sensory cells), generator potential, action potentials.

Adaptation. In considering the receptor potential we noted that even though a stimulus is held constant in time, the receptor potential may decrease (Fig. 3–1), a process called adaptation. We also observe this phenomenon in the repetitive discharge in afferent nerve fibers; as can be seen in Figure 3–1, during a maintained stimulus the time interval Δt between two sequential nerve impulses becomes greater — that is, the instantaneous frequency decreases (instantaneous frequency $= 1/\Delta t$). Adaptation can occur at all stages of the transformation of the stimulus: in the transduction process, in the receptor potential, in synaptic transmission from the secondary sensory cell to the nerve cell and in the generation of action potentials. Presumably several such mechanisms operate at the same time.

To characterize a receptor with respect to adaptation, its response to supra-threshold square-wave stimuli is studied. In such experiments, various receptors show different time courses of discharge rate. Figure 3–2A shows the discharge of slowly adapting (c), moderately rapidly adapting (b), and very rapidly adapting (a) receptors. In Figure 3–2B, the time course of instantaneous frequency is given for the receptors with slow and intermediate adaptation.

Various functional interpretations of adaptation have been proposed. The phenomenon used to be regarded as nothing more than a *fatigue* of the receptors. But in many cases the different time courses of adaptation can be interpreted as specializations to particular stimulus parameters. For example, in studies of three types of cutaneous mechanoreceptors it has been found that because of the characteristic time courses of their discharge they are transducers of amplitude, velocity and acceleration, respectively, of skin deformation (see Figs. 2–6 to 2–9 and Table 2–1).

The transformation of stimulus intensity into discharge rate. As stimulus strength increases, so does the amplitude of the receptor potential. The continuously graded values of the receptor potential induce correspondingly varying frequencies of action potentials. This situation is illustrated in Figure 3–3A. The

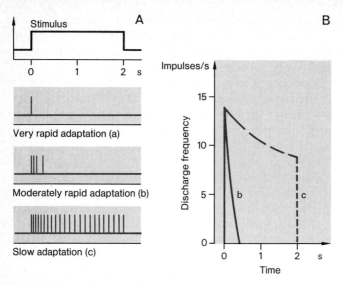

Fig. 3–2 A, B. Schematic diagram of the discharges of receptors adapting at different rates. *A* Action potentials of a very rapidly (a), moderately rapidly (b) and slowly adapting (c) receptor during a prolonged stimulus held constant in time. *B* Graph of the time course of the instantaneous discharge rate during the stimulus, in the receptors (b) and (c)

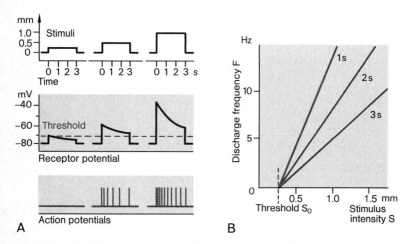

Fig. 3–3 A, B. Schematized relationship between stimulus intensity, receptor potential, and discharge frequency. *A* Receptor potentials and action potentials at three different intensities of the stimulus. Action potentials are elicited as soon as the receptor potential exceeds the threshold *(red dashed line).* *B* Graph of the instantaneous action-potential frequency F at three different times (1, 2, and 3 s) after the onset of the stimulus, as a function of stimulus intensity S. S_0 is the threshold intensity

relationship between stimulus intensity S and impulse frequency F, often called the *intensity function,* is plotted in Figure 3–3B for different times after the onset of the stimulus (the first, second, and third seconds). In this example (stretch receptor) linear relationships were found.

Since the receptor potential must be of some minimal amplitude (the threshold of the axon; cf. *Fundamentals of Neurophysiology,* Chap. 2) in order to trigger action potentials, discharge occurs only above the corresponding stimulus intensity (S_0 in Fig. 3–3B). S_0 is called the stimulus threshold of the receptor. The intensity functions in Figure 3–3B are described by expressions of the form

$$F = k \cdot (S - S_0), \qquad (3\text{--}1)$$

a linear relationship for $S > S_0$. The factor k, the slope of the line, becomes smaller for successive sample times following the application of the stimulus; this too is an expression of adaptation.

It has been shown experimentally for most receptors that the *intensity function is nonlinear.* The measured relationships can often be described by various mathematical functions, such as the logarithmic function (of WEBER and FECHNER)

$$F = k \cdot \log S/S_0 \qquad (3\text{--}2)$$

or the power function (of STEVENS)

$$F = k \cdot (S - S_0)^n \qquad (3\text{--}3)$$

We have encountered both of these expressions in the section on psychophysics (see p. 16). Intensity coding in the majority of receptor types is best described by a power function (Fig. 3–4), in which the stimulus intensity S, minus the stimulus threshold S_0, is raised to the nth power. The exponent n is a constant characteristic of each kind of receptor. For $n < 1$ and $n > 1$ the power function (on a linear plot) is convex upward and downward, respectively (Fig. 3–4A), and for $n = 1$ the intensity function is linear, like that of the stretch receptor. Most receptors exhibit exponents $n < 1$. An intensity characteristic with $n < 1$ enables the receptor to transform a particularly large range of intensity into a range of discharge rate which is limited at the upper end (the maximal discharge rate of a large myelinated nerve fiber is 500–1000 Hz, and that of thin fibers is considerably lower).

Power functions arise extensively in the description of psychophysical results (see p. 14). Comparison of the neurophysiologically measured intensity characteristic of a receptor with the subjective sensation of intensity measured in a psychophysical experiment (see Fig. 1–6) often reveals striking agreement; such comparisons are significant in research on the neurophysiologic basis of perception.

To test whether an experimentally determined intensity function can be described by a power function, the stimulus intensity and discharge rate are plotted

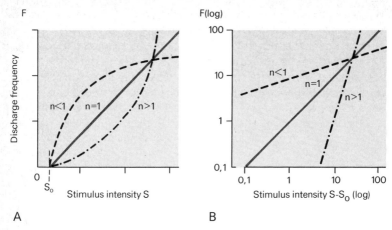

Fig. 3–4 A, B. Various power functions. **A** Discharge frequency F plotted against stimulus intensity S. Both coordinates are labeled in arbitrary units on a linear scale. Three characteristic power functions are shown, with exponents $n < 1$, $n > 1$, and $n = 1$ **(red)**. **B** The same power functions plotted in a coordinate system with logarithmic scales. On the abscissa is the stimulus intensity S minus the threshold intensity S_0

in a double logarithmic coordinate system (Fig. 3–4B). In a coordinate system of this kind a power function appears as a straight line, for if one takes the logs of both sides of Eq. (3–3) one obtains

$$\log F = \log k + n \cdot \log (S - S_0). \qquad (3\text{–}4)$$

This is the equation of a straight line with slope n, in the variables $\log F$ and $\log (S - S_0)$. If the data in a double logarithmic plot can be approximated by a straight line, then they fit a power function. The exponent n can be determined directly as the slope of this line.

Q 3.1.   What are the four groups into which mammalian receptors can be subdivided on the basis of their adequate stimuli?

Q 3.2.   The receptor potential:
a) Is an all-or-none response of a receptor cell which does not occur unless the stimulus exceeds the threshold
b) Is usually a depolarization of the receptive membrane, by a greater amount the stronger the stimulus
c) Spreads electrotonically to the axon membrane and there acts as a generator of conducted action potentials
d) Arises by way of an increased conductance specific to H^+ ions (pH value)
e) Rises slowly during a constant stimulus and lasts as long as the stimulus.
Several answers are correct.

Q 3.3. The discharge rate in the afferent axons of many receptors:
a) Increases with increasing stimulus intensity
b) Increases during a stimulus of constant intensity
c) Decreases during a stimulus of constant intensity
d) Is usually zero during stimuli of subthreshold intensity
e) Does not depend on the size of the receptor potential
Several answers are correct.

Q 3.4. In many receptors a power function describes:
a) The time course of adaptation.
b) The time course of the receptor potential as stimulus strength is increased
c) The relationship between the impulse frequency F and the amount by which the stimulus intensity exceeds the threshold S_0.
d) The relationship between the amplitude of the action potential and the size of the receptor potential

3.2 Sensory Functions of the CNS — a Survey

Peripheral nerves, spinal nerves, dorsal roots, and their innervation areas. All the receptors in a sensory system taken together are called the peripheral sensory surface, or simply the periphery. Information from the periphery is transmitted to the CNS in coded form, as action potentials or nerve impulses. The afferent nerve fibers thus perform the task of information transmission. Bundles of these fibers pass to the CNS in the peripheral nerves (skin, muscle, joint, and visceral nerves), which also contain efferent nerve fibers. From all the parts of the body, apart from the head, the peripheral nerves run to the spinal cord, which they approach as *spinal nerves.* The afferent nerve fibers then enter the spinal cord by way of the *dorsal roots* (for further discussion, and classification of the nerve fibers by diameter and conduction velocity, see *Fundamentals of Neurophysiology,* 3rd ed., Chap. 1 and Table 2–2, p. 67).

If a cutaneous nerve is accidentally cut through, there is a relatively sharply delimited region of skin in which stimuli can no longer be detected. The area of skin so affected is the *innervation area* of the transected nerve or nerve branch. The sharpness of the boundary is due to the small degree of overlap of the innervation areas of neighboring nerves (Fig. 3–5).

Another result of transection of a cutaneous nerve, in addition to the sensory deficits, is that the skin in the affected region becomes dry and hard; the innervation of the sweat glands by the sympathetic efferents — which also run in the cutaneous nerve — has been interrupted.

The afferent fibers in each dorsal root represent a particular peripheral region. But this region does not arise simply by combination of the innervation areas of the peripheral nerves. Between the spinal cord and the periphery the nerve fibers are regrouped into *new bundles,* chiefly in the plexus of the nerves to the extremities (for instance, the brachial plexus at the level of the shoulder joint). The effect of this regrouping is illustrated in Figure 3–5: Each peripheral nerve contains fibers supplying several adjacent spinal nerves and conversely, in each spinal nerve there are fibers from different peripheral nerves. Because of this rearrangement the innervation area of a spinal nerve or its dorsal root is less sharply defined than that of a peripheral nerve, and the innervation areas of adjacent spinal nerves overlap considerably (Fig. 3–5). Whereas the result of an extremely peripheral nerve transection is a clearly delimited sensory deficit (Fig. 3–5) in the organ it supplies (skin or muscle or viscera), transection of a dorsal root or a spinal nerve tends to "thin out" the innervation of all three kinds of organ simultaneously, with only slight sensory deficits.

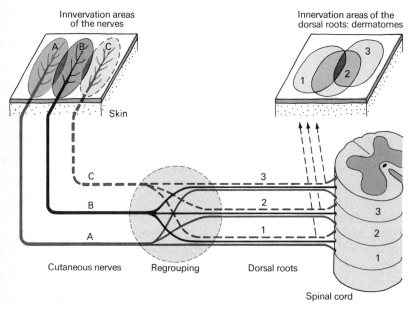

Fig. 3–5. Innervation areas of cutaneous nerves and dorsal roots (greatly schematized). The innervation areas of cutaneous nerve branches are sharply delimited and have little overlap. Because of the rearrangement of the peripheral nerve bundles to form spinal nerves the innervation areas of dorsal roots are less well defined and overlap. The regions of overlap are shown in **dark red**

The sensory innervation area of a spinal nerve in the skin is called a **dermatome.** The dermatomes are arranged on the body surface in a sequence corresponding to that of the associated spinal-cord segments. For example, the innervation of the pelvic region comes from spinal segments further away from the brain than those that innervate the shoulder. In accordance with this mapping of the body surface onto the spinal cord, the latter is subdivided into the four main sections cervical, thoracic, lumbar, and sacral. This subdivision and the approximate limits of the associated dermatomes are indicated in Figure 3–6.

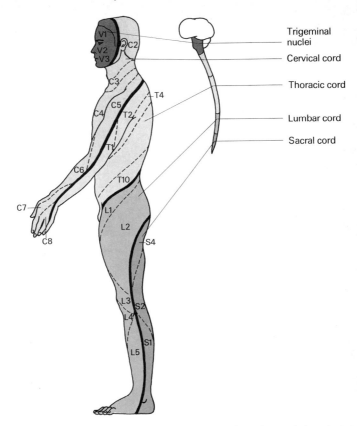

Fig. 3–6. The dermatomes. Regular arrangement of regions on the body surface and the spinal-cord levels from which they are innervated. The boundaries indicated by the ***heavy lines*** are those of the main regions of the body, each of which is associated with one of the four main sections of the spinal cord or with the trigeminal region in the brain stem. Some of the dermatomes of individual spinal nerves are shown (V: dermatomes of the trigeminal nerve; C, T, L, S: dermatomes of the cervical, thoracic, lumbar and sacral spinal cord)

The cranial nerves. The head is supplied by 12 pairs of nerves entering the brain itself, at the levels of the brain stem and diencephalon. These are summarized in Table 3–1, together with their most important functions and the organs they innervate. Some of the cranial nerves are exclusively sensory (cranial nerves I, II, VIII), whereas the others have both sensory and motor functions and in some cases also include efferent parasympathetic fibers. Nerves IX and X contain visceral afferents from receptors which act as sensors in the control circuits regulating the internal milieu (e. g., in the cardiovascular and respiratory systems).

The ***trigeminal nerve (cranial nerve V)*** carries the afferents from the face and mouth region; it innervates the skin as well as the teeth, oral mucosa, and tongue. It belongs to the somatosensory system. The trigeminal nerve occupies a special

Table 3–1. Survey of the cranial nerves, with their most important sensory and motor functions

No.	Name	Innervated organ	Example of sensory function	Example of motor function
I	Olfactory	Nasal mucosa	Smelling	—
II	Optic	Retina	Vision	—
III	Oculomotor	Eye muscles	—	Eye movements
IV	Trochlear	Eye muscles	—	Eye movements
V	Trigeminal	Face and mouth region	Somatosensory	Chewing movements
VI	Abducens	Eye muscles	—	Eye movements
VII	Facial	Face musculature, tongue	Taste	Facial expression
VIII	Statoacoustic	Inner ear, vestibular organ	Hearing, orientation in space	—
IX	Glossopharyngeal	Tongue, throat	Taste	Swallowing
X	Vagus	Internal organs	Visceral afferents	Control of heart
XI	Accessory	Neck musculature	—	Head movements
XII	Hypoglossal	Tongue muscles	—	Tongue movements

position in that its afferents operate in the newborn, to elicit feeding behavior; it is the nerve that provides the infant with its first sensory experience of its environment.

The sensory systems of skin and viscera together are called the *somatovisceral system.* This system comprises the afferents of the spinal nerves and those of the cranial nerves V, VII, IX, and X.

Central stations on the sensory pathways. After passing into the spinal cord by way of the dorsal roots, signals from the receptors are processed at several levels of the CNS. These stations of the somatosensory system are shown in Figure 3–7 (cf. central visual pathway, Fig. 5–32, and central auditory pathway, Fig. 6–16). Their interconnections should not be thought of as one-way streets; in addition to the ascending information flow there are several *descending, centrifugal influences* (not shown in Fig. 3–7), such as that of the cortex upon the spinal cord. Because of these effects, the afferent influx can be modulated at all levels (cf. Sec. 3.3).

It has proved useful in studying sensory systems — the somatosensory system in particular — to subdivide the afferent, centripetal pathways and the associated central stations into the phylogenetically young *specific system* and the phylogenetically old *nonspecific system.* Here the adjectives "specific" and "nonspecific" characterize a number of different and usually contrasting functional properties particularly emphasized in one or the other system. As an introduction, we

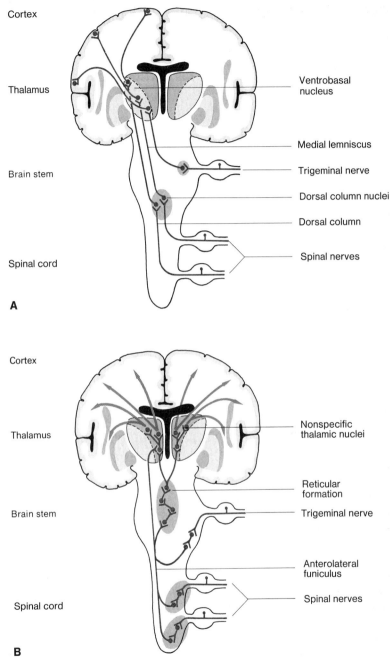

Fig. 3–7. A Survey of the anatomic arrangement of the specific part of the somatosensory system. The main connections of the spinal and trigeminal afferents with the projection fields of the cortex are shown. *B* Survey of the nonspecific somatosensory system. The most important of the known connections and processing stations are shown

propose the following definition: "Specific" is applied to those central nervous components of a sensory system with only one anatomically and neurophysiologically identifiable main input from one peripheral sensory surface. Specific systems that have been thoroughly studied so far involve the mechanoreceptors of the skin, and the receptors of the eye and of the inner ear. By contrast, in a nonspecific system the afferent input is not so clearly defined; the system is excited by convergence from several sensory surfaces (polymodal or *polysensory convergence*).

The example of the somatosensory system will now be used to illustrate the anatomy of the two subsystems; functional details will be discussed in later sections.

Anatomy of the specific somatosensory system. The specific component of the somatosensory system is called the *lemniscal system,* because the medial lemniscal tract is one of its important tracts (from the dorsal column nuclei to the thalamus). The lemniscal system (Fig. 3–7 A) consists of pathways clearly distinguishable anatomically and neurophysiologically, by which spinal and trigeminal cutaneous afferents project to two cortical regions in the parietal lobe, the first somatosensory area (SI) and the second somatosensory area (SII), respectively.

SI receives its afferent input from the skin of the opposite (contralateral) side, whereas the afferents to SII come from both sides of the body (bilateral). The ascending path (Fig. 3–7 A) passes chiefly through the dorsal column in the spinal cord and its nuclei in the medulla oblongata (the first synapse); thence it runs through the medial lemniscus to the ventrobasal nuclei of the thalamus (second synapse) and on to areas SI and SII of the cortex (third synapse). Signals are transmitted rapidly along this pathway, with a minimum of three synaptic relays. A particular characteristic of this system is its *somatotopic arrangement;* there is an orderly spatial (topographic) mapping of the skin, the peripheral sensory surface, onto all the relay stations. We could also say that the skin is projected onto these central stations. Further details of this projection will be discussed below (cf. Sec. 3.4 and 3.5).

The lemniscal system is especially highly developed in primates: the monkeys, anthropoid apes, and humans. It is the anatomic basis of the sense of touch and all the sensory abilities (conscious and unconscious) that involve discrimination of the spatial details of a stimulus.

Anatomy of the nonspecific system. This somatosensory subsystem is also called the *extralemniscal* or nonlemniscal system. It is less well defined anatomically (Fig. 3–7 B) than the lemniscal system. Its most important components are the *reticular formation* of the brain stem and certain nuclei in the medial thalamus called *nonspecific thalamic nuclei.* The chief spinal ascending tracts in the nonspecific system are the spinoreticular and paleospinothalamic, both of which lie in the anterolateral funiculus of the spinal cord.

The extralemniscal system makes connections with practically all regions of the cerebral cortex. These connections are diffuse — that is, not precisely delimited in space — and above all they show little or no somatotopic organization. In addition, there are connections to the centers for autonomic regulation in the brain stem and hypothalamus, to the limbic system, and to the subcortical centers of the motor system.

It has now become possible to improve on the anatomic and neurophysiologic categorizations of functional subsystems of the nonspecific system, by adding a neurochemical characterization. Several populations of neurons in the diencephalon and brainstem have been identified on the basis of their (presumed) neurotransmitters — for example, noradrenalin, serotonin, dopamine, opioids and other neuropeptides.

Polysensory convergence and the small degree of somatotopy are characteristics of the nonspecific system; these properties distinguish it sharply from the specific systems.

With regard to behavior and perception, the following functions are among those ascribed to the nonspecific system: affective shading of perceptions (pleasure, aversion), participation in the perception of pain, control of the state of consciousness (sleeping/waking rhythm), and orientation responses (turning toward new stimuli). The neuronal functions of the nonspecific system have been very little studied as compared with those of the lemniscal system.

The subdivision into "lemniscal" and "extralemniscal" should not mislead the reader into thinking that these are subsystems that can be activated separately, nor that clearly distinct perceptual phenomena can be assigned to them. On the contrary, the various sensory stimuli encountered in daily life activate both systems, and the interactions of the two subsystems are many and diverse.

Q 3.5. Transection of a cutaneous nerve near the extreme periphery causes:
   a) Disappearance of temperature and pain sensations only
   b) Dryness of the skin in the affected innervation area, because of denervation of the sweat glands
   c) Flaccid paralysis because of the interruption of efferent motor axons
   d) Interruption of the signals from high- and low-threshold mechanoreceptors and thermoreceptors,
   Several answers are correct.

Q 3.6. When a dorsal root is destroyed the following nerve fibers are interrupted:
   a) The efferent motor and sympathetic fibers
   b) The afferent fibers from skin, muscles, joints, and viscera
   c) Only the afferent fibers from the skin

   Those interrupted when a spinal nerve is destroyed are:
   d) Only the afferent fibers
   e) All the afferent and efferent fibers of the ipsilateral half-segment concerned.
   Several answers are correct.

Q 3.7.   The following statements apply to the concept "dermatome":
   a) Dermatome is a pathologic change in the skin (e. g., hard dryness) following transection of the associated nerve.
   b) It refers to the region of sensory deficit created when a cutaneous nerve is cut.
   c) It is defined as that area of skin in which the innervation regions of two neighboring spinal nerves overlap.
   d) It is the innervation area of the cutaneous nerve fibers of a spinal nerve.

Q 3.8.   Sketch the outlines of the CNS in longitudinal section. Mark the boundaries of the seven main regions of the CNS and label the regions.

Q 3.9.   The subdivision of the sensory system of the CNS into specific and nonspecific regions is based on the following findings:
   a) The influx of impulses in the afferent nerve fibers is carried to the cerebral cortex over rapid and clearly localizable pathways as well as over slow, diffusely distributed pathways
   b) The cranial nerves mediate clearly describable (specific) perceptions of stimuli, whereas those mediated by the spinal afferents are vague (nonspecific)
   c) There are both conscious (specific) and unconscious (nonspecific) perceptions of peripheral stimuli
   d) There are sensory regions in the CNS to which afferents come specifically from only one peripheral sensory surface, and others which can be excited unspecifically from several sensory surfaces.
   Several answers are correct.

3.3 Properties and Operation of Sensory Neurons and Aggregates of Neurons

At every station of the sensory system, afferent inputs bring about excitation and inhibition of individual neurons, as well as interaction among neurons and groups of neurons. Some of these effects are particularly characteristic of certain sensory systems. These will be described in the following paragraphs (for general properties of neuronal activity see *Fundamentals of Neurophysiology,* Chaps. 1 through 4).

Lateral inhibition. Figure 3–8 A shows schematically a neural network comprising two receptors and the associated elements at the next two synaptic levels in the central nervous system. The divergent and convergent neuronal connectivity found here, as everywhere in the nervous system, would seem to impose an avalanche-like spread of excitation at progressively higher levels in the CNS. The central nervous representation of a peripheral point stimulus would be expected to become enlarged, less precise and more diffuse at every synaptic relay station. But a situation of this type is encountered only under pathologic conditions — for example, in cases of strychnine poisoning. Strychnine blocks inhibitory synapses in the CNS. When this happens, the smallest peripheral stimulus does indeed set off an enormous chain reaction of neuronal activity. Evidently inhibition normally acts to prevent such a catastrophic spread of excitation in the central nervous system.

This inhibitory effect rests upon a characteristic spatial organization of inhibitory connections summarized by the term *lateral inhibition* or *surround inhibition;* it is illustrated in Figure 3–8 B. At the first synaptic relay in the afferent pathway, each excited neuron exerts an inhibitory effect upon nearby cells, by way of interneurons (red in the diagram). The neuron with the greatest afferent input, here the one in the middle, also imposes the strongest inhibition on its neighbors.

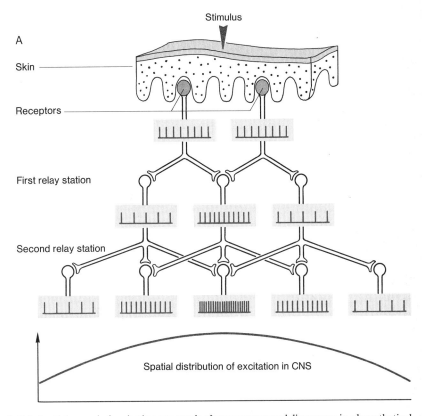

Fig. 3–8 A. Spatial spread of excitation as a result of convergence and divergence in a hypothetical CNS without lateral inhibition. The vertical marks *(red)* symbolize the axon discharges vs. time at various levels. The curve indicates the corresponding spatial distribution of excitation in the CNS; this curve can be thought of as indicating the central representation of the small-area stimulus shown at the top

This leads to a reduction of excitation at sites away from the center of excitation. In comparison to the situation of Figure 3–8 A, therefore, the spatial spread of excitation is reduced.

Lateral inhibition has been shown to exist at all levels of sensory systems; in the somatosensory system it is found in the dorsal horn of the spinal cord, in the dorsal column nuclei, in the thalamus, and in the cortex. Lateral inhibition as illustrated schematically in the diagrams of Figure 3–8 is a property of all sensory systems, the specific systems in particular. It can be regarded as a functional compensation for the neuroanatomically imposed divergence of excitation. It results in an improvement of the *sharpness of localization* of stimulus information. A special subjective effect of lateral inhibition is the phenomenon of spatial contrast enhancement in vision (cf. Chaps. 1 and 4).

Descending inhibition. In practically all sensory systems, there are inhibitory effects which originate in superordinate centers. Such *descending (centrifugal) inhibition* can act at a point as far peripheral as the receptor (Fig. 9–4), or at

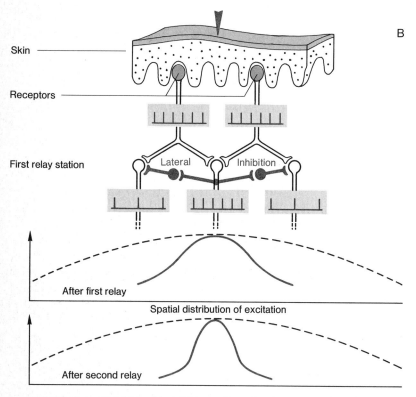

Fig. 3–8 B. By lateral inhibition (the inhibitory effect of each neuron on surrounding neurons via inhibitory neurons, shown in *red*) the spread of excitation resulting from divergence is counteracted at each synaptic level. As indicated by the excitation distributions, the consequence is a spatial sharpening of the representation in the CNS of the spatially restricted peripheral stimulus

the afferent fiber terminals in the spinal cord (Fig. 3–10). The existence of this kind of inhibition emphasizes the remark made above that sensory systems should not be regarded as one-way streets for information transfer, from peripheral to central.

Like lateral inhibition, descending inhibition can be considered to function as a means of *regulating the sensitivity of the afferent transmission channel;* superordinate parts of the brain "turn the valve" governing afferent information flow.

The receptive field. The frequency of action potentials in a central sensory neuron can usually be affected by stimuli at the periphery of the body. For example, the frequency of action potentials in a cell of the visual cortex changes when a suitable light stimulus appears in a certain region of the visual field. The totality of all points at the periphery of the body from which a cell can be influenced by specific stimuli is called that cell's *receptive field.* Figure 3–9 presents an example. On the skin of the forearm are shown the regions in which light touch can change the frequency of discharge of a particular central neuron (e. g., in spinal cord or thalamus). The region from which Neuron 1 can be excited is the excitatory receptive field (+) of this neuron for the particular stimulus "light touch". The region from which Neuron 1 is inhibited is the inhibitory receptive field (−) of this neuron. It can simultaneously be the excitatory receptive field of another neuron. The inhibitory connection shown in Figure 3–9 is a case of lateral inhibition.

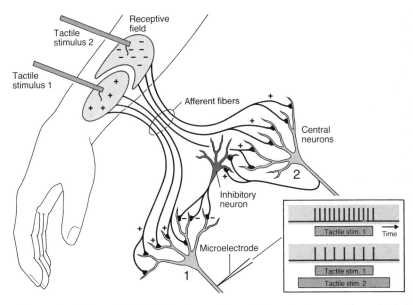

Fig. 3–9. Receptive fields on the skin of the forearm from which central neurons (e. g., in the spinal cord) can be excited or inhibited. Neuron 1 is activated by stimuli in the excitatory receptive field (+) and inhibited by those in the surrounding inhibitory field (−), as the recording of its action potentials shows. Neuron 2 is excited from the same field that is inhibitory for Neuron 1

Some cells in sensory centers have very small receptive fields. Examples include neurons in the visual cortex that are affected by light stimuli only in a part of the macula of the eye's retina measuring 0.02 mm^2. Other cells, particularly in the nonspecific systems, represent the oppposite extreme; for example, such a cell can be influenced by stimuli to the skin over large parts of the body, such as an entire leg, and will respond to touch, cold, and vibrational stimuli. In this case the receptive field is of great spatial extent and comprises various receptor modalities (polymodal or multireceptive convergence).

All an individual sensory neuron "knows" about the site of a specific stimulus is that it is somewhere within the receptive field. But more precise localization of the stimulus site becomes possible when the receptive fields of several neurons at one level of organization, which in many cases overlap considerably, are compared at the next higher level. For example, this sort of information processing in a set of neurons enables the visual system to achieve a high degree of spatial resolution even though the receptive fields of the individual neurons in the visual pathway are relatively large (cf. p. 176).

So far the only criterion given for determination of the receptive field has been the "influencing" of a central neuron by stimulation at a certain point in the periphery. But such influences can be either excitatory or inhibitory — that is, there are *excitatory and inhibitory receptive fields* or parts of fields. For example, Figure 3–9 shows the excitatory and inhibitory receptive fields of a central somatosensory neuron. Another example is given in Figure 5–27: retinal receptive fields in which an excitatory center is surrounded by an inhibitory area, and vice versa. This subdivision of the receptive field may reflect neuronal circuitry involving lateral inhibition (see above).

The *properties of a receptive field* — its localization and size, the modalities and qualities of the specific stimuli, and its subdivision into excitatory and inhibitory parts — can in principle be determined for each neuron in the sensory systems. Neighboring neurons in the different centers as a rule have characteristic, similar receptive fields. From observed differences in the receptive fields of synaptically linked sensory neurons at ascending levels one can infer the functional operation of the various centers. From one neuron to the next the size and shape of the receptive fields can change in a characteristic way, and often there are differences in the adequate stimulus. For example, in the visual system neurons at the lowest level respond to stationary stimuli of varying brightness, whereas in the visual cortex many neurons respond, for instance, only to a moving light stimulus.

Intensity-response relationships; difference thresholds. Apart from the aspects of type and localization of the stimulus, it is possible to specify the responses of central sensory neurons in relation to stimulus intensity. The relationship between frequency F of the neuron and the suprathreshold stimulus intensity $(S - S_0)$ can often be described by the power function

$$F = k \cdot (S - S_0)^n$$

as was found to be the case with many receptors (see pp. 73). Among central neurons, again, various values of n are found; there are linear relationships ($n = 1$), while in many neurons the slope of the discharge rate curve decreases as stimulus intensity increases — i. e., the exponent n is smaller than 1.

One can also determine the stimulus threshold of central neurons. The **absolute threshold**, S_0, was included in the formulation of the power function given above. It is measured by establishing the smallest stimulus intensity to which the cell responds with a change in the frequency of action potentials.

Another sort of threshold can be defined by measuring the amount by which the intensity of a suprathreshold stimulus must be changed in order to produce a barely noticeable change in discharge rate of a neuron. This threshold is called the **difference threshold.** It is found to change in a regular way with stimulus intensity, in accordance with Weber's rule describing the difference threshold in subjective sensation (see p. 21; see also Fig. 3–21).

Difference threshold can be determined for many stimulus parameters other than intensity — spatial differences, temporal differences, pitch differences, differences in frequency of vibration, and so on. In each case the above definition holds; the difference threshold is the smallest change in a stimulus parameter that produces a just measurable change in frequency of discharge of the sensory neuron.

Q 3.10. Which of the following are correct descriptions of receptive fields?
  a) The right cerebral hemisphere is the receptive field (visual field) of the left eye
  b) All points on the retina, illumination of which leads to an increase in frequency of discharge of a neuron of the visual cortex
  c) All points on the retina, illumination of which leads to a change in the frequency of discharge of a neuron of the visual cortex
  d) The region of the nasal mucosa to which local application of a dilute solution of hydrogen sulfide can affect the activity of a neuron in the olfactory lobe
  e) All points on the skin of the foot at which a painful stimulus can elicit withdrawal of the foot (flexor reflex).
  Several answers are correct.

Q 3.11. Write down from memory what is meant by the difference threshold of a neuron in the sensory system.

Q 3.12. The term "lateral inhibition" covers the following phenomena:
  a) The particular inhibitory influence that is exerted in the lateral field of view of the retina
  b) Enhancement of the contrast between the intensities of spatially separated stimuli
  c) Inhibitory action of a central neuron on its surroundings

d) An inhibitory receptive field immediately adjacent to the excitatory receptive field.

Several answers are correct.

3.4 The Somatosensory System: Spinal Cord, Ascending Pathways, and Brain Stem

Connectivity of the afferents in the dorsal horn. In the spinal cord, afferents from trunk and limbs make *synaptic connections* with spinal neurons lying in the gray matter of the spinal cord. The fibers from skin and viscera end on neurons in the dorsal parts of the gray matter, the dorsal horns (Fig. 3–10). Some of the thick myelinated (group II or Aβ) afferents send out additional branches, called *collaterals,* which enter the ascending dorsal columns (see p. 89).

The dorsal horn is the first relay and processing station in the somatovisceral system. As can be seen in Figure 3–10, from a functional point of view the dorsal horn has *four outputs:* long ascending tracts, in particular the anterolateral funiculus (discussed on p. 91), short fibers in the propriospinal tracts that provide ascending and descending connections to neighboring segments, synaptic connections with motoneurons, and finally synapses with sympathetic (preganglionic) neurons. The two outputs last mentioned imply that the cutaneous and visceral afferents are involved in the spinal motor and sympathetic reflexes. These will not be discussed here; they are presented in detail in *Fundamentals of Neurophysiology.*

The dorsal-horn neurons illustrated in Figure 3–10 represent many thousands of neurons in each segment of the spinal cord; however, an individual neuron will in general not have all four efferent connections shown there. Only a rough indication is given in this figure of the *convergence and divergence* of the afferent fibers. Each neuron makes contact with many afferent fibers, and conversely each afferent fiber has excitatory synapses with several neurons.

Within the dorsal horn there are not only excitatory synapses but also many inhibitory synapses. These and the associated interneurons are drawn in red in Figure 3–10. The two types of inhibition of particular importance in the sensory system are also represented: *afferent or lateral inhibition* and *descending inhibition* (see p. 84). The basic role of these is in control and modulation of the afferent influx; the inhibition is exerted in part postsynaptically and in part presynaptically (cf. the axo-axonal synapse on the ending of one of the two dorsal-root fibers in Fig. 3–10).

Ascending pathways of the spinal cord. Figure 3–10 shows two ascending pathways that carry information from the somatosensory afferents to the brain — the dorsal columns and the anterolateral funiculus. Like all ascending and descending spinal tracts, these are located in the white matter of the spinal cord. The fibers in the dorsal columns run on the same side as the dorsal-root afferents (i. e., they are ipsilateral), whereas those in the anterolateral funiculus are on the opposite side (contralateral).

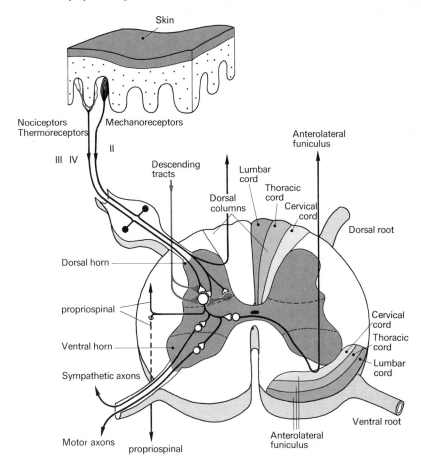

Fig. 3–10. Connectivity of the cutaneous afferents in the spinal cord. The afferents entering through the dorsal roots make synapses with dorsal-horn neurons. Nerve impulses are conducted from here along fibers leaving the spinal cord (sympathetic efferents and muscle efferents) as well as along ascending pathways. Of the latter, that in the anterolateral funiculus, leading to brain stem and thalamus, is shown. Collaterals of the group II (Aβ) afferents ascend directly in the white matter (the dorsal columns) to the medulla oblongata. Two influences with an inhibitory effect on the dorsal-horn neuron are shown *(red);* they act via descending pathways or spinal inhibitory interneurons. On the right, the topographic layering of the ascending pathways in the cervical cord is diagrammed

The ***dorsal columns*** consist of direct collaterals of the thick myelinated dorsal-root afferents (groups I and II); without exception they come from low-threshold mechanoreceptors in the trunk and limbs — in skin, viscera, muscles, and joints. All except the muscle afferents end in synapses on neurons of the ***dorsal column nuclei*** (the gracile and cuneate nuclei) in the medulla oblongata (Fig. 3–11).

The axons of these neurons cross to the opposite side and there run to the thalamus in the ***medial lemniscus.*** Neuronal processing in the dorsal column nuclei

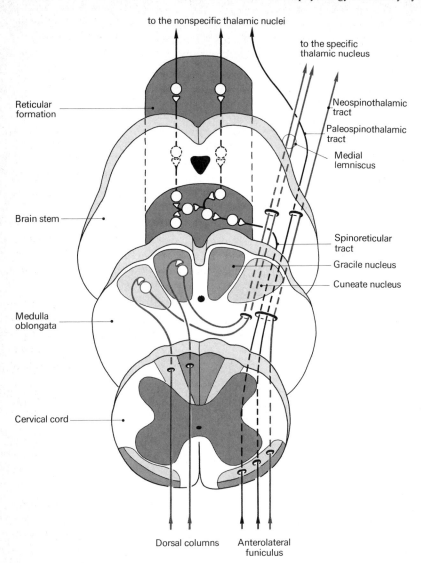

Fig. 3–11. Ascending pathways from the spinal cord. The lemniscal pathways are shown in *red* and the extralemniscal pathways in *black*. Fibers in the dorsal column synapse in the dorsal column nuclei (the cuneate and gracile nuclei), in the medulla, with neurons that send axons to the specific nucleus of the thalamus through the medial lemniscus. The phylogenetically old parts of the anterolateral funiculus run to the reticular formation (as the spinoreticular tract) and to the nonspecific thalamic nuclei (the paleospinothalamic tract). The phylogenetically young part of the anterolateral funiculus (the neospinothalamic tract) projects to the specific thalamic nucleus; it is therefore considered part of the lemniscal system *(red)*

involves both afferent and descending inhibition, as does the processing in the dorsal horn and in the thalamus (see p. 96). Dorsal columns and lemniscus are the most prominent tracts in the specific (lemniscal) part of the somatosensory system.

The *anterolateral funiculus* (Figs. 3–10, 3–11) contains axons that arise predominantly from neurons in the dorsal horn of the contralateral side (Fig. 3–10). This pathway terminates in the reticular formation of the brain stem and in the thalamus; accordingly, the anterolateral funiculus is subdivided into the spinoreticular and spinothalamic tracts (Fig. 3–11). The spinothalamic tract itself has two components, distinguished by their phylogenetic age — the paleo-spinothalamic tract (old) and the neospinothalamic tract (new). The latter is particularly well developed in primates; it is counted as part of the lemniscal system. The spinoreticular and paleospinothalamic tracts, on the other hand, are important extralemniscal spinal pathways.

The dorsal columns transmit signals exclusively from low-threshold mechanoreceptors, whereas the information carried in the anterolateral funiculus comes from mechanoreceptors, thermoreceptors, and nociceptors. In both tracts the afferent inputs come not only from skin and viscera, but from muscles and joints as well.

When one of these pathways is transected, the observed sensory deficits correspond to the arrangement of receptor types just described. *Dorsal column lesions* produce ipsilateral (on the same side of the body) impairment of abilities having to do with the spatial localization of tactile stimuli; among these are two-point discrimination (see p. 34) and the tactile exploratory movements that depend on feedback from cutaneous, muscle, and joint afferents.

After *transection of the anterolateral funiculus* temperature and pain stimuli can no longer be detected in parts of the body contralateral to the site of transection. States of severe pain that cannot be satisfactorily treated by phar-macotherapy can be alleviated by neurosurgical interruption of the anterolateral funiculus, an operation called *chordotomy.* This procedure also cuts off the transmission of thermal stimuli, whereas tactile stimuli continue to be signalled by way of the dorsal column.

In addition to the dorsal columns and anterolateral funiculus, there are *other ascending pathways* in the spinal cord. The spinocerebellar tracts transmit information from mechanosensitive cutaneous and muscle afferents to the cerebel-lum; functionally, these belong to the motor system. The spinocervical tract, which projects to the thalamus, includes predominantly cutaneous afferents from the limbs. Its function is still unclear. Apart from the long tracts mentioned so far there are polysynaptic ascending connections to the brain, comprising spinal neurons with short axons connected in series.

Within the ascending tracts, the axons coming from a particular segment run side by side. As a result, there is a *layering* of the tracts, shown diagrammatically in Figure 3–10 for the dorsal columns and the anterolateral funiculus at the level of the cervical cord. As axons enter a tract they turn to run parallel to the fibers from lower levels on the gray-matter side of the tract. The boundaries of the individual bundles are not as sharp as indicated in the diagram of Figure 3–10; actually the transitions are diffuse and overlapping. Because of this topographic arrangement, superficial damage to the anterolateral cord (such as might be caused by injury or a tumor) in the cervical region would be expected to produce symptoms first in the lower half of the body.

Trigeminal nuclei and their ascending tracts. The trigeminal nerve, the somatovisceral sensory nerve of the facial region, enters the brain at the pons. The afferents make synapses in two nuclei in the gray matter of the brainstem, the spinal nucleus and the main sensory nucleus. The spinal trigeminal nucleus corresponds functionally to the dorsal horn of the spinal cord, while the main sensory nucleus corresponds to the dorsal column nuclei of the spinal afferents. This analogy extends to the tracts leaving these nuclei. In the spinal nucleus afferents from mechanoreceptors, thermoreceptors, and nociceptors synapse with neurons sending axons to the reticular formation and/or the thalamus, like the fibers in the anterolateral funiculus of the spinal cord. In the main sensory nucleus terminate only afferents from low-threshold mechanoreceptors, and the postsynaptic axons join the medial lemniscus.

Apart from being sent on to the thalamus, the information supplied by the trigeminal afferents is integrated into the motor reflexes of the head musculature. The trigeminal system performs vital functions in infants especially — for instance, it mediates tactile recognition of the environment, feeding behavior, and sound production.

The reticular formation. The reticular formation, which occupies a considerable part of the brain stem, is an important station in the ascending nonspecific system (Fig. 3–7 B). It is involved in a great variety of afferent and efferent connections, shown schematically in Figure 3–12 A. The somatovisceral afferents run in the spinoreticular tract (of the anterolateral funiculus), probably also along propriospinal (polysynaptic) paths, as well as in corresponding tracts from the spinal trigeminal nucleus. Moreover, the reticular formation receives inputs from all the other afferent cranial nerves, that is, from all sense organs. Afferent inputs also come from many other regions of the brain, such as the motor and sensory parts of the cerebral cortex, the thalamus, and the hypothalamus. The efferent connections, too, are diverse — descending to the spinal cord, ascending via the nonspecific thalamic nuclei to the cortex, to the hypothalamus, and to the limbic system.

The diversity of afferent connections is also apparent at the level of the *individual neuron.* Microelectrode recordings in the reticular formation have shown that there is usually convergence of two or three of the afferents listed in

▶

Fig. 3–12 A, B. Reticular formation: connections and functions. *A* Diagram of afferent and efferent connections. The figure represents a combination of anatomic and physiologic findings; it is intended to give an idea of the large number of inputs and outputs. *B* The most important functions in which the reticular formation is thought to participate

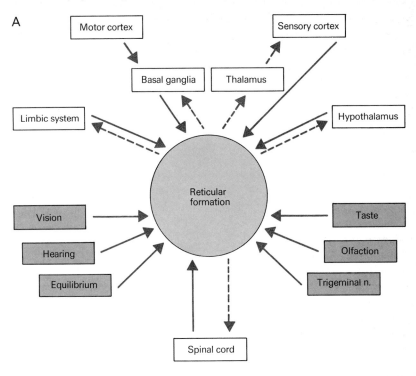

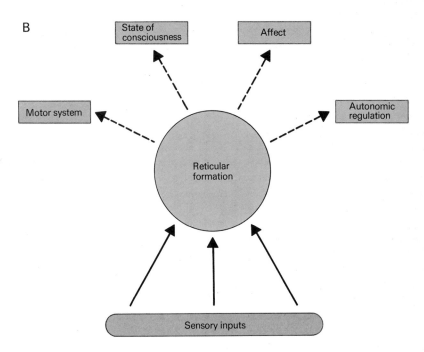

Figure 3–12 A upon a single neuron; *polysensory convergence* prevails. This is a distinguishing characteristic of reticular neurons. Other properties of these neurons are their large receptive fields, often represented bilaterally on the body surface, the long latency of the response to peripheral stimulation (i. e., multisynaptic pathways), the variability of the response (stochastic fluctuations in the number of action potentials discharged in response to repeated stimuli, or temporal facilitation with trains of stimuli). All these properties contrast with those of the neurons of specific nuclei, called lemniscal neurons in the somatosensory system (see p. 96). The neurons of the reticular formation are therefore examples of nonspecific or extralemniscal neurons.

There are still considerable gaps in our knowledge of the diverse *functions of the reticular formation.* As diagrammed in Figure 3–12 B, it is thought to participate in a number of functions that can be summarized as follows: a) control of the state of consciousness by influence on the excitability of cortical neurons, and thus participation in the sleeping/waking rhythm (the key structure in this regard is the ascending reticular activating system, or ARAS; cf. *Fundamentals of Neurophysiology,* p. 295); b) mediation of the affective-emotional effects of sensory stimuli, in particular the pain stimuli carried in the anterolateral funiculus, by sending on afferent information to the limbic system; c) vegetative regulatory functions, especially in vital reflexes (cardiovascular, respiratory, swallowing, coughing, and sneezing reflexes) in which many afferent and efferent systems must be coordinated; d) participation in the motor mechanisms for body support and directed movements, as an important element in the motor centers of the brain stem (cf. *Fundamentals of Neurophysiology,* Chap. 6).

Q 3.13. Draw a cross-section through the spinal cord, indicating the afferent fibers, with their connections to segmental efferents and to ascending tracts. Label the components of your drawing.

Q 3.14. Suppose that the spinal cord is injured in such a way that the left half is completely cut through in the thoracic region. Which of the following symptoms are observed?
  a) Temperature and pain sensations on the left side of the body are eliminated
  b) Temperature and pain sensations are eliminated in the right buttock
  c) Numbers written on the upper surface of the right foot are recognized
  d) Light touching of the left leg cannot be precisely localized.
  Several statements are correct.

Q 3.15. The reticular formation of the brain stem has the following properties and functions:
  a) It consists anatomically of a regular network of neurons with parallel axons and dendrites

b) Each of its neurons is excited by only one sense organ (monosensory convergence)

c) The general excitability of the cortical neurons, and thus also the state of consciousness, is controlled by the reticular formation

d) The afferents in the dorsal columns synapse predominantly in the reticular formation on their way to the thalamus.

3.5 The Somatosensory System in Thalamus and Cortex

Chief among the sensory centers supplying the anatomic substrate of conscious perception are those in the thalamus and cortex. They are grouped functionally as the thalamocortical system. The lemniscal system shows an especially clear somatotopic organization here, so that we may speak of a *projection* or *mapping* of the periphery of the body onto thalamus and cortex. The nonspecific system displays no such precise somatotopic arrangement.

The thalamus: general form and subdivisions. Figure 3–13 A presents a schematic, simplified view of the thalamus of the right side of the brain. It can be functionally subdivided into the following groups of nuclei: 1. specific nuclei of the sense organs of the skin, eye, and ear (red); 2. nonspecific nuclei (dark-grey); 3. motor nuclei (light-grey); 4. association nuclei (white).

The *specific nuclei* (red) each receive afferent input from the periphery that is well defined anatomically and physiologically. There is also a prominent direct fiber connection to the cortex and another conducting back from the cortex. The specific nuclei for the visual and auditory systems, the lateral and medial geniculate bodies, respectively (LGB and MGB, red in Fig. 3–13 A), are discussed in Chapters 5 and 6. The specific nucleus of the somatosensory system is the ventrobasal nucleus (VB, red in Fig. 3–13 A). Its functional properties are discussed below.

The *nonspecific thalamic nuclei,* most of which are medially situated, include (among others) the central lateral and central median nuclei, shown in dark-grey in Figure 3–13 A; these are connected functionally with the reticular formation of the brain stem (see Sec. 3.4). Like the reticular formation, they receive inputs of all sensory modalities. The fibers ascending from the spinal cord pass primarily through the anterolateral funiculus. There are efferent connections to many cortical areas, to the hypothalamus, and to the limbic system. The nonspecific thalamic nuclei are, so to speak, the subsequent distribution stations for the afferent information converging on the reticular formation (Figs. 3–7 B and 3–12 B).

Here we shall mention only briefly the nuclei of the *motor system* — the ventrolateral nucleus (light-grey in Fig. 2–13 A) and the *association nuclei* (e. g., the pulvinar, shown in white); the latter combine information from several sense organs, in collaboration with various cortical areas (the sensory cortices and association cortex).

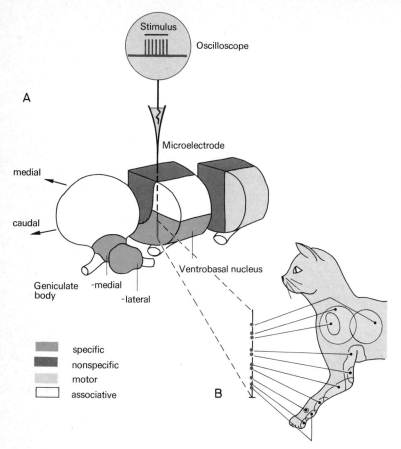

Fig. 3–13. **A** Functional subdivisions of the thalamus (schematic). The diagram shows the right thalamus, cut in two places to reveal the interior. It is subdivided into four groups of nuclei: the specific nuclei *(red)*, nonspecific nuclei *(dark-grey)*, motor nuclei *(light-grey)*, and association nuclei *(white)*. Microelectrode and oscilloscope symbolize recording from single neurons in the ventrobasal nucleus. **B** Section about 2 mm long from a microelectrode track through the right ventrobasal nucleus of a cat, showing the positions of ten neurons, of which the receptive fields on the skin of the animal are indicated. *B*: modified from POGGIO and MOUNTCASTLE: Bull. Johns Hopk. Hosp. *106,* 266 (1960)

The specific thalamic nucleus of the somatosensory system. Because of its anatomic position, this strucure is called the ventrobasal nucleus (VB) or ventrobasal complex. Here are the terminations of the medial lemniscus and the neospinothalamic tract, as well as those of the corresponding tracts from the trigeminal nuclei in the brainstem. The ventrobasal nucleus is the second synaptic relay station of the lemniscal system. The characteristic properties of VB neurons will now be discussed. They are typical *lemniscal neurons,* so that in almost all respects their responses are opposite to those of the extralemniscal neurons (see Sec. 3.4, p. 94).

Recording with microelectrodes in the VB, one tends to find neurons that discharge in response to mechanical stimulation of the skin. The electrode track through the right VB in Figure 3–13 A is enlarged in B. Each point on the track shows the position in the nucleus of a single neuron which responded to stimulation of the indicated region of skin. The most important results of this experiment are as follows: 1. Each neuron could be activated only by stimulation in the region of the left foreleg of the experimental animal (a cat); this is the *receptive field* of the neuron. 2. The receptive fields of the VB are smaller, on the average, the closer they are to the toe end of the limb. This is one of the neurophysiologic prerequisites for the high spatial resolution associated with tactile exploration using the forelimb. 3. Neighboring regions of the body project to neighboring regions in the VB. This *somatotopic* organization is still more pronounced in the subsequent projection to area SI of the cerebral cortex. 4. Each neuron is excited by only a single kind of receptor—for example, by slowly adapting pressure receptors, or by cutaneous hair-follicle receptors (see Chap. 2). 5. The intensity of a peripheral stimulus is coded in the mean discharge rate of the neurons, as it is in the receptors (see Sec. 3.1).

The neurons of the specific thalamic nuclei of eye and ear (the LGB and MGB) have equally well defined properties.

Somatosensory projection areas in the cortex. The ventrobasal nucleus (VB) of the thalamus is linked by ascending and descending axons to two cortical areas, called SI and SII (S stands for somatosensory; cf. Fig. 3–14). SI is on the *postcentral gyrus* just behind the central sulcus, a deep groove running across the cerebrum. In man SII is on the upper wall of the lateral sulcus, which separates the parietal and temporal lobes.

There is a marked *somatotopic relationship* between the periphery of the body and the contralateral SI, indications of which are already apparent at lower levels —in the tracts and nuclei of the lemniscal system, and especially in the ventrobasal nucleus of the thalamus (see Fig. 3–13 B). In Figure 3–15 the representation of the human body surface on SI is shown; this is a symbolic diagram based on the results of electrical stimulation of the cortex in the waking human (for further details see p. 101). The geometrically distorted *projection* of the body surface onto the neuronal system of SI is sometimes called the "somatosensory homunculus". This afferent projection resembles the efferent projection of the motor cortex to the musculature (see *Fundamentals of Neurophysiology*, Fig. 6–9).

It is clear in Figure 3–15 that the cortical areas associated with hand and face are each about as large as the projection area of trunk and leg together. This is a general rule; organs with particularly high densities of receptors, such as the fingers and lips, project to correspondingly large populations of neurons in SI. The consequences regarding perception are discussed below (p. 101).

In both animals and man, the somatotopic mapping of the body periphery onto the sensory cortex can be studied by peripheral stimulation and central recording of the resulting *evoked potentials* on the cerebral cortex; the latency between stimulus and evoked potential gives an indication of the number of relay stations in

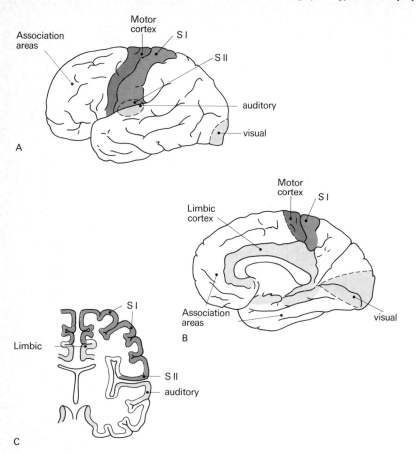

Fig. 3–14 A–C. Primary sensory projection areas of the cortex. *A* Surface view of the left hemisphere. *B* View of the right hemisphere from the midplane of the brain. *C* Frontal section of the left hemisphere at the level of the postcentral gyrus. *Dark red:* somatosensory projection areas SI, SII. *Light red:* primary projection areas of the visual and auditory systems. Also shown are the positions of the motor cortex *(dark gray),* the association areas *(white),* and the cortical parts of the limbic system *(light gray)*

the pathway (for details of this technique see *Fundamentals of Neurophysiology,* 3rd Ed., p. 280). In this way "maps" of the somatosensory projection areas of many species have been constructed. In the higher primates the SI projection is similar to that in humans, shown in Figure 3–15. In cats and rats the mouth and nose regions (especially the tactile vibrissae) have a disproportionately large representation, while the forelimb occupies a relatively small area as compared with primates.

In *SII* there is also a somatotopic organization, though it is less well marked than in SI. A peculiarity of SII is that both sides of the body are represented in each hemisphere; that is, the projection is bilateral.

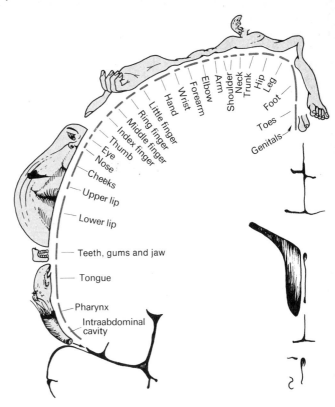

Fig. 3–15. Somatotopic organization of the somatosensory cortex SI. Symbolic representation of the mapping of the human body surface onto the postcentral gyrus, as determined by local electrical stimulation of the cortex in waking patients. Modified from PENFIELD, W., RASMUSSEN, T. (1950)

The measurement of evoked potentials can also be used to map out the primary projection regions of the visual and auditory systems. The retina projects to a circumscribed region in the occipital lobe, and the receptors of the inner ear have their projection fields in the temporal lobes. Both are shown in Figure 3–14 (cf. Figs. 5–32 and 6–16). Here, too, there are point-to-point representations of the peripheral sensory surface upon the cortical surface, comparable to a distorted map.

Neuronal processing in the somatosensory cortex. The receptive fields of the neurons lying directly one above the other in the six cytoarchitectonically distinguishable layers of SI overlap greatly, whereas those of the horizontally adjacent neurons are usually distinctly different. This finding led to the inference that the cortex is arranged in functional units consisting of **neuronal columns** oriented perpendicular to the surface, each column having a diameter of 0.2–

0.5 mm (Fig. 3–16). The anatomic basis of these columns is the limited horizontal extent of the regions in which the afferents from the ventrobasal thalamic nucleus terminate, as well as the tendency of the dendritic trees of the pyramidal cells to spread vertically (Fig. 3–16 B). The neurons in each column can be excited by receptors of only one type; that is, the column is specific not only with respect to localization but also with respect to receptor type. However, the existence of cortical columns or neurons that process temperature or nociceptive stimuli exclusively has not yet been definitely established. Both thermoreceptive and nociceptive neurons have been found in the cortical projection fields, but most of them can also be activated by low-threshold mechanoreceptors.

In theory, each cortical column, because of the large number of neurons it contains (up to 10^5), has a considerable capacity for the processing of information from the periphery. It has been proposed that a column functions — by way of a variety of excitatory and inhibitory interactions of its neurons — on a hierarchical basis (see Fig. 3–16 B). In the process, as a result of the appropriate connectivity and operations, the properties of the peripheral stimuli are encoded in various

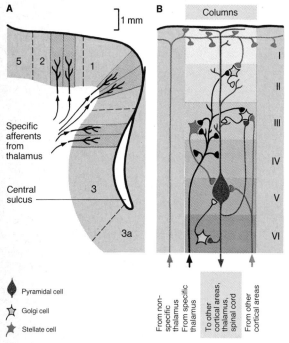

Fig. 3–16 A, B. Columnar arrangement of cortical neurons. *A* Sagittal section through the postcentral gyrus of a monkey. The numbers indicate cytoarchitectonic subdivisions (according to BRODMANN). In each of the areas 1, 2 and 3 two adjacent columns are shown, with their afferents from the ventrobasal thalamic nucleus. *B* Diagram for clarification. The functional relatedness of neurons in all cortical layers (I–VI) results partly from anatomic features: the terminations of the specific thalamocortical afferents and the dendritic trees of the pyramidal neurons *(red)* are restricted in lateral extent. The most important afferent and efferent connections are shown

neurons. The term *feature extraction* has been applied to this function of the cortical neuron aggregates. Examples of this notion are given on p. 183, for the case of the visual cortex. After such processing the information is passed on to other cortical regions — for instance, to the motor cortex on the precentral gyrus or to the association areas.

The specific thalamocortical system and conscious perception. The hand and mouth regions are represented on an especially large scale in SI of humans and other primates (Fig. 3–15). Now, these are precisely the parts of the skin with outstanding tactile abilities; the two-point spatial-resolution threshold is particularly low in these regions (cf. Fig. 2–4). The cortical projections from the skin, as well as those from the other sense organs, are involved in the process of discriminative, conscious perception. Supporting evidence is provided by a number of findings, two of which will now be described.

If the brain of a waking patient, partially exposed under local anesthetic for therapeutic reasons, is stimulated with a fine electrode in the sensory areas of the cortex, the patient reports sensations from circumscribed regions of the periphery of the body. For example, if the hand region of SI is stimulated the patient feels touch stimuli on his hand. It was by such experiments that the somatotopic organization shown in Figure 3–15 was discovered. By direct stimulation of the sensory cortex, then, conscious perception can be elicited without activation of the afferent pathways involving peripheral nerves, spinal cord, and specific thalamic nuclei. Similarly, stimuli in the projection area of the eye produce a sensation of flashes of light. However, sensations of pain cannot be produced by cortical stimulation.

In monkeys, *experimental ablation* of a circumscribed region of SI brings about sensory deficits in the associated peripheral region. For instance, before the operation the animals had learned to discriminate a cube from a sphere by touch, without looking at the objects. After removal of the cortical sensory hand region, this discriminative ability vanished and could not be relearned.

Similar observations have been made of humans with injury in a particular region of SI (as a result, for example, of gunshot wounds or tumors). Tactile stimuli are still perceived, but the ability to localize them is impaired; touch sensations have a dull, uncertain character. Pain is still recognized, but localization of the painful stimuli is less precise. Intactness of SI, then, is a prerequisite for spatially organized, conscious perception of stimuli at the body surface.

Electrical stimulation of SII in humans also gives rise to perceptions that seem to come from the associated peripheral region. Ablation of parts of SII alone, however, do not result in detectable sensory deficits. The role of SII in sensory perception remains unexplained.

Association areas of the cortex. All the sensory projection areas of the cortex, together with the motor cortex, take up less than about 20% of the cortical surface (see Fig. 3–14). The remaining areas are called association areas. They are connected to the primary projection areas by massive fiber tracts; usually each association region is linked in this way to several projection areas.

The term "association area" derives from the function ascribed to these regions; here the diverse but specific information from the sense organs is thought to be associated to form more *complex elements of consciousness.* In the parietal association area, situated between the somatosensory and visual projection areas, our subjective notion of the spatial environment and our picture of our own bodies (the "body image") are thought to arise. It has been suggested that learning processes during development in early childhood, in which somatosensory, proprioceptive, and visual information is evaluated and compared, are crucial in the formation of these concepts.

Hypotheses about the function of the association fields in man have been drawn chiefly from observation of the neurologic deficits appearing as a result of cortical destruction in circumscribed regions. An example of impairment following damage to the parietal association cortex is *visual agnosia.* A patient with this syndrome has an intact sense of sight, to the extent that he can avoid obstacles or reach for and seize objects. But he cannot recognize the significance of objects. When a person suffering from visual agnosia looks at something and is asked to name it, he cannot. But by holding it he can identify it with his sense of touch.

The relative area occupied by the association fields in primates, and especially in humans, is very much greater than in other mammals. Specifically human association areas, located in the temporal and frontal lobes, are involved in the understanding and performance of speech (speech centers; cf. *Fundamentals of Neurophysiology,* Chap. 9). Very little neurophysiologic research has been directed to the association areas.

The extralemniscal system and conscious perception. Excitation of the sensory cortex is a necessary, but not sufficient, condition for the occurrence of conscious perception. Many clinical observations and data from animal experiments support this generalization. For example, even under anesthesia and during sleep, primary cortical evoked potentials can be elicited, but these do not result in conscious perception. Moreover, lesions of the upper brain stem involving the reticular formation can produce permanent unconsciousness; conversely, electrical stimulation of experimental animals in this region causes awakening, attentiveness, and redirection of attention. The last two behavioral changes are called "arousal". On the basis of these and a great number of similar findings, the concept has been developed that a steady excitatory influx from the reticular formation to the cortex is involved in determining the degree of consciousness, over a range from deep sleep through drowsiness to attentive waking; the term "ascending reticular activating system" (ARAS) has been applied.

As diagrammed in Figure 3–17, conscious perception of, for example, a tactile stimulus requires two inputs to the neocortex — the specific projection through the lemniscal pathway (via the ventrobasal nucleus of the thalamus) and activation by the nonspecific system of the reticular formation (via the nonspecific thalamic nuclei). The lemniscal projection provides information about the object of the perception (e.g., its location, size, and the time of the stimulus); this contribution to conscious perception is labelled in Figure 3–17 as *discrimination.* The non-

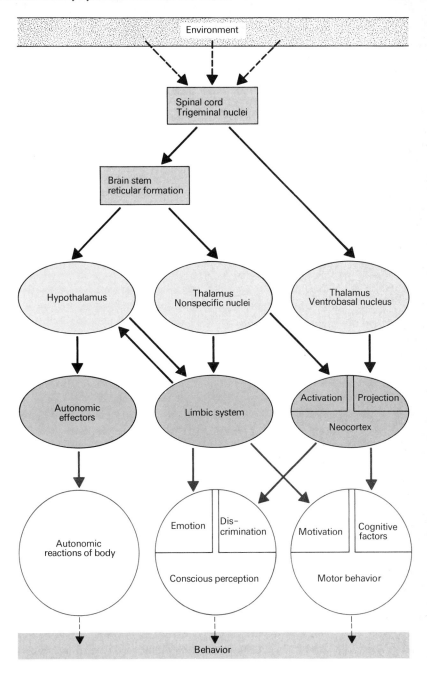

Fig. 3–17. Interaction of the specific and nonspecific systems (schematized and highly simplified) in producing three categories of behavior: conscious perception, motor behavior, and autonomic response of the body

specific activation, on the other hand, to which all sensory channels can contribute, determines the *level of wakefulness* as a condition of perception.

But we know from personal experience (introspection) that each perception has yet another aspect, that of emotion and affect or, as it is commonly called, our *feelings* about the object of perception. This dimension of perception is ascribed to the limbic system. If a cat is stimulated electrically in the limbic system, for example, rage and aggressive behavior can be elicited. The limbic system consists of a number of subcortical regions arranged roughly in a ring around the diencephalon. The reader interested in further details may consult the extensive description in *Fundamentals of Neurophysiology* (Chap. 8).

This interpretation of its function suggests that the limbic system contributes the *affective content of perceptions.* As diagrammed in Figure 3–17, the somatosensory inputs to the limbic system arrive primarily by way of the nonspecific (extralemniscal) pathway.

The limbic system has a close reciprocal relationship with the hypothalamus, the superordinate center for many control circuits in the autonomic nervous system (e. g., cardiovascular activity and body temperature) and the endocrine system (e. g., water balance). The possibility that sensory stimuli act on autonomic effectors by way of the hypothalamus is also indicated in Figure 3–17.

So far we have discussed only the interactions of the specific and nonspecific systems in Figure 3–17. In the same figure, greatly simplified, the relationship of three types of *behavioral response* to environmental stimuli is indicated. These are conscious perception, motor behavior, and the unconscious autonomic reactions of the body.

Conscious perception and motor behavior have at least two dimensions, which in each case can be ascribed to the neocortex and the limbic system, respectively. In the case of perception, we have already discussed these dimensions — discrimination and affect. In motor behavior we have on the one hand the cognitive factors (neocortical), which depend on precise signals from the sense organs. A second dimension in this case comprises the drives underlying action (motivation), which are thought to involve the limbic system. These can be roughly subdivided, according to whether the tendency is to approach or to withdraw — i. e., into the categories attraction and flight.

Autonomic reactions of the body are to a great extent unconscious. Their intensity — measurable, for example, as a change in blood pressure or skin resistance — is associated with the intensity of the affective content of perception. The strength of motivation of motor behavior is also correlated with affective content. The "common denominator" is the excitation and functional state of the limbic system.

The diagrammatic summary in Figure 3–17 should be regarded as an attempt to arrange what we know about central sensory systems in an easily surveyed scheme. It may provide the reader with a very preliminary orientation to the multitude of complex findings.

Q 3.16. "Somatotopic projection" means that:
   a) The soma of the nerve cell sends processes in certain directions
   b) The peripheral sensory surface has a point-to-point mapping onto the sensory cortex
   c) There is a representation of the periphery on the sensory cortex
   d) The neurons of the somatosensory cortex SI have a fiber connection to those of the association cortex.
   Several answers are correct.

Q 3.17. The neurons in the specific thalamic nuclei receive their afferent input:
   a) From a sense organ via at least seven synapses
   b) From several sense organs simultaneously, via at least three synapses
   c) From the thermoreceptive and pain afferents of the skin, via the dorsal column nuclei
   d) From one sense organ in each case, via at least two synapses.

Q 3.18. Which of the following statements apply to a person in whom the arm and hand regions of the right somatosensory cortex SI have been destroyed?
   a) No objects can be discriminated by tactile exploration with the right hand
   b) Painful stimuli to the left hand are perceived, but the precision of localization is reduced
   c) Lack of pain sensation in the left hand
   d) Because of the bilateral projection to SII, no detectable deficits appear.

Q 3.19. Lateral inhibition in the CNS results in:
   a) Compensation of the spatial spread of excitation caused by divergence of neuronal connections
   b) Diminishing of all impulses produced by stimulation
   c) Neuronal contrast formation
   d) A suppression of the contralateral sensory afferents.
   Several answers are correct.

3.6 The Sensory System in the Light of Information Theory

The nerve fiber can be compared, from the point of view of its function, with a cable carrying information. The approach of the communications engineer — *information theory* — can also be applied to the nervous system. This body of knowledge, together with control theory, is often called *cybernetics;* especially in Europe, its application in biology is termed biocybernetics, though such general terms are used less in the United States.

The concept of information theory. The fundamental concept from which information theory is developed is represented by the block diagram of Figure 3–18. It distinguishes the functional components that participate in the transmission of

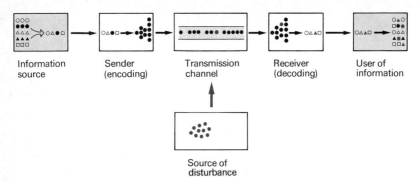

Fig. 3–18. Diagram illustrating the concept of, and terms used in information theory

information: the information source, the sender, the transmission channel, the receiver, the user, and a source of disturbance. This breakdown can be applied to all kinds of information transmission, in the realms of both technology and biology. Information theory can provide a quantitative measure of information, and thus allow one to arrive at statements that can characterize and compare information-transmitting systems.

To transmit information one requires *symbols* (such as letters or numbers); certain of these are selected or determined by the information source. These signs are encoded in the sender, usually into other signal forms more suitable for transmission. *Coding* is the general term used for such a conversion between the elements of two sets of signs; an example of coding is the association of the letters of the alphabet with the Morse symbols. In the receiver the transmitted information is decoded and passed on to the user.

Information theory is also particularly concerned with the effects of disturbances. Disturbances can be introduced in the sender (in the encoding process), in the transmission channel and in the receiver (decoding). Such sources of disturbance are considered in Figure 3–18 as element acting on the transmission channel. One of the tasks of information theory is to establish coding procedures that protect the information from degradation due to disturbances.

How can information be measured? The term "information" in information theory applies only to the aspects of a communication that are quantifiable and can be formulated mathematically. The following example shows how this usage of the term arises.

If you throw one of a pair of fair dice, one of six equally likely numbers will come up. *Before* the throw, we know only that the outcome will be one of six specific numbers. The *act* ot throwing the dice reduces this uncertainty in a quantifiable way, which we can use to define the information content of a throw. Moreover, every such event — that is, each throw of a fair six-sided dice — will have the same information content. A different kind of event — such as the act of flipping a coin (only two possible outcomes) — will have a different information content. In general, the notion is that the *information content of an event is the quantified reduction of uncertainty about a situation provided by knowledge of the outcome of the event.* Note that the communication of symbols from source to user has precise analogies with the above examples — there is a quantifiable reduction of a priori uncertainty.

It is easy to see that this reduction of uncertainty about an outcome of an event is greater, the smaller the probabilities p of the occurrences of the various outcomes; throwing a die ($p = 1/6$) rules out "more uncertainty" than flipping a coin ($p = 1/2$). A useful approach, therefore, is to define the measure of information content I in terms of the reciprocal of p — that is, $1/p$. A reasonable supplementary condition for a measure of information is that in the case of an event having only one outcome, which is certain to occur and thus has probability $p = 1$, the information content I should be zero. The condition is met by using a logarithmic function of $1/p$, since $\log 1 = 0$.

These considerations make it plausible that the measurable information content I of an event (or similarly of a communication revealing one of several equally likely symbols) has been defined as

$$I = \log (1/p) \tag{3–5}$$

In this definition the logarithm to the base 2 (written $\log_2$, or ld, for logarithmus dualis) is used, for then the situation $p = 1/2$ results in 1 unit of information, or **1 bit.** One can thus write Eq. (3–5), defining the information content I of an event having equally likely outcomes, each with probability p, as follows:

$$I = \mathrm{ld}\ (1/p) \tag{3–6}$$

For the game of dice, the information content of each throw of a die can now be computed numerically: $I = \mathrm{ld}\ (1/(1/6)) = \mathrm{ld}\ (6) = 2.58$ bits. We shall learn about the unit "bit" below. To find the function ld, a conversion formula $\mathrm{ld}(n) = \log_{10}(n) / \log_{10}(2) = 3.32 \times \log_{10}(n)$ is useful.

In introducing the measure of information we started with the assumption that all states of the information source occur with equal probability $1/p$ — as is true, for example, of a fair die. This assumption is a simplification; usually the individual signs or states of an information source are not all equally probable. The general case of unequal probabilities is outside the scope of this introductory presentation of the measure of information; the interested reader will find further literature in the list of references.

Given the special case of equal probability note that Eq. (3–6) can be written in another form; if n is the total number of possible symbols or states of the information source, it holds that $p = 1/n$.

Thus in terms of n the expression for information content of the transmission of a single symbol becomes

$$I = \mathrm{ld}\ n. \tag{3–7}$$

That is, the information content I of such a communication is the logarithm to the base 2 of the number n of all possible states that could have been communicated.

The *subjective meaning of an item of information* to the user of course depends on many factors not included in the above quantitative measure of information. In a dice game, for example, the subjective value the player puts on the numbers can vary depending on the rules of the game, unconscious motivation, his relations with the other players, whether he has just bet his last dollar, and so on. The study of such aspects of symbolic information is often called *semantics.*

Binary and nonbinary characters; the bit. Information transmission requires a set of symbols from which the information source chooses. In the simplest case the set of symbols comprises just two, called *binary symbols* (e. g., the binary digits 0 and 1). With these the information source can convey information about a *decision between alternatives.* Binary systems are particularly convenient from a technical viewpoint (e. g., switch position on/off). This is one of the reasons that the information content of the act of specifying one binary symbol has been chosen as the unit of information. This choice is implicit in Eqs. (3–6) and (3–7), for ld (2) = 1. That is, the *elementary quantity of information* that is transmitted by specifying one of two equally likely binary symbols is called *one bit.*

If extensive messages are to be transmitted with binary digits, several digits must be strung together: *words* must be formed from binary digits. The length of the words — that is, the number of binary digits used per word — is a direct measure, in bits, of the amount of information transmitted per word. A word composed of two binary digits can transmit two bits, with three digits three bits are transmitted, and so on. The number of different words that can be formed from two binary digits is $2^2 = 4$. These words are 00, 01, 10 and 11. With three digits $2^3 = 8$ words are available as follows: 000, 001, 010, 011, 100, 101, 110, 111. With m binary digits per word, it is apparent that there are $n = 2^m$ different communications; the process of specifying any one of these transmits m bits of information.

The determination of information content discussed thus far can also be applied in cases in which any arbitrary symbols serve as carriers of information. Any desired set of symbols can be represented by binary words of sufficient length. To obtain an unambiguous mapping (coding) of a set of n symbols onto binary words, the latter must have a word length, on the average, of $m = $ ld (n) binary digits.

Such a coding is illustrated in Figure 3–19. This is a diagram of a decision tree in which successive bifurcations of the branches result in precisely one branch for each symbol (here, the eight letters A through H to be presented). Each bifurcation signifies a decision between two alternatives, here labeled 0 and 1. This is a practical method of coding in binary words.

If an arbitrary sign can be replaced by a binary word, then it has the same information content (in bits) as the binary word with which it is associated. The average information content I of specifying one symbol in a set of n symbols is therefore $I = $ ld (n). This is Eq. (3–7), which we developed above as a definition of information content.

This introduction to the fundamental concepts of information theory is much simplified. More detailed and extensive presentations of information theory are listed in the references at the end of the book.

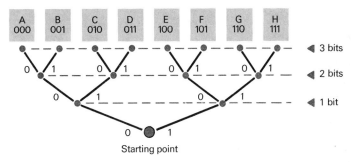

Fig. 3–19. A coding or decision tree. By successive binary decisions the set of letters A to H can be dissected into subsets. At each branch point, a decision to go left is given the sign 0, and a decision to go right is given the sign 1. Proceeding from the starting point and listing the successive decision signs in sequence, one generates a binary word corresponding to the letter at each terminal point, A through H. These binary words are shown under the associated letters

Information theory in sensory physiology. We shall now apply the concept of figure 3–18, described above in general terms, to information transmission in the nervous system. A suitable example for discussion is a receptor with its afferent nerve fiber. Here information is coded and transmitted as nerve impulses. The information source consists of environmental stimuli, the sender is a receptor cell, the transmission channel is a nerve fiber, the receiver is a synapse on a central neuron, and the latter neuron itself can be regarded as the user.

The physically measurable parameters of stimuli (for example, pressure on the skin, location of a stimulus on the peripheral sensory surface, wavelength of light and sound stimuli) are the items communicated. In the example of the stretch receptor (Sec. 3.1) we have seen how a stimulus parameter determines the response of the receptor: the rate of impulse discharge in the afferent fiber changes in the same direction as the intensity of the stimulus. In this case the variable "stimulus intensity" is coded in the variable "mean frequency of nerve impulses." This kind of coding, comparable to frequency modulation in technical communication systems, is found in receptors of all modalities; in muscle spindles, pressure receptors in the skin, chemoreceptors on the tongue, and photoreceptors of the retina, *nerve impulse frequency is the carrier of information.*

Because the afferent fibers of particular receptors project to particular corresponding cells in the CNS, the information contained in the train of impulses is evaluated appropriately. For example, Ia afferents end on homonymous motoneurons, and mechanosensitive cutaneous afferents project to the postcentral gyrus on the contralateral cortex.

Information transmission in an ideal receptor. Let us consider the coding of stimulus intensity. If, in a certain time period, the stimulated receptor responds either with no impulse or with one impulse, then it can provide information about just two levels of stimulus intensity. That is, no action potential means "stimulus intensity below threshold" and one action potential means "stimulus intensity above threshold." If the possible number of nerve impulses is 0, 1, or 2, the user element in the system receives information sufficient to distinguish between three states of stimulation. If a stimulus elicits a maximum of N impulses in the afferent fiber, the receptor can in theory signal $N + 1$ different **levels of intensity** to the CNS. This situation is illustrated in Figure 3–20. The impulse number N in the afferent fiber (ordinate) can have only integer values. For this reason the curve relating stimulus intensity S (abscissa) to impulse number has the form of a staircase. In an **ideal receptor**, which responds to a maintained stimulus with a discharge at constant frequency, the impulse number N is the product of the discharge frequency f and the observation time t: $N = f \cdot t$. The maximum number of distinguishable stimulus-intensity levels is thus

$$N + 1 = f_m \cdot t + 1 \qquad (3\text{–}8)$$

where f_m is the maximal rate of discharge of the receptor. In the case of a receptor with a spontaneous discharge frequency f_0 (in the absence of any detectable external stimulus), f_m in Eq. (3–8) and all subsequent expressions should be replaced by $f_m - f_0$.

The number of available symbols in this case, then, is the number of distinguishable states of the discharge in the afferent nerve. The information content with

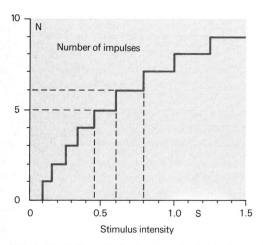

Fig. 3–20. Coding of stimulus intensity S (abscissa, arbitrary units) at a receptor into nerve impulses (ordinate). The duration of each stimulus is fixed. The characteristic curve of the coding process has the shape of a staircase **(red)**, because the receptor can produce only integer numbers N of action potentials (nerve impulses)

respect to stimulus intensity, in the example of Figure 3–20, is thus $I = \text{ld}\,(N + 1) = \text{ld}\,(10) = 3.3$ bits. In general, in an ideal receptor caused by a stimulus to discharge at the maximal frequency f_m the **information content** I with respect to stimulus intensity is

$$I = \text{ld}\,(f_m \cdot t + 1) \tag{3–9}$$

This relationship between I, f_m, and observation time t is shown graphically in Figure 3–21. It is evident that the information content I increases with both f_m and t. The maximal frequency f_m is a fixed property of the receptor. On the other hand, by prolonging the observation time t the information about intensity of a

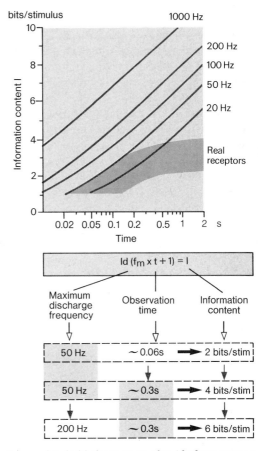

Fig. 3–21. Information content I (ordinate) associated with the response of an **ideal receptor** as a function of the observation time t (abscissa). The parameter distinguishing the different curves is the maximal discharge frequency f_m of the receptor; the curves were calculated from Eq. (3–9). The shaded region **(red)** denotes measured values of the information content of the responses of mechanosensitive cutaneous receptors, as a function of t

prolonged constant stimulus can in theory be made arbitrarily precise. In practice, however, the dynamics of the decoding processes in the CNS limit the time span over which evaluation of the afferent discharge can be extended to increase the information content. From studies of actual receptors we can get some idea of the extent to which an increase of t can be useful.

Information transmission in a real receptor. An ideal receptor, stimulated at a constant intensity, responds with an entirely regular discharge at constant frequency. This condition is not met by biological receptors.

Experimentally it is found that when the intensity of a stimulus is held constant the discharge rate of the receptor can vary in time. In Figure 3–22 A the discharge rate, here the carrier of the information "stimulus intensity", fluctuates stochastically (randomly in time for no apparent reason). Such fluctuations in signals are called **noise** by communications engineers. They cause reduced performance of an information channel — a disturbance of information transmission (cf. Fig. 3–18).

To quantify the amount of information lost due to noise in a receptor, consider the experimentally measured coding relationship shown in Figure 3–22 B. Each point on the graph represents the result of a single measurement like that in A, but here the observation time is 5 s. The number of distinguishable states can be estimated by drawing a staircase curve through the field of points; the one drawn here is found to have eight steps (the first step at 0 impulses), corresponding to 3 bits per stimulus if an ideal receiver counts for 5 s.

The rationale in drawing the staircase in Figure 3–22 B is as follows. Two stimulus intensities are distinguishable with certainty when all the impulse numbers (ordinate in Fig. 3–22 B) associated with one intensity are different from those associated with the other intensity. The "worst case", which represents the

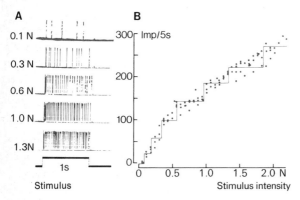

Fig. 3–22 A, B. The effect of noise on coding in a receptor. *A* Original recordings of the discharge of a pressure receptor in the sole of the cat's paw, in response to pressure stimuli lasting 1 s; the stimulus intensities (in newtons) are indicated. *B* Numbers of impulses (ordinate) discharged in response to stimuli lasting 5 s, obtained in many single experiments like that of (A) as a function of the stimulus intensity (abscissa). The staircase curve *(red)* was constructed so as to have the maximal step heights which fit within the range of scatter of the data points

minimum discriminability available, is given by the staircase curve of maximal step height that can be drawn in the point field of the coding plot of the experimentally measured responses.

If our receptor were to behave like an ideal frequency modulator (an ideal receptor, without noise), then under the experimental conditions of Figure 3–22 B at least about 300 steps of stimulus intensity would have to be distinguishable; the corresponding information content would be 8.2 bits per response (Eq. (3–9)). In this example, then, for each response 8.2 bits — 3 bits = 5.2 bits are lost due to noise!

The highest values of information content per stimulus measured so far were found in deefferented muscle spindles. Primary (Ia) endings can transmit 4.8 bits per 1-s stimulus; secondary (II) endings actually transmit 6.3 bits.

Departures from the behavior of an ideal receptor also become apparent when the observation time t is varied. As t is prolonged, the information content of transmission by the ideal receptor rises continuously, as illustrated by the curves corresponding to Eq. (3–9) in Figure 3–21. By contrast, the information content of real receptors cannot be raised infinitely. In Figure 3–21 the red shaded area indicates the region in which the experimentally measured information content per stimulus of certain cutaneous mechanoreceptors changes as a function of the observation time t. Pressure receptors in the cat's paw, for example, have essentially reached their highest value (3 bits per stimulus) after a time as short as 1 s.

Although many receptors can discharge at frequencies of several hundred per second, their performance with regard to stimulus-intensity information content is evidently little or no better than that of an ideal receptor with a maximal discharge rate of 20 per second.

Redundancy. The imprecise coding in a real receptor (due to noise) reflects a *disturbance* of information transmission. Can one find examples in the nervous system of compensation for such disturbances? In communications technology the methods available for protecting information against loss make use of the concept of *redundancy*. As an illustration of this notion, first consider an example from the field of linguistics. Try to decipher the following sequence of letters:

$$T . . . od . ng . n r . cep . . rs i .$$
$$d . st . rbe . . y . o . se$$

The information contained in this sentence is discernible even though about 40% of the letters are absent; written language contains *more symbols* than are necessary for the meaning to be detected with certainty. This excess is redundancy. It is measurable in bits.

Studies in which parts of texts have been systematically removed have shown that written German, for example, conveys on the average only 1.5 bits per letter. Theoretically, the average information content of each of the 26 letters in the alphabet is ld (26) = 4.7 bits; that is, the redundancy in this case averages 4.7 — 1.5 = 3.2 bits per letter.

This may at first appear to be an extravagant waste of symbols, but that is only one aspect of redundancy. Its advantages become clear when the *transmission channel is disturbed* — for example, with a bad telephone connection or messy handwriting. Here the redundancy in language ensures that a text can be recognized when only a fraction of the signs are identifiable. Information theory provides a general demonstration that information transmission is the more secure against disturbance, the greater the redundancy built into the coding.

Redundancy in the nervous system. One effective way of using redundancy to protect against noise consists of transmitting the information over two or more channels *in parallel.* This possibility is realized in the nervous system. In the periphery the density of the receptors is usually so high that even point stimuli excite several fibers. In such parallel transmission, the extent to which the information content is in fact utilized depends on the nature of the central nervous processing. Under the assumption that evaluation involves summation of the impulses in all excited fibers, the information about stimulus intensity available to an observer can be calculated from the variability of the summed discharge — for example, by the method sketched in Figure 3–22 B. With this process of summation, the total number of impulses per observation interval t rises approximately linearly with the number of afferent fibers involved. The variability in the discharge (noise) — that is, the width of the band of uncertainty in Figure 3–22 B — increases less. Accordingly, there is an increase in the number of steps that can be plotted in the experimentally derived coding diagram (like that of Fig. 3–22 B) as the number of afferent fibers increases. It follows that the information content of the summed discharge is greater than that of a single receptor. In general, then, *redundancy by transmission in parallel fibers compensates for disturbance of coding in the receptor.*

Redundancy is achieved by parallel transmission in the CNS as well. But here a new factor enters; because of the convergence and divergence in the synaptic connectivity, the parallel channels may act as quite complex networks, which (as information theory has shown) can in principle provide additional redundancy.

But when information about stimulus intensity is protected to this extent by parallel-fiber transmission, there should necessarily be an enormous spatial spread of excitation in the CNS, as discussed above (cf. Fig. 3–8 A). The result could be a loss of information about the site of stimulation. But lateral inhibition, as we have seen (cf. Fig. 3–8 B), can counteract such spread. Depending on the degree of such inhibition, central representations of the periphery can emphasize either the information about stimulus intensity or that about stimulus location.

Measurement of information in psychology. In experimental psychology, too, and especially in *psychophysics* (see Chap. 1), the quantitative notion of information is used. Here we shall cite a few examples, emphasizing the relationships between the neurophysiologic and the psychophysical measurements of information.

In experiments people can subjectively estimate the intensity of a stimulus (such as visual brightness or pressure on the skin) and express this estimate in some way (for example, numerically; cf. Sec. 1.3, p. 14). When such subjective estimates are plotted against stimulus intensity, the resulting graph is like that of Figure 3–22 B. In place of the number of impulses discharged by the receptor (on the ordinate in Fig. 3–22 B) one then has the numerical estimate of subjective intensity. From the scatter in the data we can estimate the corresponding information content available at the level of conscious perception, by the staircase procedure already described. In an experiment involving subjective measurement of the intensity of a pressure stimulus on the skin, values around 3 bits per stimulus were obtained; these are about the same as those derived for a single pressure receptor. For this experiment, then, the information transmitted by a single afferent nerve fiber in principle suffices for the measured subjective intensity perception; hence the contribution of all the other excited fibers — at least for this very special psychophysical question of stimulus intensity — can be regarded as redundancy.

In another experiment, the subject was required to compare two successive stimuli and determine the *differences* in intensity. Comparison of the psychophysical and receptor information contents has revealed that, at least in the case of psychophysical discrimination of cold stimuli to the skin, the information carried by all the cold fibers (cf. Fig. 2–16) of the stimulated skin area contributes to the subject's decision; in this psychophysical discrimination by the CNS all the available neuronal information is utilized to reduce difference threshold.

In conclusion we shall compare estimates of the total amount of sensory-neurophysiologic information available with those of psychophysical information. Here we shall use the maximal *information flow,* in bits per second, a measure also called the channel capacity.

The *channel capacity* of, for example, a mechanoreceptor (cf. Fig. 3–22) is determined experimentally by making the sequence of stimuli progressively more rapid and simultaneously shortening the individual stimuli. With stimulus durations less than 1 s, the information content of the discharge to the individual stimulus decreases (cf. Fig. 3–21), but because of the rise in the number of stimuli the information flow usually increases. Table 3–2 summarizes the channel

Table 3–2. Comparison of neuronal information flow (channel capacity) with that of conscious perception. On the left, estimates of the total numbers of receptors and afferents are indicated for five sensory systems, together with the maximal information flow of each. On the right side are the figures for maximal information flow available at the level of consciousness – the channel capacity determined in psychophysical experiments

Sensory system	No. of receptors	No. of afferents	Total channel capacity (bits/s)	Psychophysical channel capacity (bits/s)
Eyes	$2 \cdot 10^8$	$2 \cdot 10^6$	10^7	40
Ears	$3 \cdot 10^4$	$2 \cdot 10^4$	10^5	30
Skin	10^7	10^6	10^6	5
Taste	$3 \cdot 10^7$	10^3	10^3	1 (?)
Smell	$7 \cdot 10^7$	10^5	10^5	1 (?)

capacities of all the receptors in a sense organ, as estimated from the total number of afferent fibers and the channel capacity of each. These are compared with measurements of the psychophysical channel capacity; this is the maximal information flow at the level of conscious perception. In the case of the visual system the capacity given is that for reading, as determined in a psychophysical experiment. For the auditory system, it is the capacity associated with comprehension of speech.

As we know from our own experience, we can turn our conscious attention fully to only one sensory modality at a time. For this reason it is unlikely that more than one of the maximal psychophysical information flows given on the right in Table 3–2 could be operant simultaneously. We can therefore conclude that the maximal information flow of the process of conscious sensory perception is about 40 bits/s — many orders of magnitude below that taken in by receptors (left in Table 3–2). Our perception, then, would appear to be limited to a minute part of the abundance of information available as sensory input.

Q 3.20. For the case of coding of the information "stimulus intensity" in the receptor, the information content can be computed:
  a) As a number of discriminable states in the discharge rate of the receptor
  b) As a number of action potentials discharged per unit time
  c) As a logarithm to the base 2 of the states of stimulus intensity discriminable in the discharge of the receptor
  d) Only if there are no statistical fluctuations in the discharge rate (noise)

Q 3.21. Which (more than one) of the following statements about redundancy are correct?
  a) Redundancy, in general, involves an increase in the effort expended to transmit information, above the necessary minimum
  b) Redundancy is an increase in the information content of a nerve fiber by shortening of the refractory period
  c) Redundancy is realized in the nervous system in the form of transmission of the same information over several parallel paths
  d) In general, the vulnerability of information to disturbance increases with redundancy.

Q 3.22. The following statements apply to the concept "information content":
  a) No information content can be assigned to the words in the English language, since they have a significance which is not measurable (semantic information)
  b) The information content of each throw of a six-sided die is $I = \log_{10}(6)$ bits
  c) When an arbitrary symbol is coded into binary digits its information content fundamentally always becomes smaller (loss of information)
  d) The information content of the act of specifying a symbol depends on the probability of its occurrence.

4 Nociception and Pain

R. F. Schmidt

All humans and most animal organisms possess special receptors with thresholds so high that they are excited only by stimuli that cause, or might be able to cause, tissue damage ("noxious" stimuli, from the Latin "noxa", damage). These receptors are called *nociceptors.* In humans, excitation of such receptors ordinarily causes pain, which in turn serves as a signal that the body is endangered by stimuli originating either externally (e. g., heat) or internally (e. g., inflammation).

The reception, conduction and central nervous processing of noxious signals together are called *nociception,* and the neural structures involved in these events are the nociceptive or nocifensive system. The subjective sensation *pain,* as was just pointed out, is often a consequence of activation of the nociceptive system. However, as will be shown, pains can also occur without any excitation of nociceptors, and the excitation of nociceptors need not always result in the sensation of pain.

In the past, the concepts of nociception and pain have not been distinguished as carefully as they should have been. Noxious stimuli have been called "pain stimuli", for instance, and the terms "pain receptors", "pain nerve fibers", "pain tracts" and "pain centers" have been used for the various components of the nocifensive system. To illustrate how wrong it is to equate neuronal structures, and the electrical and chemical processes by which they function, with the subjective world of the pain experience, consider that we do not speak of "pleasure receptors", "pleasure tracts" or "pleasure centers", although the excitation of various receptors in the human skin and mucosa can certainly give rise to pleasurable sensations.

In the following four sections of this chapter we shall first describe the different qualities and components of pain (4.1), then turn to neurophysiology, especially the bases of nociception and the psychophysics of pain (4.2), discuss some of the pathophysiological aspects of pain (4.3), and finally cast a glance at the most important procedures for inhibiting nociceptive processes and alleviating pain (4.4).

4.1 The Qualities and Components of Pain

Qualities of pain. The sense of pain can be subdivided into a number of qualities with respect to the site of origin of the pain. In Figure 4–1 these qualities are given in the red boxes. The pain modality comprises the two qualities *somatic pain* and *visceral pain.*

If somatic pain derives from the skin, it is called *superficial pain;* if it comes from the muscles, bones, joints, and connective tissue, it is called *deep pain.* Superficial and deep pain are thus (sub-)qualities of somatic pain.

If superficial pain is produced by piercing the skin with a needle, the subject feels a sharp "flash" of pain, a readily localizable sensation that fades away rapidly when the stimulus stops. This sharp and localizable *initial pain* (first pain) is often followed, particularly at high stimulus intensities, by *delayed pain* (second pain) having a dull (or burning) character, with a latency of 0.5—1.0 s. The latter is more diffuse spatially and dies out only slowly; a good illustration is the pain felt in response to the squeezing of an interdigital fold.

Pains from muscles, bones, joints, and connective tissue are called *deep pain.* Like superficial pain, deep pain is an element in somatic pain. We are familiar, for example, with such pains as *headaches* — probably the most common of all forms of pain in humans. Deep pain is dull in nature, is poorly localizable as a rule, and has a tendency to radiate into surrounding regions of the body.

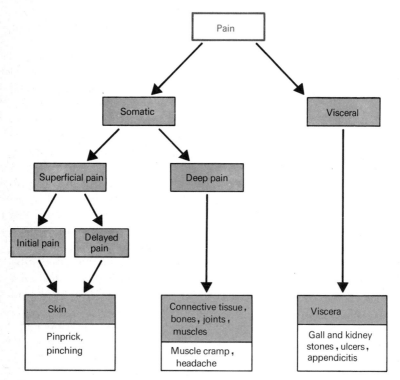

Fig. 4–1. Qualities of pain *(red background).* The localization of each quality is also indicated *(gray background),* and examples of specific forms of pain are given

In addition to somatic pain and its (sub-)qualities, an important and distinct quality, also shown in Figure 4–1, is *visceral pain.* This pain, too, tends to be dull or diffuse in character (think, for example, of gallstone pain, appendicitis, and so on). It is remarkable that when the viscera are exposed (under local anesthesia of the skin) they can be squeezed or cut without pain as long as the parietal peritoneum and the mesenteric roots are not stimulated (cf. p. 65). But rapid or extensive stretching of the hollow organs elicits severe pain. Moreover, spasms or strong contractions of smooth muscle are painful, especially when they are associated with inadequate circulation (ischemia).

Another fundamental feature by which pain is evaluated, in addition to its site of origin, is its duration. In acute pains, such as are associated with an accident, appendicitis or tooth decay, the pain is usually limited to the site of damage, we are able to locate this site accurately, and the magnitude of the pain is directly dependent on the intensity of the stimulus. These pains indicate that tissue damage is imminent or has already occured. That is, they have an unambiguous signalling and warning function. When the damage is remedied they soon fade away.

Many pains are not in the acute category; these either persist for long times (e. g., back pains, tumor pains) or return repeatedly at more or less regular intervals (e. g., migraine headaches, trigeminal neuralgia, heart pains in angina pectoris). These forms of pain — prolonged and recurrent pain — together are called *chronic pain.* In general, from the physician's point of view, a pain is not regarded as "chronic" until it has existed for more than half a year.

The sensory physiology of chronic pain is complicated by the fact that there is often no clear relation between the extent of organ damage and the intensity of the pain, especially when the pain has continued for a long time. In other words, in the course of time the experience of chronic pain frequently becomes detached from the original underlying disturbance. Because of this tendency to become "independent", *chronic pain appears as a separate, individual syndrome,* quite distinct from acute pain. In any case, from the medical viewpoint chronic pain cannot be said to serve any clear function, for in most cases it has lost all usefulness as a signal of impending or recent damage. Seen in this light, chronic pain is a "pointless" pain which should be eliminated or at least alleviated as far as possible.

In the extreme case — for example, severe recurrent headache — even the most thorough examination may fail to reveal any (still existing) physical disorder as a cause of the chronic pain. This then becomes a case of psychogenic pain (in our example a psychogenic headache). In general, the term "psychogenic pain" is not used to describe emotional states such as the grief one feels at the death of a relative or friend. Although psychogenic pains appear as the expression of psychological problems, they are experienced by the patient to be just like the pains that result from damage to the body. Accordingly, the patient cannot describe them in other than physical terms. In such cases it would be quite wrong to speak of imagined or simulated pains. For instance, back pains induced by psychological problems are felt by the patient to be just as real and severe as the back pains caused by deterioration of the vertebral joints.

Components of pain (Fig. 4–2). When a hand is immersed in water above 45 °C, nociceptors in the skin are excited. Their afferent impulses mediate information about the location of the heat stimulus, its onset, its intensity (which depends on the water temperature), and its end as soon as the hand is withdrawn from the water. This information is just as much a conscious sensation as the sensation of non-painful stimuli such as are encountered when the hand is immersed in lukewarm or cool water, which causes a sensation of warmth or coolness. We call this aspect of pain the *sensory, recognizing,* or — with regard to its interpretation in the context of experience and learning (see p. 5) — the *cognitive component* of the pain.

To stay with our example, when we dive into water at 25 °C on a hot summer day, we sense not only a cold stimulus to the skin but also a pleasant feeling of refreshment that is caused by the cooling. On a cold day in winter a bath at the same temperature would feel unpleasantly cool. That is, a sensory impression can give rise to pleasant or unpleasant feelings, depending on one's initial state and the circumstances. This is true of practically all sensations — for example, those originating in the eye, the ear, or the receptors for smell and taste. Pain is an exception. It always elicits affects or emotions with an unpleasant quality, it disturbs our well-being — in brief, the pain hurts, we suffer from it. This aspect of pain is called the emotional or *affective component.*

In cases of acute pain, feelings of *anxiety* are the most common consequences and the most important affective component, especially when we are not sure of the cause of the pain (e. g., acute abdominal pains) and we are afraid that the pain will grow stronger and stronger and finally unbearable, and that we might be seriously ill. In cases of chronic pain the anxiety gradually gives way to feelings of dejection, hopelessness and doubt that there is any point in continuing to live — that is, to *depression.* The pain experience and the depressive state seem to interact in such a way that each increases the severity of the other. However, people with chronic pain by no means always become depressives.

Immersion of the hand in hot water produces not only pain and aversion, but also causes dilation of the cutaneous vessels and hence increased blood flow, which

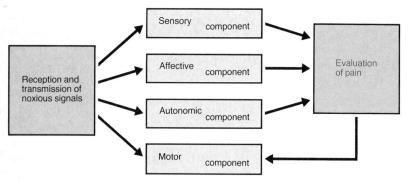

Fig. 4–2. Pain components and their role in the evaluation of pain. Extensive discussion in text

is evident in reddening of the skin. Conversely, immersion in ice water constricts the blood vessels in the skin, reducing blood flow. Both phenomena, as a rule, are accompanied by an increase in blood pressure and heart rate, dilation of the pupils, and respiratory changes. These reactions to the painful stimulus are brought about reflexly, by way of the autonomic nervous system; that is, they represent the *autonomic component* of pain. The autonomic component may be particularly well developed in cases of visceral pain. In biliary colic, for instance, it is manifest as nausea and vomiting, sudden sweating and a drop in blood pressure.

Finally, it is a familiar experience that when one's hand unintentionally makes contact with something hot, such as water or a stove, it is jerked back long before we become conscious of heat pain and could have reacted voluntarily. This *motor component* of the pain appears as an escape or protection reflex in many contexts. It is particularly important with regard to noxious stimuli of external origin. But even deep pains and visceral pains can be found to have motor components — for example, in the form of muscular tension. In a broader sense still other behavioral manifestations of pain, such as facial expressions, moaning or voluntary movements resulting from the evaluation of the pain (see below), can be regarded as motor components of the pain.

Usually all four components of pain appear together, although their magnitudes may vary. Because the central pathways they employ are in part very different, and because highly diverse parts of the nervous system (e. g., autonomic nervous system, motor system) participate in producing them, they are basically very loosely interrelated and it is entirely possible for them to *appear in isolation.* For example, a sleeping person may pull his hand away from a painful stimulus even though he has no conscious sensation of the pain, and chronically decerebrate animals can be observed to give motor and autonomic responses to pain just like those of intact animals, even though the possibility of their feeling pain is ruled out by the fact that they have no cerebrum.

The evaluation of pain. Pain is evaluated — that is, judged as mild, unpleasant, disturbing, violent or intolerable — on the basis of the sensory, affective and autonomic components to varying degrees, depending on the cause of the pain and on the circumstances (Fig. 4–2). For example, in cases of acute superficial pain the sensory component will often predominate, in acute visceral pain the autonomic component will play a major role, and in chronic pain the affective component often crucially influences the evaluation.

The evaluation of pain and the resulting expressions of pain (facial, vocal, demands for painkilling medicine, and so on) also involve a number of other factors that can be mentioned only briefly here. The degree to which a patient complains of pain depends greatly on his character and personality. The more extroverted a sick person is, the more willing he is to give expression to his pain; the more introverted he is, the less he will say about it. Family origins, upbringing, social position and surroundings and, in particular, ethnic origins also influence the manner and extent of expression of pain. A North American Indian being martyred at the stake behaves entirely differently with regard to the expression of pain than does a Southern Italian houswife with biliary colic — even if both are suffering pain at the same intensity. Furthermore, the circumstances in which a pain arises often decisively affect the evaluation. It is well known that soldiers wounded in action need far less treatment with painkillers than is required for comparable injuries in civilian life. Apparently the feeling that one is lucky to have survived the battle at all considerably reduces the perception of pain and causes it to be evaluated as less severe.

Finally, it should be pointed out that appropriate behavior and emotionally **normal responses to painful stimuli** are apparently to a large extent not innate but **must be learned** by the young organism at an early stage in its development. If such experiences are missed in early childhood, the responses are very hard to learn later. Young dogs prevented from encountering harmful stimuli for the first 8 months of their lives were found to be incapable of responding appropriately to pain, and subsequently learned to respond only slowly and incompletely. They would sniff repeatedly at open flames and allow needles to be stuck deep into their skin without showing anything more than local reflex twitches. Comparable observations have also been made of young rhesus monkeys.

Itch. Another modality of cutaneous sensation, about which we know too little, is at least related to pain and will therefore be mentioned here — itching. It may be that itch is a special form of pain sensation that appears in certain stimulus conditions. This interpretation is supported by the fact that a sequence of itch stimuli at high intensity leads to sensations of pain; moreover, an interruption of pain conduction in the anterolateral funiculus is accompanied by a loss of itch sensation, whereas a disturbance of the senses of pressure and touch (transmitted in the dorsal columns) leaves the itch sensation unaffected. It has also been shown that the skin is sensitive to itch only at discrete points, and that these **itch points** correspond to the pain points.

But other findings make it appear possible that itch is a sensation independent of pain, perhaps mediated by special receptors. For example, the sensation of itch can be elicited only at the outermost layers of the epidermis, whereas pain is produced in the deeper layers of the skin as well. It is also possible, using suitable techniques, to generate all degrees of itch without pain, and vice versa. Finally, it should be mentioned that a prerequisite for the occurrence of an itching sensation appears to be the liberation of a chemical substance, perhaps **histamine.** An intradermal histamine injection elicits severe itching, and in skin injuries that lead to itching histamine is set free in the skin.

Q 4.1.   Headaches are in the category of
   a) Superficial pain
   b) Deep pain
   c) Initial pain
   d) Visceral pain
   e) Delayed pain

Q 4.2.   In clinical practice pain is regarded as chronic if it has continued, either uninterrupted or recurrently, for longer than
   a) Two weeks
   b) Four weeks
   c) Three months
   d) Half a year
   e) One year

Q 4.3.   List the four components of pain.

Q 4.4.   What is the most important affective component of chronic back pain?

Q 4.5.   Which of the following substances that occur naturally in the body is thought to enhance the sensation of itching:
   a) Acetylcholine
   b) Bradykinin
   c) Histamine
   d) Noradrenalin
   e) Serotonin

4.2 Neurophysiology and Psychophysics of Pain

Experimental research on pain in humans and animals encounters many special problems not encountered in studies of other sensory modalities. These begin with the fact that one cannot specify unambiguously an adequate stimulus for pain. Moreover, because of the injurious nature of painful stimuli, the constancy of stimulus conditions usually demanded in experimental procedures cannot always be achieved. Comparisons of subjective sensations in humans with physiologic correlates measured in animals are also difficult. In both man and animals, experimental pain can obviously be induced only within relatively narrow limits. Finally, it must be kept in mind that the emotional and motivational components of pain are often more important to patient and physician than the physiologic aspects, with which we are chiefly concerned here. Nevertheless, in recent years (particularly in the past decade) much has been learned about the neurophysiology of nociception and the psychophysics of pain, and our understanding of these processes has considerably increased.

Nociceptors. In the course of the last century three main hypotheses have been proposed regarding the mechanism of peripheral coding of noxious stimuli. They are the intensity, pattern, and specificity theories; of these, only the last has received sufficient experimental support.

The intensity and pattern theories were formulated because the variety of noxious stimuli — that is, the absence of a single adequate stimulus — led to the assumption that there were no special nociceptors. Rather, it was thought, pain always occurred when the low-threshold mechanoreceptors and thermoreceptors were stimulated above a certain intensity. According to the **intensity theory,** nociceptive stimuli elicit volleys of impulses at particularly high frequencies in the low-threshold receptors; according to the **pattern theory** such stimuli produce special temporal patterns of impulses, differing from those discharged in response to noninjurious stimuli. In both proposals, the central nervous system would decode the altered afferent input as a sensation of pain. By contrast, the **specificity theory** postulates (as with the other sensory modalities) the existence of special nociceptors which respond only to high-intensity stimuli, giving rise directly to the pain sensation.

A first indication of the existence of special nociceptors was the finding shown in Figure 4–3 — that the skin contains distinctly more **pain points** than pressure points (the ratio is 9:1 in Fig. 4–3). Because the cold and warm points in the skin are even less dense than the pressure points, the ratio of pain points to thermal points is greater than 10:1. This finding alone made it most unlikely that nociception occurs by way of mechano- or thermoreceptors.

More recently, electrophysiologic methods have been used successfully to record, in both experimental animals and humans, from receptors which — as the specificity theory demands — respond not to low-intensity stimuli but only to those of tissue-damaging intensity. These, then, must be regarded as special **nociceptors. In the skin,** so far, purely mechanosensitive, purely thermosensitive, and mechano- plus thermosensitive nociceptors have been found. The latter, called **polymodal** nociceptors, apparently are considerably more common than the other two types in human skin.

Examples of the **responses of polymodal nociceptors** to warm stimuli are shown in Figure 4–4. The receptors do not respond to cold or warm stimuli below 41°C.

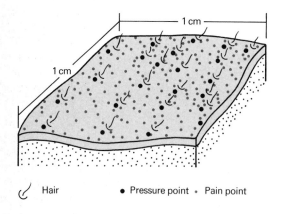

𝒸⟋ Hair   • Pressure point · Pain point

Inside of the forearm

Fig. 4–3. Pain and pressure points on the human skin. The location of the pain points was determined with von Frey bristles. Modified from STRUGHOLD: Z. Biol. **80,** 376 (1924)

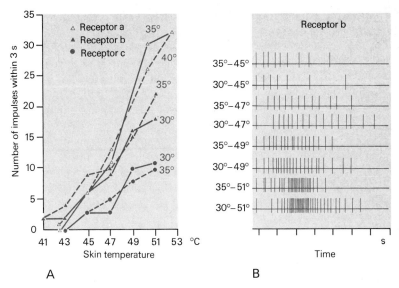

Fig. 4–4 A, B. Responses of polymodal nociceptors of the monkey's facial skin to heat stimuli. **A** Dependence of the discharge of three receptors upon the final temperature of heat stimuli within the associated receptive field. The ordinate indicates the number of impulses discharged within the 3 s following the first impulse after application of the stimulus. The starting temperatures for each of the six experiments are indicated at the **right** of the curves. **B** Discharge patterns of the receptor *b* in response to the indicated heat stimuli (starting temperatures 30 °C and 35 °C). Each row begins with the first impulse elicited by the stimulus. Modified from BEITEL, DUBNER: J. Neurophysiol. **39,** 1160 (1976)

But if the skin is warmed to about 45°C or more the receptors discharge, at a rate that clearly increases as the temperature rises. Because painful heat sensations occur at skin temperatures above 45°C (see p. 127), these receptors, like the purely thermosensitive nociceptors, can also be called *heat receptors.*

Histologically, the nociceptors in the skin (as well as those of the viscera and skeletal muscles, to be mentioned below) are *free nerve endings* with thin myelinated (group-III, conduction velocity ~ 11 m/s) or unmyelinated (group-IV, conduction velocity about 1 m/s) nerve fibers. By graded electrical stimulation of human cutaneous nerves it has been shown directly that excitation of the (low-threshold) thick myelinated afferents (group-II) does not give rise to sensations of pain, whereas excitation of the (high-threshold) group-III and group-IV afferents does cause pain. It appears that in the case of superficial pain the transmission of the initial pain (see p. 118) is via group-III fibers, while the delayed pain is signaled by group-IV fibers (C fibers). This view is supported by the following findings: a) When a nerve is blocked by mechanical pressure, activity disappears first in the thick fibers and later in the thin fibers. If only the group-II fibers are blocked, both qualities of superficial pain persist. But as soon as the blocking extends to the group-III fibers the initial pain vanishes, and only the delayed component is felt.

b) When the nerve is blocked with a local anesthetic (such as novocaine) to which group-IV fibers are more sensitive than those of group III, the reverse phenomenon is observed — the delayed pain disappears before the initial component. c) Electrical stimulation of exposed cutaneous nerves at intensities such that group-III fibers are excited produces sharp pain sensations. But if the myelinated fibers are blocked and a stimulus intensity appropriate to group IV is used, the result is a dull burning pain, subjectively very unpleasant; indeed, subjects describe it as difficult to endure. The time difference between the appearance of the initial and delayed pain appears to be caused primarily by the difference in conduction velocities of the fiber concerned.

Pain sensations can arise from all the internal organs. Mechanosensitive *visceral nociceptors* with group-IV afferent fibers are found in the smooth-muscled *hollow organs of the viscera.* Some of these receptors respond to passive stretch, and some to active contractions of the smooth musculature. When such contractions occur isometrically (i. e., with no change in length), as they do when the exit of contents from a hollow organ is obstructed, the visceral nociceptors are especially strongly excited. The most severe pains experienced occur under these conditions — for example, during obstruction of the bile duct or a ureter (disorders known as biliary or renal colic, respectively). A local deficiency of blood (ischemia) can also produce severe visceral pain; it is not known whether this is due to the associated mechanical effects or to the chemical changes in the tissues. The *lung,* too, contains numerous nociceptors, activated by irritant gases or dust particles; their group-III and group-IV afferents run centrally in the vagus nerve.

Pains in the skeletal musculature (which most have experienced in the form of acute cramp) are also mediated by nociceptors with free nerve endings and afferents of groups III and IV. Little is known of their physiology. Apparently they comprise purely mechanosensitive and purely chemosensitive nociceptors, as well as many polymodal endings. In heart muscle, nociceptors are especially responsive to local inadequacies in the blood supply; the resulting painful condition is termed *angina pectoris.* Here, too, it is not known which of the tissue alterations caused by the ischemia (e. g., abnormal contractions, oxygen deficiency, increased concentration of metabolic products) activates the cardiac nociceptors.

To conclude this discussion of the nociceptors in the diverse tissues of the body, it should be emphasized that by no means all free nerve endings are nociceptive. In the sections on mechanoreception and thermoreception it was pointed out that many receptive units with group-III (thin myelinated) and group-IV (unmyelinated) afferent fibers are specifically sensitive to mechanical or thermal stimuli at low intensity; probably all of these have free nerve endings as well. Thus free nerve endings can have different adequate stimuli. The absence of histologic differentiation does not at all imply an absence of *functional specificity.* Such specificity is probably associated with corresponding *molecular properties of the receptor membrane* which are inaccessible to the light and electron microscopes.

Central conduction and processing. Within the spinal cord, the nociceptive afferents end on neurons of the dorsal column. These nerve cells are the origin of the anterolateral funiculi, described in detail in the preceding chapter, which ascend to the brainstem and there join the nociceptive afferents (most of which come from the trigeminal nerve) from the head region on the way to the thalamus. For discussions of the operation of these ascending systems, their projections at further centripetal levels, and the involvement of the reticular formation, thalamus and cerebral cortex in the processing of nociceptive signals, see the corresponding sections in Chapter 3.

Here we shall only mention, in regard to the participation of the cerebral cortex in nociception and pain, that in the first half of this century clinical and experimental findings had led to the view that the cortex was not absolutely necessary for the production of conscious sensations of pain. The thalamus was regarded as the crucial center for conscious pain sensations. But careful observations, especially of people who suffered brain injury in the Second World War, have caused this view to be revised. Bullet wounds to certain areas of cortex deep in the central sulcus of the parietal cerebrum were found to produce contralateral insensitivity to pain, which proved to be permanent. In some cases only part of the contralateral half of the body was affected — an arm or leg, for instance — and in others the whole body half remained analgesic. These findings have since been corroborated by experiments in which local electrical stimulation of this part of the brain in humans elicited sensations of pain. It is now accepted that pain, like all the other conscious sensations — hearing, seeing, touch and so on — is impossible without the participation of the cerebral cortex.

Measurement of pain. A major problem encountered in psychophysical studies of pain is to find a reliable measure of the pain sensation. Measurement of the intensity of superficial pain has been attempted by various methods. One example was illustrated in Figure 1–7, where the intensity of the pain produced by electrical stimulation of the skin was quantified by an intermodal psychophysical comparison. The absolute threshold and the difference thresholds for dull superficial pain caused by pressure stimuli (mechanical pain) have also been measured. When such stimuli are applied to the forehead the threshold is about 600 g/cm^2, and about 15 discrimination steps can be detected up to the level of maximal sensation. Warmth stimuli — warm radiation in particular, which can be applied without simultaneous mechanical stimulation — have also been used extensively to measure pain thresholds. The first sensation of such *heat pain* appears at skin temperatures between 43° and 47°C, usually near 45°C. When skin temperature is raised further, as many as 21 intensity steps can be discriminated, until the maximal sensation of pain is reached. *Chemical stimuli* as a rule are not effective when applied directly to the skin. To test these experimentally a blister is first formed by application of an irritant. When the skin over the blister is then removed, its floor (formed by the stratum basale) is exposed and can be rinsed with test solutions. This procedure has attracted great interest, particularly because of the possibility that a "pain substance" might be found — a material common to all pains, liberated from the tissues by the noxious stimulus. So far such experiments have revealed a number of substances normally found in the body which, in the appropriate concentration, give rise to pain. Taken together, these findings are evidence *against the existence of a single pain substance.*

Deep pain, quantitatively graded, can be experimentally induced in the form of *ischemic muscle pain.* The blood supply to one arm is cut off by applying a tourniquet, after which the subject carries out rhythmic gripping movements of the hand (fist closure, etc.). Muscle pains soon appear and become more severe, the more frequently and powerfully the muscles are tensed. Ultimately the muscular work becomes impossible to continue because the *pain-tolerance limit* has been reached; the "tourniquet test" is stopped by removing the obstacle to blood flow. In cases of pathologically inadequate muscle perfusion, as in advanced arteriosclerosis, everyday muscular effort can produce comparable ischemic muscle pains which may, for example, cause a walking person to limp or come to a stop (intermittent claudication).

Adaptation to pain. In addition to the character and intensity of pain, a clinically important aspect is whether pain adapts. Subjective experience tends to indicate a

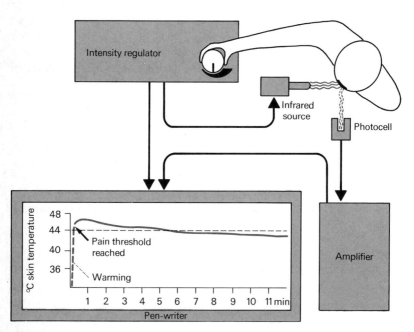

Fig. 4–5. Thermal pain thresholds can be studied with this arrangement. Infrared rays warm a blackened area on the skin of the forehead of the subject. The skin temperature is monitored by a radiation sensor and recorded on a pen-writer. Modified from HARDY: J. Appl. Physiol. *5,* 725 (1953). The *red curve* shows the dependence of the pain threshold (average values) on the duration of the heat stimulus. The subjects are required throughout the experiment to regulate the intensity of the radiation themselves, to a level such that the temperature of the forehead is just felt to be painful. The initial overshooting of skin temperature, beyond the pain threshold, is caused by the inertia of the equipment. Modified from GREENE, HARDY: J. Appl. Physiol. *17,* 693 (1962)

lack of adaptation; think, for example, of the hours-long persistence of headaches and toothaches. An experiment designed to measure adaptation of pain is illustrated in Figure 4–5; with this device, pain caused by thermal stimulation of the skin is measured. An adjustable source of radiation (an infrared lamp) irradiates the blackened skin of the subject's forehead. An infrared sensor (photocell) is used to measure the temperature of the skin, and both its output and the intensity of the radiation are recorded on a pen-writer. This procedure makes it possible to apply pain (heat) stimuli without simultaneous mechanical stimuli. In this situation, the question of adaptation to pain can be examined as follows: The subject is allowed to control the intensity of radiation himself, but with no information as to the setting of the intensity regulator. He is required to adjust the radiation intensity to a level such that it remains at the threshold for pain. The skin temperature is a measure of the pain threshold; that is, a progressive increase in skin temperature in this situation would imply an increasing threshold — or adaptation.

The average result of such measurements is shown in Figure 4–5 (lower left). After the pain threshold has been established in the first minute of the experiment, the skin temperature and thus the *pain threshold shows little change.* In fact, a slight decrease of skin temperature is detectable during the experiment, showing that the subjects needed less intense radiation to just sense pain. This finding implies that rather than adaptation there is a progressive *sensitization* of the stimulated area of skin. We can thus state that neither everyday experience nor the results of experiments on heat pain give any indication of the existence of adaptation to pain.

Q 4.6. Which of the following assertions is (are) correct?
On the skin, as a rule:
a) Pain points are more common than warm points
b) Warm points are more common than pressure points
c) Cold points are rarer than warm points
d) Pressure points are more common than pain points
e) There are no sensory points; the sensitivity is uniformly distributed over the skin

Q 4.7. The histologic substrate of the nociceptors consists as a rule of:
a) Pacinian corpuscles
b) Merkel's cells
c) Meissner corpuscles
d) Free nerve endings
e) Hair-follicle receptors

Q 4.8. Which of the following hypotheses about the peripheral mechanism of nociception accounts best for the known facts?
a) The intensity theory
b) The pattern theory
c) The specificity theory

Q 4.9.   The afferent nerve fibers subserving nociception belong to the fiber group(s):
a) Ia
b) Ib
c) II
d) III
e) IV

Q 4.10. The tourniquet test is a method for experimental pain research in which
a) the number of pain points per cm² of skin is determined
b) the time course of adaptation to the heat pain is measured
c) the pain threshold for visceral pain is found
d) sensitization of the nociceptors is achieved
e) ischemic muscle pain is produced.

4.3 Pathophysiology of Pain: Special and Abnormal Forms of Pain

The physiology of nociception, presented in the preceding section, will now be supplemented by certain particular aspects of clinical and psychologic importance. Projected and referred pain, for example, are special forms often observed; we shall also consider peripheral disturbances of pain reception and mention a few examples of disruption of the central processing of pain signals.

Projected pain. A sharp blow to the ulnar nerve, which passes superficially over the elbow, produces unpleasant sensations, difficult to describe (tingling, tickling, and the like — giving rise to the expression "to hit one's funny bone"), in the areas supplied by this nerve, the ulnar parts of the lower arm and hand. Evidently the activity elicited in the afferent nerve fibers at the elbow is *projected* by the CNS (that is, by our consciousness) into the regions served by these afferent fibers. We have learned that normally such sensory impulses come from the receptors in this region. We find it difficult to interpret the resulting sensations (tingling and so on), because the pattern of impulses produced by direct mechanical stimulation of the nerve is not ordinarily encountered. Similar atypical sensations occur when, for experimental or therapeutic reasons, skin nerves are stimulated via electrodes applied externally or introduced into the nerve. In such cases, intensity and nature of the sensation depend on stimulus conditions (cf. p. 126).

In principle, projected sensations can occur within all sensory modalities. In the ulnar-nerve example of projected pain the effects were transitory, but much projected pain is clinically important. The way it arises is diagrammed in Figure 4–6. Abnormal stimulation of the afferent fibers is transmitted, as usual, to the brain way of the lateral spinothalamic tract (see p. 91); there it gives rise to a *sensation in the area supplied by the afferent fibers.* A common cause is compression of the spinal nerves at their points of entry into the cord, resulting from damage to the intervertebral disk (the well-known "slipped disk"). The

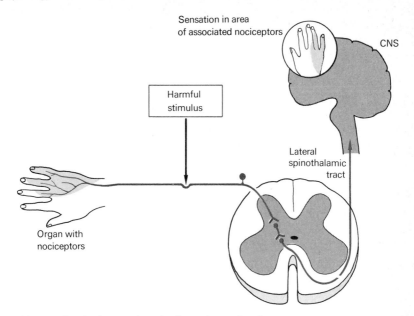

Fig. 4–6. Diagram showing how projected pain can be produced

centripetal impulses thus produced abnormally in nociceptive fibers generate pain sensations which are projected into the area supplied by the stimulated spinal nerve. (There may, of course, also be pain at the site of the slipped disk.) Projected pain is distinguished from referred pain (see below) in that it is caused by direct stimulation of nerve fibers, rather than the receptive endings.

Neuralgia. When a noxious stimulus (e.g., tension, pressure, crushing) acts on a nerve for a long time, the eventual result is "spontaneous" pains that occur in waves or sudden attacks. As would be expected from the above considerations, these *neuralgic pains* are restricted to the region supplied by the affected nerves or nerve root (segment). In a manner of speaking, then, the projected pain just described is the "acute model" of neuralgia. Typical examples of neuralgic pain are the leg pains in the region supplied by the ischiatic nerve that occur in association with the slipped-disk syndrome (ischialgia), and attacks of facial pain in the region supplied by the trigeminal nerve (trigeminal neuralgia). Similarly, some time after infection of a nerve with the herpes zoster virus (shingles) very severe neuralgic pains may appear. Neither for this disease nor for the other neuralgias is it known which particular pathophysiological mechanisms cause excitation of the nociceptive afferents and their central neurons.

Causalgia. Occasionally nerve injuries, especially bullet wounds, can give rise to a special form of neuralgia, the cause of which is unknown. Agonizing pain is produced in the area supplied by the damaged nerve, with simultaneous trophic and circulatory disturbances in the affected region. This syndrome is called causalgia. The circulatory and trophic effects indicate involvement of the sympathetic nervous system.

Referred pain. Nociceptive signals from the viscera are often felt not only (or not at all) at the internal organ itself but also at distant superficial sites. Such pain is called referred pain. The referral is always to parts of the periphery supplied by the same segment of the spinal cord as the affected internal organ — that is, with respect to the skin surface, the *pain is referred within the associated dermatome* (see p. 76). A well-known example is that of pain originating at the heart but appearing to come from the chest and a narrow strip along the inside of the arm. Because the relationship between dermatomes and internal organs is known, such referred pain is an important aid to diagnosis.

The *production of referred pain* probably occurs as illustrated in Figure 4–7, left. Some of the nociceptive afferents from the skin and the internal organs which enter a given spinal segment are connected with the same dorsal horn neurons. Excitation of such cells is interpreted as pain at the periphery, because this interpretation is usually appropriate in the body's experience.

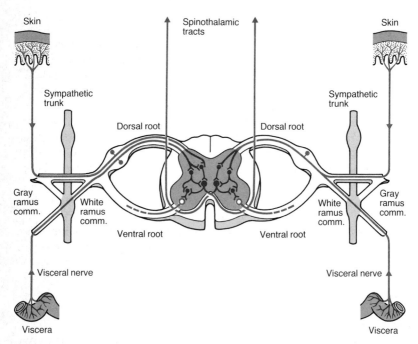

Fig. 4–7. Pathways by which referred pain is produced. The left part shows that some of the nociceptive afferents from the viscera end on the same dorsal-horn neurons as do nociceptive afferents from the skin. On the right, a single nociceptive afferent can in some cases innervate both superficial and deep tissue

Recently it has been shown that in rats, cats and monkeys there are certain afferent nerve fibers in the dorsal roots that have peripheral arborizations in both the skin and deeper tissues (Fig. 4–7, right). If such nerve fibers also exist in humans, they will presumably be involved in the production of referred pain, because they would be excited both by skin stimulation and by stimulation of the deep tissue.

In the case of a diseased internal organ, there is a further consequence of the convergence of nociceptive afferents from the dermatome and the associated internal organ upon neurons in the nociceptive pathway; this is a *hypersensitivity of the skin* (hyperpathia) in the associated dermatome. The reason is that the excitability of interneurons is raised by the visceral impulses, so that a given nociceptive stimulus to the skin causes greater central activity than in the normal condition. This form of enhancement of excitability is called "facilitation".

Other interactions between the somatic and autonomic nervous systems. There appear to be still other interactions between the somatic and autonomic systems, apart from referred pain, which we do not yet entirely understand. An example is the therapeutic effect of heat application to the skin, in certain cases of internal illness. The warmth does not act directly on the internal organ (the blood serves as a coolant to prevent warming of the deep tissues), but probably has a reflex effect by way of the warm receptors in the skin (see p. 58).

Stimulation of visceral nociceptors often produces an increase in muscle tension (or tone), and in extreme cases can lead to *reflex spasms of the muscle.* The visceral afferents can thus also excite motoneurons (via polysynaptic arcs). These reflexes involve not only motoneurons of the same segment, but also those of other, functionally related muscles. Under conditions of pain in the abdominal cavity (e. g., appendicitis) the abdominal muscles are tense. At the same time, the patients often lie with knees drawn up, partly because the flexor muscles of the thighs are excited by the same afferents, and partly to reduce the tension in the abdominal muscles, for such a marked, prolonged increase in muscle tonus produces *muscle pain* and *tenderness* of the muscle. Pains of this kind are found not only in cases of organic illness, about which they can provide important evidence, but also during psychological stress. A typical example is headache, with painful tension of the dorsal neck musculature, which disappears once the source of psychological stress is resolved or when the patient is given appropriate psychotherapy. The mechanism by which such pain arises in the muscles is unknown. High muscle tone reduces blood flow through the muscle, which probably plays a role in the production of pain (perhaps via the accumulation in the tissue of metabolic products with nociceptive effects).

Peripheral disturbances of nociception. A few hours after the skin has been damaged by intense ultraviolet radiation, "sunburn" appears; the skin is reddened and the sensitivity to mechanical stimuli is increased. These phenomena are also observed after damage to the skin by heat, freezing, X rays, or abrasion. This hypersensitivity is called *hyperalgesia.* The pain threshold is lowered, and even ordinarily painless stimuli (such as the friction of clothing) are perceived as unpleasant or painful. Hyperalgesia and reddening (the latter caused by expansion of the local blood vessels, or vasodilation) can last for days. Hyperalgesia, reddening, swelling and often spontaneous pain (with no touching or movement) are also among the basic symptoms of inflammation of deep tissue, such as joint inflammation. In these cases, as in skin inflammation, it is plausible that hyperalgesia, spontaneous pains and vasodilation are caused by the local release of chemical substances from damaged cells in the tissue. According to the evidence so far available, the chief candidates are various prostaglandins, bradykinin, serotonin, histamine, potassium ions and hydrogen ions (acidification of the tissue). These substances are called *algesic substances* ("painful substances") because of their sensitizing and excitatory actions on nociceptors.

The opposite of hyperalgesia — that is, an increase in the pain threshold — is called *hypalgesia,* and a complete loss of pain sensitivity is called *analgesia.* Both usually occur only in combination with disturbances or deficits in other sensory modalities. For example, in the simplest case transection or blockage (e. g., with Novocain) of a skin nerve causes analgesia of the region it supplies but also eliminates all the other modalities of sensation in the skin; that is, it causes complete *local anesthesia.*

Occasionally humans are found to be *completely insensitive to pain at birth.* In some of these cases a clear defect in the nervous system can be demonstrated, and in others either the nociceptive afferents in the peripheral nerves or the first higher-order neurons in one of the ascending tracts of the spinal cord (Lissauer's tract) are absent. Although the congenital pain insensitivity can result from either peripheral or central disturbances of nociception, the symptoms in all cases are the same: the patients do not perceive injurious stimuli as such. Typically, therefore, from earliest childhood they are constantly being seriously hurt or hurting themselves. As a rule, these mutilations result in an early death.

When nerves are cut — for example, when a limb is amputated — outgrowths at the ends of the nerve fibers often form more or less thick knots of fibers, called neuromas. Frequently the neuromas are painful, spontaneously and in response to pressure, because the fine fibrous outgrowths are both spontaneously active and highly sensitive to touch. *Neuroma pains* are thus a special case of neuralgic pain (cf. p. 131).

But it may also happen that after an amputation very severe pains develop that seem to come from the amputated limb. With these *phantom pains* the patient almost always feels that his phantom limb is in a cramped, stiff position. Unlike neuroma pains, phantom pains are often essentially uninfluenced by sensory inputs from the stump. That is, they amount to chronic pains that have become "independent" by way of some unknown changes in the central processing of pain.

Disturbances of central pain processing. We have now encountered three examples of pains produced not only by changes in peripheral nerves but probably also by changes in central nervous structures involved in the origin of pain. These are phantom pain (see above), herpes zoster neuralgia (p. 131) and causalgia (p. 131), though the central involvement was not mentioned explicitly in the last two cases. There are also pains in which disturbances of central pain processing predominate, so that these can be regarded as *central pains* in the strict sense. For example, when accidents have torn the dorsal roots in the cervical and upper thoracic levels of the spinal cord, a common result is agonizing pain in the arm that receives its sensory innervation from these dorsal roots, even though the arm is entirely without sensation. This paradoxical condition, reminiscent of phantom pain, is called *anesthesia dolorosa.* It appears that when the dorsal roots are torn out the nociceptive neurons in the spinal cord become hyperexcitable and discharge continually at a higher rate, with sporadic bursts at especially high frequencies.

Disturbances in structures of the nociceptive system at a more central level tend less to cause deficits than to alter the pain sensation, because normal experience of pain is possible only with simultaneous, undisturbed activation of the cortical and subcortical central components of the system (see p. 127). For example, in disorders of the parts of the thalamus involved in pain processing, nociceptive stimuli cause especially unpleasant pain sensations, which subjectively give the impression of oversensitivity to pain (hyperpathia). Moreover, the patients often experience spontaneous, almost unbearable pain in the associated (i.e., contralateral) half of the body, which is difficult to treat *(thalamus pain).*

One's affective attitude to pain can also be changed by central damage. For instance, patients with severe frontal-lobe injury in many cases hardly notice their pains as long as they are distracted and kept occupied. The pain thresholds, however, are entirely unchanged. In *pain asymbolia,* which usually occurs with simultaneous defects in frontal lobe, insula and parietal lobe, the affective evaluation of and motor reactions to nociceptive stimuli are so greatly diminished that the patients repeatedly expose themselves to the same injurious stimuli and often mutilate themselves. This situation is reminiscent of congenital pain insensitivity (p. 134), though here it is more a matter of *indifference to pain* — probably because the brain areas responsible for the pain experience have become less active or inaccessible to the normal inputs.

Q 4.11. In many cases of female breast cancer pressure on the brachial plexus in the region of the armpit produces severe pain in the area innervated by these nerves. This symptom is an example of
a) Projected pain
b) Analgesia
c) Sympathetic-trunk irradiation
d) Referred pain
e) Spreading pain

Q 4.12. Chronic tension or pressure on a dorsal root in the spinal cord (disk malformation) can cause tormenting pain in the region it supplies. These pains are in the category of
a) Hyperpathic pain
b) Neuralgic pain

     c) Psychogenic pain
     d) Referred pain
     e) Central pain

Q 4.13. In disease of the renal pelvis or the ducts through which urine leaves it the patient often reports, in addition to other symptoms, pain in the groin (testicles, vulva). This symptom is an example of
     a) Hypalgesia
     b) Referred pain
     c) Projected pain
     d) Initial pain
     e) Delayed pain

Q 4.14. In cases of sunburn, vasodilation (reddening) is accompanied by
     a) Analgesia
     b) Lumbar anesthesia
     c) Hypalgesia
     d) Local anesthesia
     e) Hyperalgesia

Q 4.15. Which of the following pain syndromes is due chiefly to a disturbance in peripheral nociception (I), and which to disturbed central processing of pain (II)?
     a) Anesthesia dolorosa
     b) Inflammation pain
     c) Hyperalgesia in sunburn
     d) Ischialgia
     e) Neuroma pain
     f) Pain asymbolia

4.4 Factors that Affect Pain; Pain Therapy

Although here we are chiefly concerned with the sensory physiology of pain, we cannot ignore the fact that for the person suffering pain the unpleasant affective and autonomic components usually dominate the pain experience to such an extent that there is a strong incentive to eliminate the pain — either by one's own efforts or by consultation with a physician. The first hope is that whatever is causing the pain can be eliminated, in which case presumably the pain will also disappear. But in many cases, especially when there is chronic pain, this approach to treatment is not successful — at least, not immediately. Then the physician must treat the pain itself by choosing one or more of the large arsenal of available methods, depending on the nature of the pain.

    A survey of the most fundamental procedures for pain treatment is given in Figure 4–8. The pharmacological procedures (1 to 4) serve either to prevent the

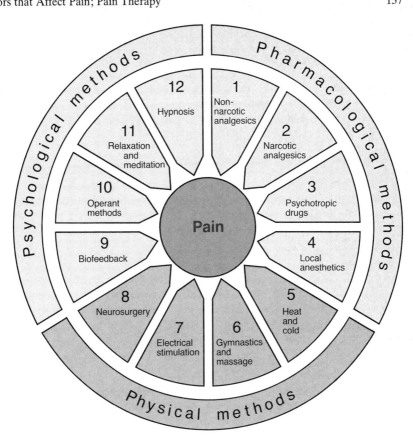

Fig. 4–8. Spectrum of the main pharmacological, physical and psychological methods for the treatment of pain. Extensive discussion in text

reception (1) and conduction (4) of noxious signals or to inhibit central processing (2) and diminish affective participation in the pain event (2,3). The physical procedures (5 to 8) act against pain by extremely diverse routes and at quite different sites. A third category includes the psychological procedures (9 to 12), which in general can be described as strategies for "coming to terms" with the pain. In the following the manner in which treatments in these three categories act will be considered briefly, in the same order as in Figure 4–8. As elsewhere in this book, the somatic aspects — the methods employing medication and physical treatment — will receive most attention.

Pharmacological treatment of pain. Under the rubric ***non-narcotic analgesics,*** or weak analgesics, are a number of substances and their derivatives that reduce pain without appreciably restricting, changing or abolishing (narcosis) consciousness. The best-known group of these analgesics are derivatives of salicylic acid, and by far the most commonly used of these is ***acetylsalicylic acid*** (aspirin, also sold under various other trade names); indeed, aspirin is taken more often than any other analgesic in the world. In addition to inhibiting pain, acetylsalicylic acid and the other salicylates have anti-inflammatory and antipyretic (fever-reducing) actions. Therefore they are particularly useful medications for pain associated with fever and inflammation, such as rheumatic pains.

Other *analgesic acids,* apart from the salicylates, include indomethacin, naproxen, piroxicam and so on; these also have anti-inflammatory and antipyretic in addition to analgesic properties. All of them exert their analgesic and anti-inflammatory effects mainly at the periphery, in the inflamed, painful tissues. The molecular mechanism of action is thought to be inhibition of prostaglandin formation. The prostaglandins are products of the breakdown of unsaturated fatty acids from cell membranes, which build up to especially high concentrations in inflamed tissue and are a major cause of the symptoms of inflammation and pain. But it is not yet clear whether the pain-inhibiting action of analgesic acids is based entirely on inhibition of prostaglandin formation or whether other, unknown effects may also be involved.

The *narcotic analgesics* (2 in Fig. 4–8), or strong analgesics, comprise a large number of substances that are capable of alleviating even the most severe pain but as a side effect have such a strong sedating, even somniferous action that at high concentrations they can induce a narcotic state. All these substances have an "ancestor" which even today is used as a standard for comparison; this is *morphine,* at one time also called morphia or morphium. Morphine is the principal active constituent of opium, which was used as an analgesic even in antiquity. It was not until the beginning of the 19th Century that opium was refined to give pure morphine. It is because of these relationships that substances with actions comparable to that of morphine are called *opiates* or *opioids.*

Morphine and the other opiates reduce the activity of those structures in the brain that are involved in receiving and, in particular, in processing nociceptive signals. Their chief action in humans is on the limbic system, which is responsible for the forms of behavior with emotional overtones that are characteristic of the species. The limbic system is also the site of the neural events underlying our affective participation in pain — our perception of its unpleasantness. In view of this central target site of the opiates, in the limbic system, it is understandable that patients given opium report not only that the pain is less severe (inhibition of the sensory components) but also that they are less troubled by the remaining pain (emotional indifference to the pain event).

The standard dose of morphine, which normally is effective in reducing pain, is 10 mg; this is so little that for decades it seemed puzzling that such clear effects on the body could result. The explantation is that morphine and the other opiates act in the same way as substances produced by the body itself. These substances, which inhibit pain just as morphine does, are called endorphins because of their endogenous (within the body) production. The category includes several polypeptides — *beta-endorphin,* the *enkephalins,* and *dynorphin.* They all share the property of binding to special receptor molecules embedded in the cell membranes of neurons in the nociceptive and pain-processing systems, so as to inhibit temporarily the activity of the neurons. The more receptor molecules are occupied in this way, the stronger is the inhibition of the individual nerve cell and the whole complex of neurons to which it belongs. This inhibition is the basis of the analgesic action of all opioids, whether endogenous or introduced to the body from outside. (The physiological role of the endorphins is not yet well understood. It may be that an "endorphinergic basal tone" is involved in setting the sensitivity level of the pain system.)

Many mixed preparations to treat pain contain substances such as barbiturates or caffeine. These substances do not directly inhibit pain, but are intended to potentiate the actual analgesic by their sedating (barbiturates) or stimulating (caffeine) action — in a sense, to produce a favorable climate for the analgesic. That is, they are used to influence the mental state of the patient, as (weak) *psychotropic drugs* (3 in Fig. 4–8).

Of the medications regarded as psychotropic in the strict sense, because of their strong effects on mental state, two groups play a special role in pain therapy, the *tranquilizers* and the *antidepressants.* In the former group, the benzodiazepines in particular have many applications in addition to the management of pain; they are used to abolish or alleviate anxiety, tension and agitation. Of the benzodiazepines, diazepam is the best known and, under the name Valium, currently the most frequently prescribed. The antidepressants are used primarily to treat endogenous depression. Because such depressives often complain of pain, and because, conversely, chronic pain often leads to a depressive state, in these cases antidepressants can be used with considerable hope of success. Some antidepressants actually seem to have a direct analgesic action, in addition to elevating the mood.

Local anesthesia (4 in Fig. 4–8) of body tissues can be achieved either by surrounding the associated nerve with a local anesthetic (*nerve blocking* by a dentist, for example, in the region of a jaw-nerve branch) or by injecting the local anesthetic at many places in the tissue itself, where it diffuses and transiently inhibits all the receptors *(infiltration anesthesia).* On mucous membranes, but not on the skin (which repels water), a local anesthetic can be applied *topically* by spraying or brushing it onto the surface. On the other hand, when a small area of skin is to be anesthetized briefly, one can spray it with ethyl chloride. This is a volatile substance, which extracts heat from the skin so rapidly as it evaporates that the receptors are inactivated by the cold. Examples of local anesthetics include procaine, lidocaine and mepivacaine. All of these are synthetic compounds related to the only naturally occurring local anesthetic, cocaine.

In the treatment of pain in a well-defined region, nerve block can bring considerable relief temporarily (for some hours, as a rule). It is a disadvantage that not only the pain but all sensations from the region supplied by the nerve are abolished. Furthermore, if motor fibers in the nerve are blocked, the associated muscle is paralyzed. The autonomic nerve fibers to the blood vessels are also blocked, which eliminates most of the regulation of blood flow in the affected region. In rare cases pain is relieved for longer than would be expected from the duration of action of the local anesthetic on the nerve, perhaps because the nerve block has opened reflex circuits that were reinforcing the pain-producing process (for instance, by way of muscle tension). Local anesthesia can also be used not only to alleviate pain temporarily but in the hope of positively influencing the disease process itself, in which case it is called *therapeutic local anesthesia.*

Physical treatment of pain. The physical measures taken to relieve pain (5 to 8 in Fig. 4–8) rely on several quite different actions, ranging from the simple application of cold or heat through massage and gymnastics to electrical stimulation and neurosurgery. These methods, except for the last, have been used to combat pain for centuries and in some cases millennia. A very ancient physical treatment is also the simplest, *rest and immobilization;* it is often extremely effective in relieving joint pain and the pains associated with bone fractures and muscle cramps.

Heat is probably the physical treatment in most frequent use. It has three basic actions. First, it produces a feeling of comfort, which in turn leads to relaxation. Second, it dilates the blood vessels, and the resulting increase in blood flow washes pain-inducing substances away more rapidly. And third, stimulation of the warm receptors in the skin sends a stream of afferent impulses into the spinal cord and brain, which apparently inhibits the incoming nerve impulses from the nociceptors. In any case, the sensory signal "warmth" somehow obscures, to a greater or lesser extent, the nociceptive signals. Locally applied heat warms only the superficial layers of the skin. Nevertheless, circulation of the blood through deeper organs can be increased reflexly. It is also possible to heat deeper tissues directly by diathermy (high-frequency electromagnetic irradiation). Heat application is most effective on pains caused or exacerbated by insufficient blood flow.

On the other hand, some pains (e. g., those resulting from acute inflammation or the headache of a hangover) are associated with dilation of the vessels. This can be counteracted by application of *cold.* The excitability of nociceptors is also reduced by cold, or entirely suppressed (consider, for example, the analgesic effect of cold water on burns and scalds). Finally, immediate application of cold to burns, bruises and other injuries can slow the development of inflammation by temporarily reducing both blood flow and the local rate of metabolism.

Therapeutic exercises are widely used to promote healing of joints, muscles, tendons, ligaments and bones, to repair damage resulting from defective posture or movement, and to prevent the ill effects of insufficient movement — not only in muscles and bones, but also in the cardiovascular and respiratory systems. Therefore the contribution of therapeutic exercise to the alleviation of pain is usually indirect. The same is true of the various forms of massage. Classical *muscle massage* loosens cramped muscles and improves blood flow through them. These effects can reduce or eliminate the pain of muscle cramp. *Connective-tissue massage* is done for another purpose; here the skin and the underlying tissue layers ("connective tissue") are manipulated with pressing and shearing movements so as to stimulate the local receptors, which then reflexly affect the function of internal organs.

Electrical stimulation for the treatment of pain (7 in Fig. 4–8) was used even in antiquity; in pre-Christian Greece shocks from electric fish were applied to relieve chronic pain. Like this old method, the more recent stimulation procedures take advantage of the observation that pains are often distinctly reduced by other, simultanous sensations produced by stimuli such as rubbing, scratching, heat and cold (see above). In all these cases of "masking" or "counterirritation", the stream of nerve impulses from the nociceptors continues as before, but is no longer able to reach the brain structures necessary for a conscious sensation of pain. Somewhere on the way the nociceptive impulses are inhibited. The inhibition may occur in the spinal cord, but it can also be brought about at higher levels, perhaps in the brainstem or thalamus. Although we do not yet fully understand the mechanism of this *afferent inhibition,* the efforts being made to find ways of activating the inhibitory processes as a means of relieving pain are quite justified.

The electrical current is usually applied through the skin. In this *transcutaneous electrical nerve stimulation (TENS),* pulses (duration 0.5 ms, repeated at 40–100 per second) are presented at an intensity such as to produce sensations like vibration and tingling, and even slight contractions of the muscles below the two knoblike electrodes, but no pain. A variant of this method is *dorsal-column stimulation,* for which the electrodes are surgically implanted in the vertebral canal. The intention is to achieve especially intense stimulation of the afferent fiber bundles in the dorsal column of the spinal cord and hence especially strong afferent inhibition. However, the long-term results with this method have, on the whole, been disappointing. A third approach is to attempt direct activation of the afferent inhibitory centers in the brain, and especially in the brainstem, by implanted electrodes. This *electrical brain stimulation* is the most precise application so far devised of a phenomenon known for some time in animal experiments: "stimulation-produced analgesia" (SPA), a state resembling narcosis which can be brought about by electrical stimulation of the brainstem, particularly in the places at which the action of opiates is exerted. It is therefore conceivable that the analgesic effects of SPA and of electrical nerve and brain stimulation are mediated by the same neuronal systems that are influenced by the opiates and endorphins.

All the *neurosurgical procedures for pain relief* (8 in Fig. 4–8) are used only as a last resort, because of their serious disadvantages. For example, when a cutaneous nerve is transected, the skin it supplies becomes insensitive to all stimuli (anesthetized). It is therefore very vulnerable to damage and injury of all kinds. Moreover, the innervation of the blood vessels and sweat glands is eliminated, so that skin nutrition is impaired. Transection of a muscle nerve has the additional disadvantage that the associated muscles are permanently paralyzed. All nerve transections present the risk that neuromas will develop, and these can become a new source of pain (see p. 134). Some of these disadvantages can be avoided by cutting dorsal roots at the spinal cord, because these contain only afferent fibers, but complete anesthesia of the affected part of the body cannot be avoided. In addition, the operation is often followed by the development of unpleasant sensations reminiscent of anesthesia dolorosa (see p. 135). Transection of the ascending nociceptive tracts in the anterolateral funiculus of the spinal cord (chordotomy; cf. 91) can be quite successful in the short to medium term (weeks to months). This operation is therefore most suitable for seriously ill patients who are not expected to live more than a few months. Surgery within the brain itself — for example, in the thalamus (thalamotomy), in the cingulate gyrus of the limbic system (cingulotomy) or in the white matter containing connections to the frontal lobe (leukotomy) — appeared highly promising when it was first attempted. The results, however, have been entirely unsatisfactory, and this approach is now hardly ever considered.

Psychological methods of pain management. When pain exists mainly or entirely on the subjective level (psychogenic pain, p. 119), psychological treatment would probably be chosen as a matter of course. But there are many situations in which pains associated with organic disorders respond better to psychological than to somatic treatment — for example, when previous pharmacological and physical therapy did not make a long-lasting improvement, or when the affective component of the pain strongly predominates. In all conditions of chronic pain, supplementary psychological therapy is useful; it will take a form dependent on the patient and the nature of the complaint. Important examples of such therapeutic procedures are given in Figure 4–8 under 9 to 12. All these methods have been used with impressive success, although it is not yet possible to predict with the desired reliability which patient should be treated with which method.

Q 4.16. What is the mechanism to which the action of acetylsalicylic acid and other non-narcotic analgesics is ascribed?
a) Inhibition of prostaglandin synthesis
b) Inhibition of transduction and transformation in nociceptors
c) Inhibition of conduction in afferent nerve fibers
d) Inhibition of the nociceptive dorsal-horn neurons
e) Inhibition of thalamic neurons in the pain-processing system

Q 4.17. Which of the structures listed below is regarded as the main target site of opiates?
a) Cerebellum
b) Limbic system
c) Nociceptors
d) Primary sensory cerebral cortex
e) Anterior funiculi of the spinal cord

Q 4.18. Which statement is false? In a conduction (nerve) block with a local anesthetic
a) all sensations in the affected area are abolished.
b) the nervous supply to the blood vessels in the affected area is also eliminated.
c) in the case of a muscle nerve, the muscle is paralyzed.
d) the nociceptive afferents (groups III and IV) are blocked selectively.
e) the effect usually persists for only a few hours.

Q 4.19. The main form of electrical stimulation currently used in pain therapy to produce afferent inhibition ("masking", "counterirritation") is
a) electric shocks from electric fish.
b) transcutaneous electrical nerve stimulation.
c) diathermy.
d) electrical brain stimulation by implanted electrodes.
e) dorsal-column stimulation in the cervical region of the spinal cord.

5 Physiology of Vision

O.-J. Grüsser and U. Grüsser-Cornehls

In our environment we see a large number of three-dimensional objects. These can be described as moving or stationary, or having a particular spatial arrangement. They may differ in **brightness, color, size, shape** or **movement.** Visually perceived objects can have special **significance** to us or they may be irrelevant; they can make an emotional impression or elicit no subjective response at all. Physiologists have become accustomed to saying that visual perception occurs **because** an image of the environment is cast onto the retina. This image gives rise to certain signal-detection and processing events in the receptors and the higher-order nerve cells, which eventually — at the level of "consciousness" — result in perception (cf. p. 5). But everyone is aware from his dreams that visual perception can occur in the absence of retinal images. On the other hand, it is a common experience that when "daydreaming" one does not see much, even with eyes open. In seeing, as in any form of perception, the direction of attention (i.e., a central nervous selection process) plays an important role.

In this chapter we shall intentionally limit ourselves to the "simple" mechanisms of vision, those that can be explained in terms of present-day physiologic knowledge. More complicated phenomena such as form perception, space perception, and the visual processing of symbols, letters, and words will not be discussed in detail. Nor shall we consider the everyday experience that each perception is associated with an "expectation" on the part of the perceiver, which is to some

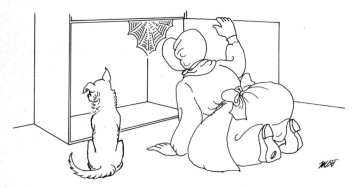

Fig. 5–1. "Old Mother Hubbard went to the cubpoard to get her poor dog a bone ..." (Did you spot the misspelled word?)

extent dependent on emotional state. Look at Figure 5–1 to demonstrate the effect of expectation on what is perceived.

As an introduction to visual physiology, here are a few simple observations you can make yourself. Cover your left eye with your hand, *fixate* an object with the right eye, and notice what you can see in your surroundings while fixating. You will find that only part of your environment is included in the *monocular field of view* of your right eye. When you then fixate the object with both eyes (binocularly), there is not only an improvement in your perception of spatial depth, but you also see a larger part of your environment. The *binocular field* of view, for obvious reasons, is larger than the monocular field. The binocular field consists of the central *overlap area* (the area seen by both eyes) and two regions at the sides, each of which is seen by only one eye. Figure 5–2 shows the schematized result of measurement of the *limits of the visual fields,* made with the perimeter apparatus ophthalmologists use for diagnosis.

Fixate some object again, and now try to decide how *distinctly* you can see the other objects in the binocular visual field. You will notice that the further away an object is from the fixation point, the less distinct it is. The distinctness of visual perception is correlated directly with a quantitatively measurable value, the *visual acuity* (see p. 158). The place being fixated is the part of the visual field for which your acuity is greatest, when viewing normally in daylight. If you want to see clearly an object in a part of the visual field not being fixated, you normally shift your direction of gaze toward that object, which moves the previously fixated object into the periphery of the visual field.

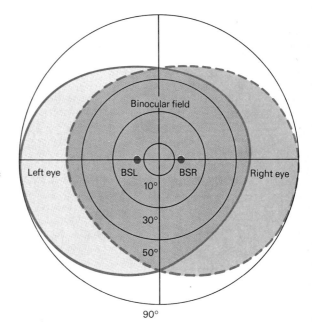

Fig. 5–2. Visual fields of the left *(continous outline)* and right *(dashed outline)* eye. The binocular overlap area, where the two are superimposed, is *dark red. BSL,* blind spot for the field of view of the left eye; *BSR,* that for the right eye. The *circles* demarcate angles of 10°, 30°, 50°, and 90° from the fixation point

The eyes can deviate at most about 60° to either side of their central position, and 40° up or down. Therefore when the head is not moved but the eyes are, the total visible field is greater than the visual field of the stationary eye in Figure 5–2 by 120° in the horizontal direction and 80° in the vertical direction. Obviously, though, one can view one's entire surroundings by moving the head and/or the body. When one looks around in this way, the movements of body, head and eyes are coordinated by central nervous mechanisms.

But *eye movements* have importance beyond their function of shifting the direction of gaze. The displacement of the image on the retina that occurs when the eyes move is actually essential for normal visual perception. If a suitable optical system is used to "stabilize" a stimulus pattern within the visual field, so that it is not displaced at all over the retina even when the eyes move, the contours and colors of the stimulus pattern fade and disappear within a few seconds. (Very small movements, hard to suppress even during steady fixation, serve to prevent this fading, so it is hard to demonstrate without special apparatus). It is evident that in visual perception, as in some of the other modalities, the sense organs and the associated central perception systems are not simply passive "receivers"; rather, *active motor components* play an important role in perception. We may say that we "see" passively, but we also "look", "scan", "view" — all words that emphasize the active component in vision. Even in the state of apparently passive seeing we "sample" our visual environment by voluntary and involuntary eye movements; the *amplitudes and directions* of these depend not only upon the internal state of the CNS (attentiveness, interest) but also on the visual stimulus patterns.

For simplicity the sensory and motor aspects of the visual apparatus will be introduced separately. Section 5.1 is concerned with the optical system of the eye, the formation of images on the retina and retinal structure. In Section 5.2 elementary observations and some "laws" in the area of visual psychophysics are described, and the underlying neurophysiologic events and some theoretical consequences are discussed in Section 5.3. Section 5.4 deals with the physiologic basis of oculomotor performance and the coordination of the sensory and motor components of vision.

5.1 The Eye

When you look at your eyes in a mirror you see the *conjunctiva,* white connective tissue infiltrated by small blood vessels, which at the anterior pole of the eyeball merges with the transparent *cornea* (Fig. 5–3). Behind the cornea is the *iris,* which looks blue, grey, or brown depending on the number and distribution of pigment cells. Centered in the iris is the *pupil,* an opening that is normally round; its diameter is variable like that of a camera aperture. Between the cornea and the iris lies the anterior chamber of the eye, filled with a clear liquid called the aqueous humor.

Cornea and conjunctiva are covered with a thin film of lacrimal (tear) fluid. The tears are formed in the *tear glands,* located in the outer (temporal) part of the eye

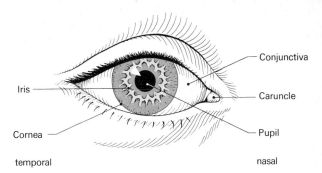

Fig. 5–3. Right eye as
seen in a mirror;
discussion in text

Iris

Cornea

temporal

Conjunctiva

Caruncle

Pupil

nasal

socket above the eyeball. The ducts of the tear glands end in the conjunctiva behind the eyelids, above the outer "corner" of the eye. Movements of the eyelids (blinking) distribute the tears uniformly over cornea and conjunctiva, and this thin film of fluid improves the optical properties of the corneal surface. The lacrimal fluid is produced continuously in very small quantities. Part of the water evaporates into the air, and the rest flows into the nasal cavity through the lacrimal duct.

Tears taste salty, because their composition is approximately that of an ultrafiltrate of blood plasma. The tears protect the cornea and the conjunctiva from desiccation and act as a "lubricant" between the eyes and lids. When a small foreign body such as a grain of sand lodges between eyelid and eye, there is a reflex increase in tear production and blinking. In this case the tears function as a rinsing fluid. Tears contain enzymes that act against bacteria, protecting the eyes from infection. Finally, the tears of humans — in "crying" — are a means of expressing emotion.

The optical system of the eye. Figure 5–4 is a diagrammatic cross section through the right eye of a human. The optical system — the *dioptric apparatus* — is a compound, not-exactly-centered lens system that casts a reversed, much reduced image of the environment onto the retina. The cornea, anterior chamber, and iris are the anteriormost parts of the dioptric apparatus. Just behind the iris is the narrow posterior chamber of the eye and the biconvex lens. The elastic lens is surrounded by the lens capsule; the fibers of the zonula ciliaris fan out into the latter. The zonal fibers are connected to the ciliary muscles and the outer vascular layer of the retina (the chorioid layer), and thus are indirectly attached to the outer wall of the eyeball.

The space inside the eye behind the lens is filled by the vitreous body. This gelatinous structure, as transparent as water, is formed by the colloidal solution of hyaluronic acid in extracellular fluid. The posterior, inner surface of the eye is lined with the *retina;* this is composed of layers of pigment cells, receptors, and nerve cells (cf. Fig. 5–10). The visual axis (Fig. 5–4), which diverges from the optical axis of the eye by a few degrees, intersects the retina at the fovea centralis, a small indentation in the retina. The fovea is the region of *greatest visual acuity.*

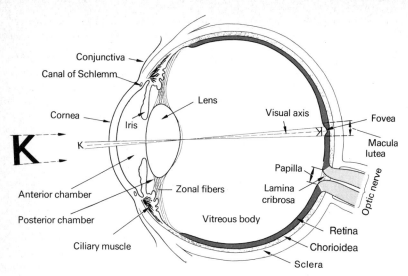

Fig. 5–4. Horizontal section through the right eye

Between the retina and the sclera is the chorioid layer, a network of blood vessels supplying the pigment cells and receptor cells. The remaining nerve-cell layers in the retina, which are closer to the vitreous body, are supplied by the vascular system of the **central retina artery,** which enters the eye through the papilla of the optic nerve.

Regulatory processes in the dioptric apparatus. The principles of physical optics and of image formation in the eye will not be discussed in this introductory text (for the details of these see SCHMIDT and THEWS, Chapter 2). Most readers will remember from their high-school physics that the refractive power of a lens is measured in terms of its *focal length* f. The focal length is the distance beyond a lens at which parallel incident light is focused to a point. Refractive power is expressed in diopters (D) and related to f as follows:

$$\text{Refractive power} = \frac{1}{f}\ [\text{D}], \qquad (5\text{–}1)$$

where f is the focal length in meters. In the normal eye the overall refractive power of the dioptric apparatus is about 58.6 D when the eye is focused on a distant point. Most of the refraction occurs at the interface between air and cornea; this surface acts like a strong lens of 42 D. In the normal eye with a refraction of 58.6 D an *infinitely distant pattern* (for example, the stars or for practical purposes, very distant objects) is sharply imaged on the retina. In order for a sharp image of an object at *finite* distance to be formed, the optical system must be *refocused.* There are two "simple" ways of doing this — shifting the lens relative to the retina or increasing the refractive power of the lens. In the human eye the second method is used, whereas in the frog eye, as in a camera, the lens is shifted relative to the sensitive surface.

In a human eye with normal sight, if the refractive power of the lens is increased by x diopters, the plane of best focus moves inward from infinity to a distance of approximately $1/x$ meters from the eye. When a person with normal vision (sharp focus at infinity) wants to read a book held 30 cm from his eyes, the refractive power must increase by $1/0.3$ m $= 3.3$ D. The increase in refractive power when one focuses on a nearer point is called **accommodation.** The increase in refractive power of the lens during accommodation is achieved by an increase in the curvature of the lens surface. That is, the lens becomes "more spherical".

Certain anatomic details are needed for an understanding of the change in form of the lens during accommodation. In the unaccommodated eye the ciliary muscle (Figs. 5–4 and 5–5) is not contracted; the zonal fibers *passively* transmit the tension in the chorioid and the wall of the eye to the lens capsule, so that the elastic lens becomes relatively flat. The tension in the wall of the eye is maintained by the intraocular pressure (18–20 mm Hg). In **accommodation** the ciliary muscle contracts and, because of its connection with the zonal fibers, counteracts the elastic forces of the chorioid. As a result, the tension in the lens capsule decreases (right in Fig. 5–5). The intrinsic structure of the lens is such that, with the reduced

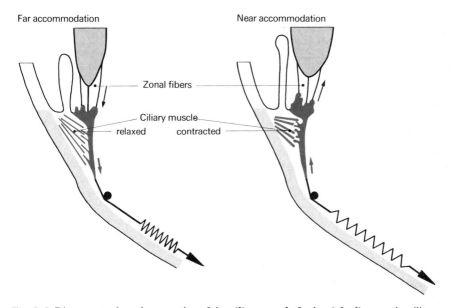

Fig. 5–5. Diagrams to show the operation of the *ciliary muscle.* In the *right diagram* the ciliary muscle is contracted. This brings about a reduction in the elastic tension transmitted from the chorioid and sclera via the zonal fibers to the lens capsule. Because of the reduction in tension in the lens capsule, the curvature of the lens increases *(near accommodation).* In the *left diagram* the ciliary muscle is relaxed. The pull of the elastic tissue in the chorioid is transmitted by the zonal fibers to the lens capsule. As a result the lens becomes flatter *(far accommodation)*

tension, curvature is increased particularly at its anterior surface; the focal length is reduced. The state of contraction of the ciliary muscle is controlled by autonomic nerve fibers, chiefly by parasympathetic fibers from the oculomotor nerve (see p. 193).

The elasticity of the lens decreases with age, so that as a person grows older the lens becomes less able to accommodate. A 10-year-old can accommodate 10 D on the average, but by the age of 50 accommodation has often decreased to 2 D and at 70 it is only about 0.5 D. For this reason older people with otherwise normal vision need glasses with convex lenses to see nearby objects sharply and to read (a condition called *presbyopia*). Humans of any age who do a great deal of close work or reading, and whose accommodation is inadequate, should wear corrective lenses. Otherwise there can be great strain on the neuronal accommodation system, which can cause tiredness and headache.

Pupillary responses. The size of the pupil, like the aperture setting of a camera, determines the amount of light that enters. For a given brightness of the environment, the quantity of light entering the eye per unit time is proportional to the *area* of the pupil. If a person in a lighted room shuts his eyes for about 10–20 s and looks into a mirror when he opens them again, he sees that both pupils constrict immediately after the eyes are opened. An interesting property of this pupillary *light response* can be demonstrated by illuminating each eye separately with a flashlight (Fig. 5–6). When light is shone into one eye only, the pupils of both eyes constrict. The constriction of a pupil when the contralateral eye is illuminated is called the *consensual light response,* while the term *direct light response* refers to the constriction of the pupil of an illuminated eye.

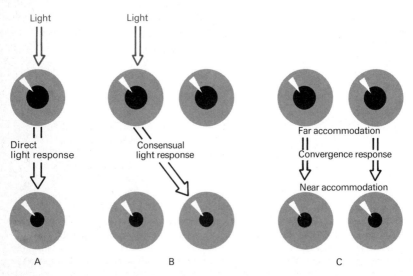

Fig. 5–6. Diagram of the *pupillary responses;* discussion in text

The *pupillary light response* is a regulatory mechanism that reduces the amount of light incident on the retina when the environmental light intensity is high (for example, in bright sunshine); it results in an increase in relative light acceptance, by increase in the size of the pupil, when the environment is dimly illuminated. The pupillary response cannot compensate for the enormous range of environmental luminance, but it is a major factor in regulation of light reaching the retina when brief changes in luminance occur. The diameter of the human pupil also depends on the *distance* of the object being fixated. If one changes focus from a distant to a nearby object, the pupils become smaller (near-point-reaction). Because the axes of the two eyes converge when focused on a near object, this response of the pupils has also been called a *convergence response.* The quality of the image in the eye is affected by the aperture as it is in a camera; that is, the "depth of focus" increases when the pupil constricts.

Constriction of the pupil is brought about by contraction of the ring-shaped *sphincter muscle* in the iris, which is innervated by parasympathetic fibers. Contraction of the *dilator muscle,* with radial fibers in the iris, causes pupillary expansion; this muscle receives sympathetic innervation. The autonomic innervation of the iris muscles explains why pupil diameter varies with psychological factors, fatigue, and with the consumption of even common drugs (alcohol, caffeine, nicotine). Children and adolescents have, on the average, relatively larger pupils than adults.

Refractive anomalies. As a rule the cornea is not perfectly spherical; its curvature is somewhat greater in one direction than in the others. This optical error is called *astigmatism.* Usually the refractive power of the cornea is somewhat stronger in the vertical than in the horizontal direction. Astigmatism can be measured simply with a device designed by PLACIDO (Fig. 5–7). The optometrist looks at the patient's cornea through a hole in the center of the disk, and on the cornea he sees a small reflection of the concentric pattern. In cases of astigmatism the rings in this reflected picture are deformed — they no longer appear round, but may be elliptical or irregularly bent.

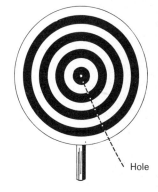

Fig. 5–7. Placido's disk for determining corneal astigmatism. The physician looks through the hole in the disk at the mirror image of the circles produced by the cornea of the patient. The diameter of the disk is about 20 cm

Hole

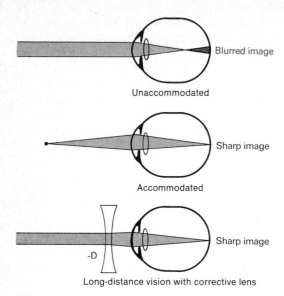

Blurred image

Unaccommodated

Sharp image

Accommodated

Sharp image

-D

Long-distance vision with corrective lens

Fig. 5–8. Myopia (near-sightedness) and its correction by a concave lens

In an eye of normal refractive power (58.6 D) a sharp image of a far-away object is formed on the retina only if the distance between the front surface of the cornea and the retina is about 24.4 mm. If — because of the shape of the eye or the refractive power of the dioptric apparatus — the cornea-to-retina distance is larger than the cornea-to-focal-plane distance, then the eye is *near-sighted (myopic);* if smaller, the eye is *far-sighted (hypermetropic).* In the condition of myopia objects at a distance cannot be sharply focused on the retina, because even in the unaccommodated state the refractive power of the dioptric apparatus is too large (Fig. 5–8). Therefore a myopic person must rely on the concave lenses in his glasses to reduce the overall refraction of the dioptric apparatus, if he is to see distant objects sharply. The refractive power of concave lenses is given in negative diopters.

A far-sighted person, on the other hand, can accommodate so as to see sharply objects at infinity and at great distances (Fig. 5–9). But his range of accommodation is usually not sufficient to focus sharply on nearby objects. Such a person needs convex lenses to compensate his hypermetropia. When a far-sighted child tries to perform the accommodation necessary to see sharply at short distances there is usually an abnormally large convergence of one eye, producing an inward "squint". A correctly designed pair of glasses often prevents squinting in a hypermetropic child.

The retina. Figure 5–10 is a simplified diagram of the retina in the eye of a primate, which closely resembles the human eye. The retina consists of the *photoreceptors,* four different classes of *nerve cells, glial cells* (Müller's supporting cells), and

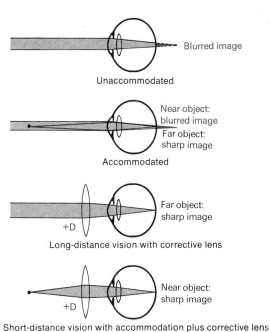

Fig. 5–9. Hypermetropia (far-sightedness) and its correction by a convex lens

pigment cells. The light-sensitive part of the retina is the layer of photoreceptors. In the human eye, two classes of photoreceptors can be distinguished morphologically, the *rods* (about 120 million of them) and the *cones* (about 6 million). In the region of most acute vision (the fovea centralis) the retina contains only cones. Each photoreceptor has a slender outer segment consisting of about 1.000 membrane disks (in rods) or infoldings (in cones). The molecules of the *visual pigments* (which absorb the light and trigger receptor response) are embedded in these membrane structures in a regular arrangement. The rods and cones are linked by *synaptic contacts* (cf. *Fundamentals of Neurophysiology,* 3rd Ed., Chapter 3) to bipolar cells and horizontal cells. The bipolar cells transmit the signals from the photoreceptors into the layer of ganglion cells and to the amacrines. Horizontal cells and amacrines function in "horizontal" signal transmission, at right angles to the main direction of signal flow (receptors → bipolar cells → ganglion cells → CNS). The *pigment cells* are bounded at their outer ends by the external vascular system (the chorioid, Fig. 5–4). The pigment cells serve an important function in the regulation of the content of visual pigment in the outer segments of the photoreceptors. As can be seen in Figure 5–10, the spreading arrangement of synaptic contacts of the neuronal elements provides for considerable *divergence and convergence* of the signals (cf. diagrams in Fig. 3–8 A, p. 84).

All the neuronal elements anatomically and functionally connected (whether directly or indirectly) to a single nerve cell of a sensory system are called the *receptive unit* of this nerve cell. The receptive unit of a ganglion cell in the retina, then, consists of all the receptors, horizontal cells, bipolar cells, and amacrines functionally connected to it.

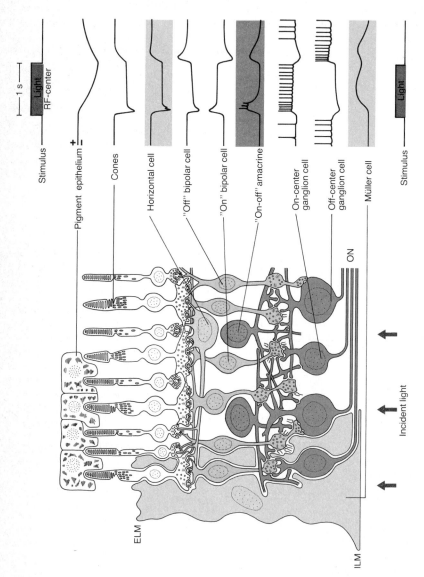

Fig. 5–10. Structure of the *primate retina* [redrawn schematically from an illustration by BOYCOTT and DOWLING, Proc. Roy. Soc. (Lond.) *166,* 80–111 (1966)] and diagram of the responses of single neurons in the retina to a light stimulus [GRÜSSER, Fortschr. Ophthalmol. *80,* 502–515 (1983)]. ELM: external limiting membrane; ILM: internal limiting membrane; ON: axons of the optic nerve

In the inner region of the fovea centralis there is a 1:1 connectivity between receptors and ganglion cells. Each cone in this region makes direct contact with a single bipolar cell, and this in turn synapses with just one ganglion cell. However, because of the arrangement of horizontal cells and amacrines, the receptive unit of a ganglion cell associated with the fovea includes a fairly extensive indirect, *lateral signal convergence* which, as discussed on p. 177–179, has a predominantly inhibitory function.

On the average, convergence predominates in the retina. The information received by about 125 million receptor cells is represented in the activity patterns of about 1 million ganglion cells, the axons of which form the optic nerve (Fig. 5–4).

Q 5.1. At what distance does a person with *normal eyes* see objects sharply, when the refractive power of the lenses of his eyes has been increased by 4 D by near accommodation?

    a) 40 cm
    b) 5 cm
    c) 25 cm
    d) 4 m

Q 5.2. Old people often need glasses to (read/see at a distance). But many people, regardless of age, need glasses to see at a distance. These people are .....; their glasses have (concave/convex) lenses.

Q 5.3. Which of the following are correct? The pupils of a human with normal sight are

    a) The same size in daylight as in the dark
    b) Smaller in daylight than in the dark
    c) Normally equally large in the left and the right eye
    d) Smaller when looking at a nearby than at a far-away object
    e) Smaller in the illuminated eye only, when one eye is illuminated
    f) About the same size in both eyes during monocular illumination

Q 5.4. Match the functionally corresponding parts of a camera and the eye in the following lists:

Camera	Eye
1. Lenses	a) Change of pupil diameter
2. Diaphragm	b) Retina
3. Light-sensitive layer of film	c) Sclera
4. Focusing by moving the objective	d) Iris
5. Case	e) Accommodation
6. Reduction of incident light by selection of smaller aperture	f) Cornea
	g) Lens
	h) Constriction of the pupil

Q 5.5.   Which of the following statements apply to the *receptive unit of a retinal ganglion cell* associated with the region of the fovea centralis?
a) In the fovea centralis there are only rods.
b) In the fovea centralis there are only cones.
c) In the region of the fovea centralis there is convergence of many receptors onto one bipolar cell.
d) In the inner region of the fovea centralis there is 1:1 connectivity between receptors, bipolar cells, and ganglion cells.
e) In the foveal region there are no horizontal cells or amacrines.

5.2 Psychophysics of Visual Perception

In the section on general subjective sensory physiology (p. 2) time, place, quality, and intensity were presented as the *basic dimensions* in the description of any perception. In the following paragraphs these basic dimensions of vision will be discussed in the light of certain examples. The influence of the spatial and temporal aspects of visual stimuli upon seeing are considered; the *qualities* of visual perception treated are brightness, color, movement, and the impression of spatial depth.

"Intrinsic light" (Eigengrau). If an experimental subject stays in a completely dark room for a long enough time, and then tries to describe his visual perception, he says he perceives not "black" or "dark" but rather a medium gray, in which there are lighter "fog patches", dots of light and even some orderly structures, all varying in space and time. The description of the medium gray (sometimes called the intrinsic light of the retina) is highly reproducible among different subjects, whereas there is great variation among the accessory visual perceptions. Eidetically predisposed subjects easily detect structures in the gray, and relatively often these take the form of human figures or faces. Aristotle recognized this phenomenon and suggested that it might be a reason for "seeing ghosts". The gray sensation is assumed to be a subjective correlate of the *spontaneous activity* of the nerve cells of the retina and the central visual system (see p. 176).

The gray scale. Suppose that there is a chessboard in front of a subject seated in a dark room, describing the perception of "intrinsic light". If the board is suddenly illuminated by a light source dim enough not to blind the subject, he immediately sees the chessboard "correctly"; the black squares appear darker than the gray previously seen and the white squares lighter, even though now more light is falling on all parts of the retina than during the preceding period of total darkness. This simple observation tells us that the perception of black, gray, or white depends not only on the amount of light striking each photoreceptor per unit time, but also on the relative illumination of adjacent regions of the retina. Under the lighting conditions prevailing in normal daylight it is possible to distinguish 30–40 different *steps of gray,* from the deepest black to the brightest white.

Because the perception of intrinsic light evidently characterizes the "resting state" of the visual system, Ewald HERING more than 100 years ago proposed that the perceptions *black* and *white* (in the example of the chessboard) be interpreted in terms of two neuronal systems acting in opposition; these "antagonistic" systems could be either in the retina or in the higher visual centers. In this view the relative degrees of activation of the *darkness system* (black system) and *brightness system* (white system) would determine the subjective impression of brightness at any point in the field of view. The neuronal systems postulated by HERING were in fact found in both the ganglion-cell layer of the retina and in higher visual centers. These entities are described on p. 176–185; they are the *on-center neurons* (brightness system) and *off-center neurons* (darkness system).

Simultaneous contrast. Figure 5–11 illustrates visual simultaneous contrast. A gray area on a white background appears darker than an identical gray area on a black background. That is, the properties of the background determine the subjectively perceived brightness of the gray fields, even though physically they are the same. Along the light/dark boundary the lighter part appears especially bright, and the darker part seems darker than it does further away from the boundary. This effect is called "edge enhancement", and the regions of altered perception are known as "Mach bands". The Mach bands in Figure 5–11 can be seen best by fixating the middle of one of the gray disks from a distance of about 50 cm. With the left disk fixated, its rim appears brighter then the central part of the disk, and the dark zone just beyond the rim appears darker than the rest of the background.

The phenomenon of simultaneous contrast shows that the subjective response to input at a certain place on the retina depends on the illumination of its surroundings. It will be shown later that this dependence can be explained by the functional organization of the *receptive fields* of the "on"-center and "off"-center neurons (see pp. 177 and 179).

Successive light/dark contrast; afterimages. The response to excitation of a particular spot on the retina depends not only on the simultaneous excitation of adjacent regions (as above) but also on the spatial distribution of illumination during the immediately preceding time. A change in sensitivity limited to a

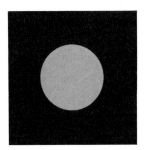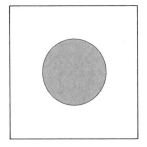

Fig. 5–11. Simultaneous contrast; discussion in text

 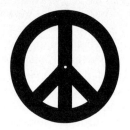

Fig. 5–12. Patterns used to observe *afterimages*

restricted region of the retina is called *local adaptation.* To observe local adaptation in your own retina, fixate with one eye the white dot in the center of the geometric pattern on the right in Figure 5–12 for about 30 s, and then fixate the dot in the middle of the circle next to it. What you see now is an "afterimage". The parts of the original picture that were dark appear, in the afterimage, brighter than the background in the white area and the parts that were light now appear darker. Those places on the retina where the dark parts of the fixated pattern were imaged have apparently become more sensitive than the adjacent more strongly illuminated retinal regions.

Visual acuity. The image of a binocularly fixated object is projected, as was mentioned above, onto the *fovea centralis of each eye.* Under daylight conditions *visual acuity* is greatest in this part of the retina, and decreases progressively toward the periphery of the retina. In clinical practice visual acuity is tested with charts like those in Figure 5–13, by determining the smallest symbols the subject can see clearly. When Landolt rings are used, visual acuity is expressed (as in Figs. 5–14 and 5–15) by $1/a$, where a is the angle (in minutes of arc) subtended by the smallest detectable gap. Another measure of acuity is the Snellen fraction. Its numerator is the distance between the subject and a test chart with letters, usually 20 feet. The denominator is calculated from the size of the smallest letters read,

Fig. 5–13. Various charts to test vision, with numbers, letters, Landolt rings, Snellen hooks, and pictures of objects. From LEYDHECKER: 1975

and represents the distance at which the black bars forming the letters subtend an angle of 1 min of arc. For people with "normal" vision this is the same as the test distance; hence their acuity is given as 20/20.

Visual acuity can be measured for various parts of the retina if the subject fixates monocularly a point away from the chart. The **measured relationship between visual acuity and position on the retina** is shown in Figure 5–14. It must also be

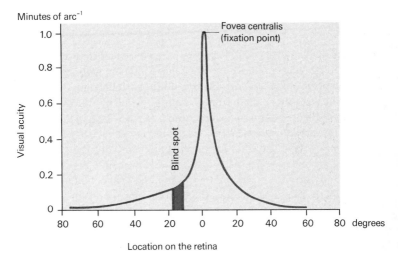

Fig. 5–14. Dependence of **visual acuity** on the location of the test symbol on the retina, as measured under photopic conditions

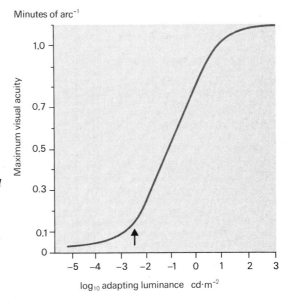

Fig. 5–15. Dependence of **visual acuity** (ordinate) on the state of adaptation of the retina. The abscissa indicates the mean luminance of the viewed surface. The region of transition from photopic to scotopic conditions of adaptation is marked by the **arrow**

mentioned that acuity is affected by the brightness of the viewed pattern. In Figure 5–15 the dependence of acuity in the region of the fovea (near the fixation point) upon the *mean luminance* of the test pattern is illustrated. Everyone knows from ordinary experience that visual acuity depends on the lighting conditions:

you could not read this small print without enough light

Proper choice of illumination is important not only for reading, but in industrial and domestic work areas as well.

The blind spot. Close study of Figure 5–4 will reveal that part of the inner back surface of the eye is not covered by retina; this is the *papilla,* the exit of the optic nerve. The part of the field of view (Fig. 5–2) projected onto the papilla is the *blind spot.* In the region of the blind spot "nothing" is seen. To examine your own blind spot look at Figure 5–16 and fixate monocularly, with the right eye, the upper cross from a distance of about 25 cm. You will find that the black disk on the right "disappears"; its image is falling on the papilla of your right eye.

But the lower part of Figure 5–16 shows that even though stimulus patterns in the blind spot are not seen, the region of the blind spot is "filled in" perceptually by extrapolation from the pattern in the surrounding area. When you fixate the *lower* cross in this figure (with the right eye alone, at about 25 cm) you will find that the mouse disappears in the blind spot but the vertical grating does not appear to have

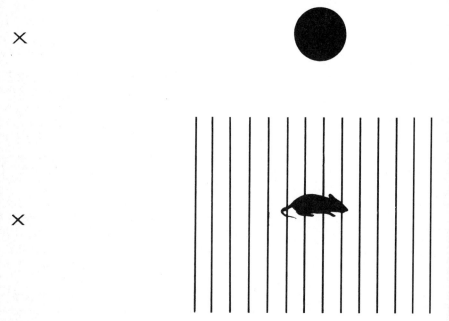

Fig. 5–16. Patterns to determine the *blind spot* of the right eye; discussion in text

a hole in it. This "perceptual impletion" can be explained neurophysiologically by the rather large "complex" receptive fields of orientation-sensitive cortical visual neurons (p. 184).

Photopic and scotopic vision. Most readers will remember from their school biology courses that the *cones* are the receptors with which we see predominantly under daylight conditions *(photopic vision)*, while the *rods* are used preferentially under conditions of lighting corresponding to a clear night *(scotopic vision)*. In twilight neither of the two receptor systems is dominant *(mesopic vision)*. Visual acuity is best under photopic conditions and colors are clearly seen; the position of greatest visual acuity is centered in the fovea. Temporal resolution of rapidly changing patterns is also better in photopic than in scotopic vision (see p. 163). In scotopic conditions, visual response times are prolonged.

In scotopic vision with the rod system, functional color-blindness prevails ("at night all cats are gray"), and the visual acuity in the region of the fovea is considerably poorer than in photopic vision. Moreover, the position of greatest visual acuity and greatest sensitivity under scotopic conditions is not the middle of the fovea but rather its edge. This shift of the point of maximal sensitivity away from the fixation point can easily be demonstrated by watching the starry sky at night. When you try to fixate a very pale star you will note that as soon as you try to do so the star vanishes, only to reappear when you choose a fixation point slightly to the side.

The time course of light/dark adaptation. When you leave a brightly lit room at night and walk into a garden lighted only by the stars, at first you see practically nothing. But gradually the sensitivity of your visual system adjusts to the low light intensity in the environment *(dark adaptation)*. As dark adaptation progresses, your visual acuity gradually improves and objects in the garden become visible, at least in rough outline.

The time course of dark adaptation can be quantified by measuring the threshold intensity of stimuli presented at different times following the transition from light to dark (Fig. 5–17). The *dark-adaptation curve* so obtained shows that the eye does not reach its maximum sensitivity until one has spent over 30 min in the dark. The normal dark-adaptation curve consists of two parts; the first is interpreted as the *cone component,* and the second as the *rod component.* The cone component can be measured separately with small red light spots focused in the foveal region. Although the initial adaptation occurs more rapidly than in rods, the final sensitivity of cones is considerably lower (i.e., the thresholds are higher) than that of the rods (as measured with white or blue light outside the region of the fovea).

The process opposite to dark adaptation is *light adaptation.* You can easily observe the rapid course of light adaptation by entering a brightly lit room after spending considerable time in the dark. If the difference in intensity is very great, you are temporarily blinded; then, within 15–60 s, your visual system adjusts to the new light intensity. This sort of blinding is associated with a lowered sensitivity and a disruption of form perception. A similar state can occur when one is driving at night and a car with bright headlights approaches.

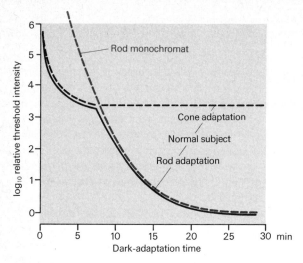

Fig. 5–17. Dark-adaptation curves. On the ordinate is the relative stimulus intensity (luminance) of a just suprathreshold light stimulus; on the abscissa is the dark-adaptation time. The **dashed red curve** corresponds to data from a totally color-blind person (a rod monochromat). The **dashed black curve** was obtained with red light in the fovea, and the **continuous black curve** with white light in the extrafoveal region of a normal subject

The temporal properties of visual perception. When you look at the spokes in the wheels of a fast-moving bicycle you see a "transparent" gray area. The temporal alternation between light and dark in the moving images of the spokes on your retina is too rapid to be perceived distinctly. This everyday observation indicates that there is an upper limit to temporal resolution in vision, called the *flicker fusion frequency* or critical flicker frequency. An intermittent light stimulus, flashing at a rate above the flicker fusion frequency, cannot be distinguished from a maintained light at the same average intensity. The flicker fusion frequency can easily be measured with a disk divided into black and white sectors, like that shown in Figure 5–18. The subject watches part of this disk while increasing its rate of rotation, until eventually he perceives it as being a uniform gray. The flicker fusion frequency increases with both the average luminance and the area of the fluctuating light stimulus (Fig. 5–18). There are two distinct sections of the curve in Figure 5–18; the part rising more slowly is associated with rod vision and that with the steeper slope, with cone vision. Flickering light is perceived as such at frequencies below 22 Hz under scotopic conditions of adaptation and stimulation. The higher fusion frequency of the cone system implies that signal transmission by the cones occurs considerably more rapidly than in the rods.

Ordinarily when flicker fusion frequency is measured, a particular part of the field of view is examined in each trial. But if the successive light stimuli are projected in alternation onto *different* parts of the retina, both the temporal and spatial aspects of signal processing in the retina and in the visual system are

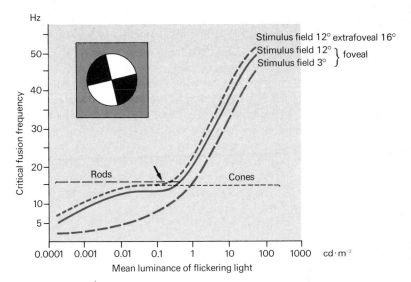

Fig. 5–18. Dependence of *flicker fusion frequency* (ordinate) on the mean luminance of the flickering light stimulus (abscissa). Measured with sinusoidally modulated light; amplitude of modulation 70%

involved. Suppose that at time t_0 a light stimulus appears at point A in the visual field and at time $t_0 + t_r$ it is switched off; the stimulus then reappears later (at time $t_0 + t_r + \Delta t$) at point B. Under these conditions the subject perceives an ***apparent movement*** of the light from A to B, which cannot be distinguished from a real movement if $\Delta t < 120$ ms. Alternating illumination of regions A and B gives rise to the impression that the light stimulus is moving back and forth between A and B. The phenomenon of apparent movement, described here for the case of two simple lights, is turned to advantage in motion pictures. The projected film consists of a sequence of stationary pictures differing in configuration; these appear in succession on the screen at a rate between 18 and 24 per second. This frequency is high enough to elicit apparent movement in the visual system, so that the succession of images cannot be distinguished from real movement.

Color vision. To a person with normal eyes, the objects in his surroundings exhibit a great diversity of color qualities or valencies, the ***chromatic series.*** It is convenient to consider the steps of gray (mentioned on p. 156) as an equivalent series, also called the ***achromatic series.*** The achromatic series ranges from the brightest white to the deepest black, which is produced by simultaneous contrast. The perceptible colors of the surfaces of objects can be characterized by three phenomenal quantities: hue, saturation, and lightness. The ***hues*** are arranged in a natural, closed sequence (the "color circle", Fig. 5–19): red, orange, yellow, green, blue, violet, purple, red. The ***saturation*** of a color depends on the relative magnitudes of the chromatic and achromatic components. (The ***chromaticity*** or shade of a color is determined by hue and saturation. A mixture of spectral red with black, for example, is a shade of brown, while the shades of pink are produced by mixing red with white). The *lightness* indicates the relative position of the achromatic component of a shade on the gray scale, between black and white.

All the hues in the color circle either correspond to certain colors in the spectrum of visible sunlight or can be produced by an *additive combination* of two spectral colors. An additive combination of colors occurs when light of different wavelengths falls on a *single part of the retina* (Fig. 5–20). For a person with normal color vision *any* color that can be produced by luminous objects can be duplicated by a particular additive combination of *three* appropriately chosen monochromatic stimuli C_1, C_2, and C_3. This situation is described completely and unambiguously by the sensation equation or color matching equation:

$$a\{C_1\} + b\{C_2\} + c\{C_3\} \cong d\{C_x\} \tag{5-2}$$

In this expression the symbol $\cong$ signifies "equivalence of sensation" or "matches".

By international convention, three particular wavelengths, the *primary colors,* have been assigned to C_1, C_2, and C_3. These are the spectral colors with wavelength 700 nm (red), 546 nm (green), and 435 nm (blue); certain proportions of these can be used to specify any shade.

Colors can also be generated by a process which is the opposite of additive combination. This *subtractive combination* occurs when a white light from a source is sent through one or more filters of different colors (Fig. 5–20). When a painter mixes pigments (for example, blue and yellow to make green), he creates a subtractive combination of colors, since the individual granules of the blue and yellow pigments act as color filters. But when one observes the colors in mosaics and paintings, additive combination can also play a role, if two different small points of color are imaged on the same cone. In the "dot technique" of some impressionist painters and in works of the pointillist school this effect was systematically turned to advantage. Color fusion is produced only if the distance between painting and viewer is great enough.

White and black as colors. For every color C_1 in the color circle there is a second color C_2 which, when additively mixed with C_1, gives the color white; that is,

$$a\{C_1\} + b\{C_2\} \cong w\{white\} \tag{5-3}$$

In this color matching equation, the constants a and b depend on the definition of "white". The hues C_1 and C_2 are in all cases *complementary colors.* White light can be emitted from luminous sources, but black and the various shades of gray cannot; a contrast mechanism (see p. 157) is necessary for these to be elicited.

The term *color solid* is applied to representation of the perceived colors in a three-dimensional continuum. In the simplest of these, the color spindle, the axis black/white is "perpendicular" to the plane of the color circle representing the pure hues.

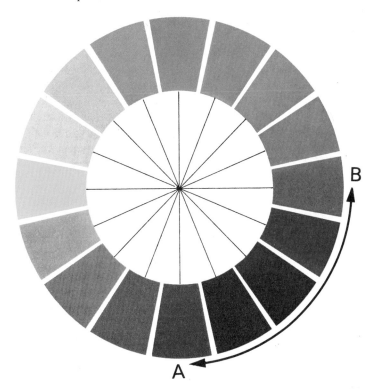

Fig. 5–19. Arrangement of the hues in a *color circle.* The hues between (A) and (B) are not spectral colors, but rather were produced by mixture of red and blue

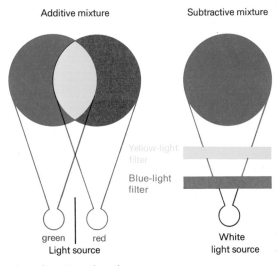

Fig. 5–20. Diagram of an *additive* and a *subtractive* color mixture

The results of experiments in sensory psychology involving the additive combinations of luminous colors [Eqs. 5–2) and (5–3)] are represented geometrically by the two-dimensional "color triangle" (or chromaticity diagram, Fig. 5–21). If two of the hues included in the triangle are combined additively, the resultant color lies on the line between the two hues. The color complementary to any hue lies on a line passing through the *white point* (E in Fig. 5–21). For a person with normal color vision all the hues of luminous colors [as expressed by Eq. (5–2)] are sufficiently specified by at most three constants. This observation gave rise to the term "trichromatic vision". The values of the constants a, b, and c in Eq. (5–2) required to produce any given hue in the color triangle are practically identical for the great majority of the population; these people are called *normal trichromats*. A small percentage have deviant constants and are called *anomalous trichromats*. About 1% of humans, the *dichromats,* perceive all luminous hues in a way that can be described by an equation with *two* constants:

$$a\{C_1\} + b\{C_2\} \cong d\{C_x\}. \tag{5–4}$$

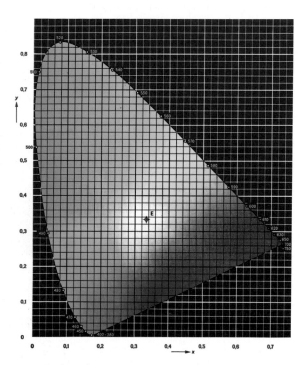

Fig. 5–21. Chromaticity diagram based on the German standard DIN 5033. The white region surrounds the point (E). The base of the "color triangle" is formed by the purple tones, which do not occur in the spectrum but are produced by an additive mixing of the spectral colors blue and red

The color diagram describing perception by these people is considerably less differentiated than that of trichromats. These dichromatic departures from normal color vision, as in the case of the anomalous trichromats, are genetically determined. The most common form is "red/green color-blindness" (for details see SCHMIDT and THEWS). Less than 0.01% of people are *totally color-blind.* They perceive only different shades of gray, and are called "monochromats". In most of the totally color-blind patients their genes provide them with only one pigment system; their rods and cones contain only the pigment rhodopsin (see p. 173).

The two most important *theories of color vision* deserve mention here. The *trichromatic theory* of YOUNG and HELMHOLTZ postulates three different types of cones, which operate as independent receiver systems in photopic vision, their signals being jointly analyzed in a neuronal brightness system and a neuronal color system. This theory is supported by the color-fusion relationships (Eq. (5–2)], by the discovery of three different cone pigments (cf. p. 173), and by the spectral sensitivities of the receptor potentials of different cones (Fig. 5–26).

The *opponent color theory* ("four-color theory") of E. HERING postulates antagonistic neuronal processes with the opponent colors green/red and yellow/blue, in addition to a black/white system, which is also antagonistically organized. The known organization (cf. p. 180) of the receptive fields of color-specific neurons of the retina and lateral geniculate body, together with considerable data from experiments in sensory psychology, corroborate this theory. The trichromatic theory of color vision and the opponent-color theory are thus both "correct", at different levels of the afferent visual system. That a synthesis of these two most important, competing theories of color vision is possible was pointed out as early as the beginning of this century, in the *zone theory* of the Freiburg physiologist J. VON KRIES. The opponent color theory has been developed further in the color theory of LAND. With a pattern consisting of many different colors, he showed that the color one perceives depends primarily on the chromatic reflection of a color field relative to the sum of all adjacent chromatic contrasts. This relationship explains the remarkable constancy of the colors of objects in our natural surroundings, in spite of extreme variation in the chromatic composition of the light.

Binocular vision. An object in the visual environment appears to us to be essentially the same object, regardless of whether it is viewed monocularly with the right or left eye, or binocularly. The unification of the two monocular images of an object is called *binocular fusion.* In binocular viewing of a nearby three-dimensional object the *impression of spatial depth* is enhanced as compared with monocular vision. Because the eyes are located at different positions in the head, there are slight geometric differences in the representation of the world visualized on the two retinas. These differences between the images formed by a single fixated object on the right and left retinas are greater, the closer the object. The disparity between the two images is in fact a prerequisite for depth perception *(stereoscopy).* With just one eye, one can use size differences, amount of overlap, haze effects, and parallactic shifts during head movements to achieve a certain degree of depth perception, particularly for objects at a considerable distance.

You can easily see for yourself the difference in the images of the visual environment on the two retinas by the following experiment: Stretch your right arm all the way out, point the thumb upward and fixate it first binocularly and then monocularly with the left and right eye in alternation. As you change between the two eyes the thumb appears to shift its position with respect to the background. It follows that the representation of the world on the left retina is distinctly different from that on the right.

Binocular fusion is ***disrupted by changing the position of an eye in its socket*** while an object is being fixated, by pressing on the eyelid lightly with a finger. Here the object is imaged "incorrectly" on the displaced retina; you "see double", because binocular fusion is prevented.

A binocularly fixated object is seen as a single object only when its images fall on very specific parts of the retina in the two eyes, the ***corresponding retinal areas***. With maintained binocular fixation on a given point (e.g., the fixation point

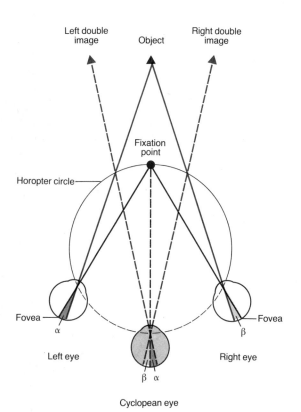

Fig. 5–22. Diagram of ***binocular vision*** and the construction of a ***cyclopean eye.*** The object viewed is here positioned outside the horopter surface. Its image is projected to the right of the fovea in the left eye. In binocular vision uncrossed double images of the object are produced, the positions of which can be determined by projection of the retinas of the left and right eyes onto the imagined retina of the cyclopean eye

marked in Fig. 5–22), these corresponding areas can be defined by moving a test object and finding positions in space at which it is seen as single. It turns out (as you can convince yourself by measuring it or by making more detailed geometric drawings) that all such positions in space fall on a three-dimensional curved surface which includes the fixation point. This surface is called the *horopter,* and there is of course a different horopter for each fixation point. In the horizontal plane only, the situation is simpler — the resulting section of the horopter surface is the "horopter circle" shown in Figure 5–22.

Objects positioned an appreciable distance off the horopter are seen "double". For example, in Figure 5–22, with binocular fixation on the point indicated, the marked object is outside the horopter. Its images in the two eyes clearly fall on *non*-corresponding areas — in fact they fall on opposite sides of the foveas, by the angles a and β in Figure 5–22.

One way of thinking of the "two eyes — one world" problem in such situations is to imagine a "cyclopean eye", positioned on the extended horopter halfway between the two eyes. As illustrated in Figure 5–22, when the two eyes, fixating the point marked on the horopter, view an object further away, the cyclopean eye would see two apparent objects, one on either side of the real object. Whenever the cyclopean eye sees only one image, it must be on the horopter — i. e., pairs of corresponding areas in the two eyes are by definition mapped onto single areas in the cyclopean eye.

The fundamental distinction between images of objects located inside and outside the horopter is easily illustrated with the "two-finger experiment". Hold your right index finger in front of your eyes at a horizontal distance of about 20 cm, and your left index finger behind it, about 50 cm from your eyes. First fixate the closer finger; you will see the further finger double. Then close your left and right eyes in alternation, and note that the double images are *"uncrossed"*. That is, it is the left eye that sees the left image and the right eye the right image. The far finger (like D in Fig. 5–22) is outside the horopter defined by fixating the near finger. Next fixate the more distant finger. Now the nearer finger appears double, and when you close your eyes sees the left image and vice versa. Here the near finger is inside the horopter defined by fixation on the far finger. Try drawing this situation to construct the positions of the images formed, in analogy with Figure 5–22.

From the observations noted so far one might conclude that all the objects in the visible surroundings that are not imaged on corresponding retinal positions — because they lie inside or outside the horopter — must cause double images to be perceived. But when you look around in a well-structured visual environment, disturbing double images do not appear. Apparently there are mechanisms that prevent seeing double. One of these is the low visual acuity in the periphery of the retina (see p. 159). A second is thought to be a *binocular inhibitory mechanism* in the central visual system, suppressing perception of one or the other of two disparate images. By looking at different objects with the *foveae centrales* of the left and right eyes you can observe the binocular inhibitory mechanism. To do this, make two tubes about 30 cm long and 3–4 cm in diameter; through one of them look with one eye at a stamp, and through the other (with the other eye) at a coin.

With these drastically different stimulus patterns, binocular fusion does not occur — you do not see a unitary "stamp-coin". Because of the binocular inhibitory mechanism there is a "binocular rivalry", an alternating perception of either the stamp or the coin. Parts of each stimulus pattern may be visible simultaneously, but only *next to one another* and not superimposed. In this binocular rivalry, contours, as a rule, are more effective than uniformly shaded surfaces. This result can be explained by the known marked activation of neurons in the afferent visual system by contrasting boundaries (discussed on pp. 178–179), as compared with the activation by homogeneous surfaces.

Stereoscopic vision. Despite the fact that any fairly large three-dimensional object viewed binocularly throws somewhat different images onto the foveas of the two eyes because of the geometric situation considered above, we normally do not see "two" of such an object; we perceive it as a single, *spatially extended* entity. The discrepancies in the horizontal plane between the images on the two retinas (with the head in the normal position) — that is, the departures from the exactly corresponding retinal areas — are called the *horizontal receptive-field disparity.* Horizontal disparity is an important prerequisite for binocular three-dimensional vision. The amount of the disparity determines the strength of the impression of depth. The previous discussion of functional significance of corresponding retinal areas must therefore be modified; it is only when a certain horizontal disparity is exceeded that the perception of a binocularly viewed object as a single entity gives way to a double image. In other words, perception of an object as single in stereoscopic vision does not require functional analysis of corresponding *points* in the retinas of the two eyes, but rather there is an analysis of associated images, covering *areas* that extend over a few degrees of arc. The horizontal disparity of the two images of an object decreases, for geometric reasons, with the distance of the object from the eyes. This is why accurate depth perception becomes impossible for objects at great distances. An optical range finder functionally increases the distance between the eyes, in addition to enlarging the viewed objects, and thus improves depth perception. The influence of horizontal disparity on depth perception can be studied using Figure 5–23. Fixate an imagined point

Fig. 5–23. Figures to illustrate stereoscopic perception based on *horizontal disparity.* For explanation see text

behind the book so that the two large circles fuse binocularly. When you have achieved this, you will see three large circles, the middle one with both eyes. In the middle circle the small circle will appear to hover in space ca. 1–2 cm in front of the larger circle. Its images in the two eyes are horizontally disparate, because of the asymmetric arrangement of the figure.

Form vision. When we glance about in well-structured surroundings we perceive not isolated "stimuli" but rather objects and their relationships to one another. "Dissecting" the mechanisms of visual perception into simple processes ("sensory impressions"; see p. 5) as in the preceding sections has proved useful in sensory physiology; it is an obvious approach to quantifying and understanding the function of the peripheral sense organs. The hypothesis implied by this procedure — that the perception of a complex form can be attributed to elementary physiologic mechanisms in the retina and afferent visual system — has been supported by direct neurophysiologic measurements in certain systems (see Sec. 5.3, p. 173).

On the other hand, the way in which *perception of a solid form* (Gestalt) arises, from the elementary mechanisms found so far, has not yet been explained. Nor have we any explanation of the "phenomenal invariance" of perceived objects. By this we mean the familiar fact that (for example) a teapot is perceived as being the same teapot regardless of lighting conditions, its position and orientation, and whether it is seen with one or two eyes. The teapot is perceived as a whole even though only part of it is visible.

In form perception, as in the elementary mechanisms of color and light/dark perception, numerous processes of contrast evaluation and impletion are involved. Under certain conditions these give rise to illusions. Some such illusions are demonstrated in Figure 5–24. The perceived length and curvature of a line are determined not only by its "objective" characteristics but also by the length and the angle of lines in its vicinity (Fig. 5–24 a, b). The contours of simple shapes are filled in, so that an edge may be seen to continue through an "objectively" blank area

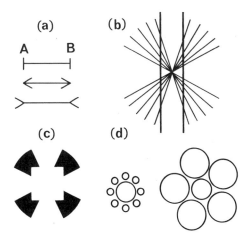

Fig. 5–24. Examples of illusions in form perception. (a) The distance *A B* is objectively the same in the drawings of the double arrow and the double fork, but it appears to be different. (b) The two thick vertical lines are parallel and straight, as you can confirm with a ruler. (c) The *white square* in the middle is produced by subjective "filling in". (d) The central circles are the same size in each of the two figures

(Fig. 5–24 c). The perceived size of a figure depends upon the size of neighboring figures (Fig. 5–24 d). Systematic studies in the field of Gestalt psychology, particularly in the first quarter of this century, have revealed many of the rules governing the visual perception of complex forms. Because neurophysiologic findings to date offer only inadequate explanation of these rules, or none at all, they will not be presented here. However, on p. 188 some neurophysiologic results are described which allow a first approach to an understanding of the perception of complex visual forms.

Q 5.6.   Simultaneous contrast in light/dark vision is:
  a) An error of judgment that can be easily prevented by concentration
  b) Caused by a disturbance in the dioptric apparatus of the eye
  c) A mechanism acquired by learning
  d) An effect brought about by lateral inhibition in the retina and in the central visual system

Q 5.7.   Which of the following statements apply to the visual acuity of a human with normal sight?
  a) Acuity is greatest in the fovea under light-adapted conditions.
  b) Acuity is greater in the light-adapted state than in dark adaptation.
  c) The place on the retina where resolution is sharpest varies with the state of adaptation.
  d) The acuity in the region of the blind spot is 1.0 (min of arc)$^{-1}$.
  e) Acuity can be determined with Landolt rings.
  f) When the eyes are blinded by bright light, acuity is reduced.

Q 5.8.   What is the visual acuity of a subject who correctly recognizes a Landolt ring with opening $a = 0.8$ min of arc?

Q 5.9.   Which mechanisms are necessary for normal stereoscopic vision (with two eyes)?
  a) Binocular fusion
  b) Light adaptation
  c) Dark adaptation
  d) Binocular inhibition of disturbing double images (binocular rivalry)
  e) Horizontal disparity
  f) Identical color impressions in the two eyes

Q 5.10.   By *corresponding retinal areas* we mean:
  a) The relationship between receptive field center and receptive field periphery
  b) The areas in the two retinas that are associated in normal binocular vision
  c) The areas in one retina that are at equal distances from the fovea
  d) Retinal areas in which only cones are present

Q 5.11. The *horopter* is:
   a) The region of the visual field projected onto the fovea
   b) The region of the binocular field of view projected onto both foveas
   c) An imagined surface in space, each point in which is projected onto geometrically corresponding places on the two retinas
   d) The region of the environment lying outside the binocular field of view
   e) None of the above is correct

Q 5.12. Which of the following statements is correct?
   a) If three different monochromatic light stimuli fall on one photoreceptor in the eye, additive combination of colors occurs.
   b) If two different monochromatic light stimuli fall on one photoreceptor in the eye, subtractive combination of colors occurs.
   c) When a painter mixes red and yellow to make orange, he has produced a subtractive combination of colors.
   d) When a painter mixes yellow and blue to make green, he has produced an additive combination of colors.
   e) The set of all hues of luminous light sources perceived by a normally sighted person can be adequately and unambiguously described by a color-combination equation comprising three spectral colors (the primary colors).

5.3 Neurophysiology of Vision

The primary process: a photochemical reaction. The dioptric apparatus of the eye focuses onto the retina an inverted and reduced image of the environment. If this image is well structured, different numbers of light quanta (photons), of characteristic wavelength, fall on different portions of the receptor mosaic in each interval of time. Some of the photons are absorbed by the molecules of visual pigment embedded in the membranous disks (cf. Fig. 5–10) of the photoreceptors. Each molecule of pigment can absorb just *one* photon, as a result of which it assumes a state of higher energy. The probability is then about 0.5 that this state will give way to a particular configurational change leading to a multi-step *process of decomposition* of the pigment molecule (this probability is called the "quantum efficiency"). The visual pigment in the rods (rhodopsin) consists of a protein (opsin) and retinene 1, the aldehyde of vitamin A_1. In terms of photon wavelength, the *absorption maximum* of the rhodopsin molecule is at about 500 nm. The decomposition of rhodopsin produces the colorless opsin and vitamin A_1. The composition of the cone pigments has not yet been entirely clarified. They are thought, however, to have a structure similar to rhodopsin. In the cones of the human retina three different pigments have been demonstrated. Their absorption maxima are at about 445, 535, and 570 nm. In the human retina each cone evidently contains only *one* pigment.

The breakdown of the pigment molecules initiated by photon absorption is the first step in the *transduction process* (see p. 70) of vision, upon which all the other neurophysiologic processes of excitation depend. The configurational changes in the pigment molecule presumably increase the *calcium conductance* of the disk membrane, so that calcium ions (or another, as yet unknown, intracellular transmitter substance) diffuse out of the interior of the membrane disks into the intracellular space of the outer segment of the photoreceptor. There an interaction with the molecular receptors at the "sodium channels" of the *outer membrane* of the outer segment brings about a decrease in the sodium conductance of the membrane. This conductance change is responsible for the *receptor potential* of the photoreceptors, which will be discussed below.

The decomposed pigment molecules are reassembled, in various intermediate steps, by *chemical, energy-consuming* processes. A "membrane pump" returns the calcium to the interior of the membranous disks. Under *steady illumination* an *equilibrium* is reached between the photochemical decay of the pigments and their chemical resynthesis. This *reaction balance* represents the physiochemical component of light/dark adaptation; as the level of adapting illumination decreases, the concentration of visual pigments in the photoreceptors increases.

The receptor potential. If a microelectrode is positioned at the surface of or inside a single photoreceptor during total darkness, it records a relatively large electrical current flowing through the cell membrane (the "dark current"). In the dark the resting potential of the photoreceptor is only -20 to -40 mV. Upon illumination of the photoreceptor a *hyperpolarization* of the membrane potential appears; that is, there is a greater electrical negativity of the cell interior as compared with the extracellular space. At the same time, the flow of electrical current through the membrane decreases. The photoreceptor membrane resistance has thus been increased by illumination. This hyperpolarization of the receptor potential in response to the adequate stimulus is a peculiarity of the photoreceptors in the vertebrate retina. In all the other receptors so far investigated, excitation is associated with *depolarization* of the membrane; the "resting potential" in other receptors lies between -60 and -80 mV (cf. Sec. 3.1, pp. 69ff.).

The amplitude (A) of the hyperpolarizing receptor potential in response to illumination is greater, the higher the light intensity I relative to the threshold intensity I_0 in the preceding state of adaptation (Fig. 5–25):

$$A = k \cdot \log\frac{I}{I_0} \text{ [mV],} \qquad (5\text{–}5)$$

in which k is chosen to give units of mV.

The *spectral sensitivities* of the receptor potentials of single photoreceptors in the vertebrate retina have been determined by stimulation with monochromatic lights of different wavelengths, matched for equal energy. In such measurements microelectrodes are used to record intracellularly from single photoreceptors. Figure 5–26 shows the way receptor-potential amplitude depends on wavelength in a large sample of receptors studied in such experiments. In these data, again, it is

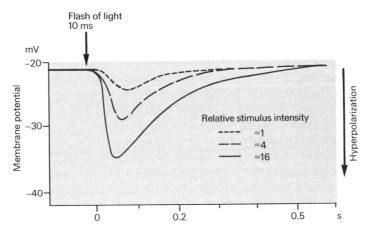

Fig. 5–25. Receptor potential of a single cone in the turtle retina. Response to brief flashes of light at three different intensities. Modified from Baylor, Fuortes,: J. Physiol. (Lond.), **207,** 77–92 (1970)

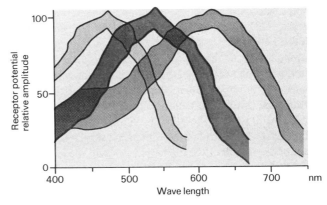

Fig. 5–26. Spectral sensitivity curves of the three cone types in the fish retina (carp). On the ordinate is the relative amplitude of the receptor potential (normalized, with the maximal response = 100%); on the abscissa is the wavelength of the monochromatic stimulus flash (all stimuli have the same energy). Despite the considerable scatter in the individual results, three different types of cone can be distinguished; the ranges of scatter are represented by the shaded regions. Modified from Tomita et al.: Vision Res. **7,** 519–531 (1967)

possible to distinguish three different classes of cones. The response maximum of the rods lies at about 500 nm, the wavelength of maximum absorption by rhodopsin. These neurophysiologic results corroborate the above-mentioned evidence of the existence of different visual pigments in rods and cones, and the presence of three different cone types in the vertebrate retina. Taken together, they confirm the ***trichromatic theory*** of color vision discussed on p. 167.

Signal processing in the horizontal cells, bipolar cells and amacrines. In experiments on animals it is possible to penetrate retinal nerve cells with micropipettes and measure the membrane potential intracellularly. Via varied synaptic contacts, the retinal neurons form a close-meshed neuronal network (Fig. 5–10). Within this retinal network two *directions of signal flow* can be distinguished: the *main* signal flow (from receptors to bipolar cells to ganglion cells) and the *lateral* signal transmission (in the layers of the horizontal cells and amacrines). In the horizontal cells, bipolar cells, and amacrines, signal processing is done by slow changes of membrane potentials; trains of action potentials are not generated. Here the amounts of synaptic transmitter substances released (see *Fundamentals of Neurophysiology,* Chap. 3) evidently depend upon the membrane potentials of the synaptic terminal structures. Figure 5–10 shows diagrammatically the "processing" of the signals in the network of the retina. The end result of this processing is reflected in the functional organization of the receptive fields of the retinal ganglion cells — the „output elements" of the retina.

Neurophysiology of retinal ganglion cells. The term *receptive unit* is applied to the set of afferent neuronal elements that influence *one* nerve cell of a sensory system. The receptive unit of a retinal ganglion cell thus consists of all the receptors, bipolar cells, horizontal cells, and amacrines directly or indirectly linked to this ganglion cell. Examination of Figure 5–10 will show that the receptive unit of a ganglion cell covers quite a large area of the retina. The receptive unit is the anatomic basis of the stimulus-defined *receptive fields* of retinal ganglion cells. Whereas the membranes of the receptors, horizontal cells, and bipolar cells exhibit exclusively slow potentials, the membranes of the ganglion cells can generate *action potentials.* The action potentials are transmitted to the CNS along the ganglion-cell axons. These axons constitute the *optic nerve,* which runs from the socket of the eye through the wall of the skull into the cranial cavity; it enters the brain in the region of the diencephalon, and the ganglion-cell axons synapse with cells in the lateral geniculate body, the superior colliculi, and the pretectal region.

   The functional organization of the receptive fields of retinal ganglion cells can be analyzed by recording the action potentials of their axons in the optic nerve with microelectrodes. For each ganglion cell in the eye there is a small region of the overall *visual field* (see p. 145) within which suitable light stimuli can elicit excitatory and/or inhibitory responses. This area is called the *receptive field* (RF). The receptive fields of neighboring ganglion cells in the retina overlap considerably. When the responses of many retinal ganglion cells are tested with white-light stimuli projected into different parts of their respective fields, it first becomes apparent that there are two large classes of neurons — the *"on"-center neurons* and the *"off"-center neurons.* Each of these classes comprises two subtypes: neurons with phasic responses (on I, off I) and neurons with tonic responses (on II, off II). In the light-adapted mammalian retina "on"- and "off"-center neurons have receptive fields within which stimuli in the center elicit different responses than stimuli in the periphery (Fig. 5–27). In the case of an "on"-center neuron, illumination of the *RF center* produces excitation (that is, an increase in the rate of

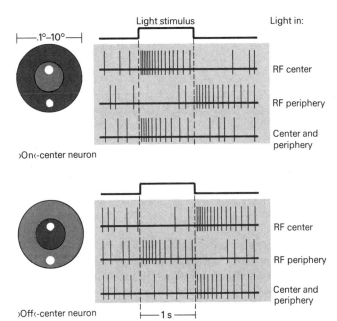

Fig. 5-27. Functional organization of the receptive fields of the ganglion cells in the mammalian retina. To analyze the receptive fields white light spots are projected onto either the center or the periphery of the receptive field, or to both

discharge of action potentials), whereas illumination of the **RF periphery** causes inhibition, a decrease in action potential frequency (Fig. 5-27). When center and periphery are illuminated simultaneously, the response associated with the center ordinarily predominates. When the small light stimulus is turned off, the result is inhibition if it is in the center and activation if it is in the periphery — the reverse of the responses to "on".

The receptive fields of the "off"-center neurons also have an "antagonistic" organization, about the converse of the receptive fields of the "on"-center neurons; illumination of the RF center causes inhibition, and turning off of the light in the center, excitation of the ganglion cell. As one might predict, illumination of the RF periphery elicits activation, and "light off" in the periphery results in inhibition (Fig. 5-27).

Neurophysiology of simultaneous contrast. From the functional organization of the retinal receptive fields it is possible to work out the way simultaneous contrast (as discussed on p. 157) can arise. Figure 5-28 shows diagrammatically the change in response of a retinal "on"-center neuron when a light/dark boundary, or edge, is projected into different parts of the receptive field. The numbers given in the figure indicate relative levels of neuronal excitation or inhibition. If the edge is in position A, both periphery and center of the RF are uniformly illuminated by the bright region of the stimulus. In an "on"-center neuron, the neuronal activation

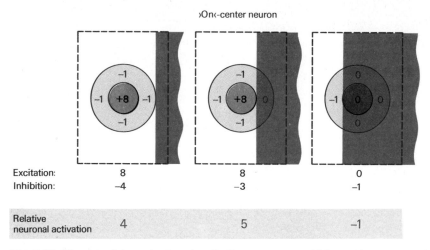

Excitation: 8   8   0
Inhibition: −4   −3   −1

Relative
neuronal activation   4   5   −1

Fig. 5–28. Diagram of the activation of an "on"-center neuron which would account for the phenomenon of simultaneous contrast; further explanation in text

from the field center predominates (net excitation = 4). But if the edge is in position B, only part of the inhibitory surround is illuminated. Therefore the inhibition is less than when the stimulus is in position A, and the net excitation of the ganglion cell is greater (= 5). If the edge is in position C, only a small part of the inhibitory surround is illuminated, and the center of the RF is dark. The net result in this case is inhibition of the spontaneous activity of the cell. Activation is thus greatest when the edge is just at the boundary between center and periphery of the receptive field (position B). On the well-founded assumption that the subjectively perceived degree of "brightness" is positively correlated with the impulse frequency in "on"-center neurons, such ganglion-cell responses would predict the phenomenon of simultaneous contrast (Fig. 5–11).

The change in receptive field organization with dark adaptation. The antagonistic RF organization can be explained by the superposition of excitatory and inhibitory processes within the receptive unit of a retinal ganglion cell. The reasoning here is based on the assumption that the *lateral excitation processes* are transmitted predominantly by the *convergence* of signals from several bipolar cells upon a single ganglion cell, while the *lateral inhibitory processes* are mediated by horizontal and amacrine cells. The relative strength of excitation and inhibition within the receptive unit of a retinal ganglion cell depends on the *state of adaptation* — that is, the average amount of light incident upon a fairly large area of the retina.

Figure 5–29 illustrates the fact that the functional RF center becomes smaller, the higher the mean luminance of the stimulus pattern; the connections of the neurons within a receptive unit are of course still the same, so that the area of the RF remains constant. As dark adaptation progresses the RF center enlarges, and

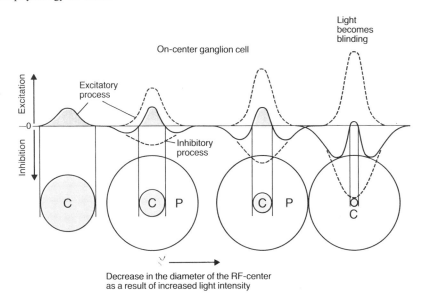

Fig. 5–29. The spatial organization of the receptive field of an "on" ganglion cell can be explained by superposition of the spatial distributions of an excitatory and an inhibitory process. The excitation has a lower threshold than the inhibition. As luminance is raised in the above-threshold region, if inhibition increases more than excitation the result is a functional reduction of the RF-center. With very strong lights, which are perceived as dazzling, inhibition predominates; the light response of the "on" ganglion cell is inhibited and visual form perception is impaired. In optimal light adaptation the RF-center is smallest and hence visual acuity is greatest [from GRÜSSER, Fortschr. Ophthalmol. *80*, 502–515 (1983)]

when dark adaptation is complete the antagonistic organization of the receptive fields disappears altogether. Under these conditions an "on"-center neuron responds to illumination in any part of its receptive field with activation at "light on", and the "off"-center neuron responds throughout its RF with activation at "light off".

Receptor density and RF size as a function of eccentricity in the retina. Retinal *eccentricity* denotes the distance of a site on the retina from the *fovea centralis.* The receptor density (number of receptors per square millimeter of retinal surface) varies with eccentricity. In the cone system, receptor density is greatest in the fovea. Rod density, on the other hand, is greatest in the parafoveal region; the fovea contains no rods. Rod density also decreases toward the periphery of the retina. At the extreme edge of the retina the receptor layer consists almost entirely of rods. Since rods do not distinguish colors, the extreme periphery is functionally color-blind.

Receptive-field size increases from the region of the fovea to the extreme periphery of the retina. Data from ganglion cells in the light-adapted monkey retina show that the receptive field centers of the ganglion cells are a few minutes of arc in diameter in the foveal region, become larger with increasing eccentricity, and can be as much as several degrees of arc in diameter in the periphery of the retina. Comparison of actual receptor density from anatomic measurements with the sizes of receptive fields suggests that the *signal convergence* from receptors to ganglion cells also increases with retinal eccentricity. From the close correlation between the diameters of the RF centers and the visual acuity at different places in the retina, one may conclude, as expected, that visual acuity (see p. 159) is correlated not only with receptor density but with the arrangement of the receptive field as well. This conclusion is supported by the change in acuity with change in mean luminance (see p. 179); in this case, too, the diameter of the receptive field centers is very closely correlated with visual acuity, whereas the receptor density is of course independent of the state of adaptation.

The responses of retinal ganglion cells to colored light stimuli. Behavioral measurements imply that the color vision of animals such as the rhesus monkey is

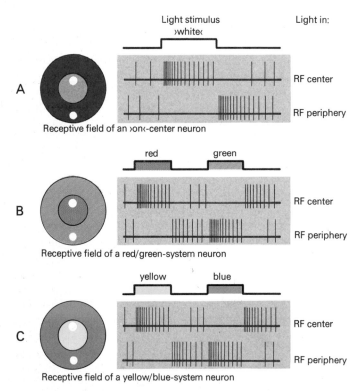

Fig. 5–30 A–C. Diagram of the spatial organization of three receptive fields in the ganglion-cell layer of the retina and in the lateral geniculate of a mammal with color vision. **A** Nerve cell in the light/dark system; **B** Nerve cell in the red/green system; **C** Nerve cell in the yellow/blue system. In the color-specific receptive fields (B and C) the center and periphery are antagonistically organized. *(B)* and *(C)* are highly schematized. There exist also nerve cells which have an opponent color RF-center but no RF-periphery.

similar to that of humans. The functional organization of the receptive fields of retinal ganglion cells in these animals, however, is more complex than the "on"-center or "off"-center pattern described above. In the light-adapted retina, as well as in the lateral geniculate body and the visual cortex of these animals (see p. 186), nerve cells can be found which have partially *color-specific* responses. Simplifying the situation somewhat, we can distinguish three classes of such cells (Fig. 5–30).

The *ganglion cells of the light/dark system* react in *qualitatively* the same way ("on"-center or "off"-center properties) regardless of the wavelength of the monochromatic light stimulus, in the visible spectrum ($\sim$ 400–700 nm). The spectral sensitivity is not different in the center than in the periphery of the receptive fields of ganglion cells in this class.

The ganglion cells of the *red/green system* have in part a color-specific antagonistic RF organization. Monochromatic light stimuli in the red region of the spectrum elicit activation in the RF center and inhibition in the periphery, whereas monochromatic stimuli in the green region of the spectrum produce the reverse responses.

The ganglion cells of the *yellow/blue system,* when the RF center is stimulated monochromatically, are activated by yellow light and inhibited by blue; conversely, in the periphery a yellow light inhibits and a blue light excites.

The retinal and geniculate neurons thus perform a transformation relevant to color vision. By way of the bipolar cells, horizontal cells and amacrines the signals from the *three different cone types* are directed so as to provide the ganglion cell layer with a neuronal system for "achromatic vision" and two color-specific, antagonistic neuron systems. The latter constitute a *four-color opponent system* with the opponent color pairs yellow/blue and red/green (p. 167).

Projections of the retina in the CNS. The optic nerves of the two eyes join at the base of the skull to form the *optic chiasm* (Fig. 5–31). In the human optic chiasm, about half of the 1 million optic nerve fibers cross to the contralateral side; the other half remain ipsilateral and, with the crossed axons of the other optic nerve, form the *optic tract.* On each side, then, about 1 million axons of retinal ganglion cells pass along the optic tract to the first central relay stations of the visual pathway — the *lateral geniculate body,* the *superior colliculus,* the *nucleus of the optic tract,* the *hypothalamus* and the *pretectal region of the brain stem.* Crossing of the nerve fibers in the chiasm is governed by a strict rule: The axons of the ganglion cells in the *temporal part* of the left retina and the *nasal part* of the right retina proceed into the left optic tract, while those from ganglion cells in the nasal part of the left eye and the temporal part of the right eye form the right optic tract (Fig. 5–31). The axons of most nerve cells in the lateral geniculate pass through the optic radiation to the primary visual cortex (area 17 or V1) in the occipital lobe of the cerebrum. This cortical region is connected to the secondary and tertiary visual regions as well as to the higher visual association regions, also located in the occipital part of the cerebral cortex or in the parietal cortex. From these visual regions there are pathways to the subcortical relay stations of the afferent visual system shown in Figure 5–31, to the regions of the brain stem responsible for

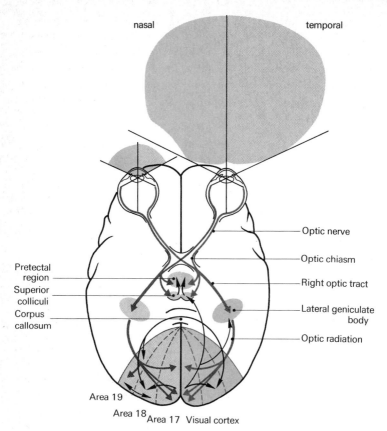

nasal   temporal

Optic nerve

Optic chiasm

Pretectal
region
Superior
colliculi
Corpus
callosum

Right optic tract

Lateral geniculate
body

Optic radiation

Area 19
Area 18 Area 17 Visual cortex

Fig. 5–31. Diagram of the visual pathway in the human brain. Some of the efferent connections between the visual cortex and subcortical structures are also shown on the *right.* The visual cortices of the left and right halves of the brain are joined by axons passing through the corpus callosum. The delimitation of area 17, 18, and 19 is very much simplified. The arrow to the pretectal region indicates several destinations of optic-nerve axons: the actual pretectal area, the nucleus of the optic tract (NOT) and the other projection regions of the accessory optic tract, and the hypothalamus

control of the eye movements (see p. 193) and to the association regions in the parietal and temporal lobes which function in speech. Visual centers of the left and right cerebral hemispheres communicate with one another by way of the corpus callosum (Fig. 5–31).

The central visual pathway is *topographically organized.* That is, just as the spatial relationships in a particular geographic region are preserved on a map of the region, the spatial pattern of excitation in the ganglion-cell layer of the retina is "mapped" onto the spatial patterns of excitation of neurons in the lateral geniculate, superior colliculus, and visual cortex. But the details of this mapping differ somewhat from the geographic standard. Whereas a map is drawn to a particular scale (e.g., a reduction of 1:100,000), so that each kilometer of horizontal distance in the natural terrain corresponds to a fixed distance on paper, the topographic projection of the retina is ***nonlinear.*** The small area of the fovea is projected onto many more central neurons than is an area of equal size in the retina periphery. This nonlinear retinotopic projection ("retino-cortical magnification factor") reflects the greater functional importance of the fovea as compared with the periphery, and the decrease in visual acuity with distance from the fovea (see p. 159).

Neural processing in the lateral geniculate body. The nerve cells of the lateral geniculate body, the first relay center between the retina and the cerebral cortex, usually have simple, concentrically organized receptive fields (as measured by stimulation of the retina by light), like those of the retinal ganglion cells. ***Binocular interaction*** between the signals from the left and right eyes is detectable here only as a slight reciprocal inhibition. In three of the six nerve-cell layers of the geniculate body one eye is "dominant", while the other eye is dominant in the other three layers. Thus signal processing in each of the two sets of three layers is primarily determined by one eye. The actual ***binocular integration of the visual information*** from the two eyes first occurs in the visual cortex. The function of the lateral geniculate is still rather unclear, despite extensive research on it. There is evidence that the lateral-inhibition processes so important in contrast discrimination (see p. 178) are especially pronounced in some of the lateral-geniculate nerve cells. And as was mentioned above, information related to color is represented in at least three different nerve-cell classes in the lateral geniculate (the light/dark, yellow/blue, and red/green systems). The excitability of the nerve cells in the lateral geniculate body changes greatly with the transition from the waking to the sleeping state. In deep sleep, signal transmission in the lateral geniculate is probably very much reduced.

The neurons of the visual cortex. Principles of receptive-field organization not found at lower levels appear in the nerve cells of the primary and secondary visual regions (V1, V2) of the occipital cortex. The arrangement typical of retinal and lateral geniculate neurons, with concentric excitatory and inhibitory areas, is found in only some of the neurons of the primary visual cortex. Other cortical visual neurons have receptive fields with "on" or "off" zones arranged in parallel (Fig. 5–32). Diffuse illumination of the entire receptive field ordinarily causes little change in the spontaneous activity of these cells. But if a "bar" of light in the "correct" orientation and position is projected into the receptive field, there is strong activation. This occurs, for example, with a bar oriented as in position C of Figure 5–32. Receptive fields with such parallel "on" and "off" zones are called "simple" receptive fields, because it is easy to establish their functional organization by projecting small spots of light onto different parts of the receptive field; that is, the response to bars is comprehensible from the response to spot stimuli.

Still other cortical visual neurons, however, have "complex" receptive fields. To activate these neurons one must project light/dark contours with specific spatial orientation and extent, interruptions of outline, corners and so forth into the

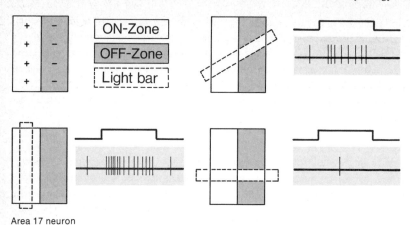

Area 17 neuron

Fig. 5–32. Organization of a "simple" receptive field of a nerve cell in the primary visual cortex. Schematized from HUBEL, WIESEL: J. Physiol. (Lond.) *160,* 106–154 (1962)

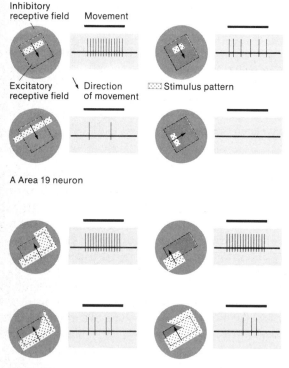

A Area 19 neuron

B Area 18 neuron

Fig. 5–33 A, B. Diagram of the responses of two neurons in the visual cortex (areas 18 and 19 of cat) with complex receptive fields. The stimulus pattern is shown by *gray stippling,* and the *arrows* indicate the direction of motion. Schematized from HUBEL, WIESEL: J. Neurophysiol. *28,* 229–289 (1965)

receptive fields. Those regions of the receptive field in which stimulation with the "correct" pattern elicits neuronal activation are together called the *excitatory receptive field* (ERF). The usual finding is that the ERF is surrounded by a region in which light/dark patterns elicit only inhibition. This region is called the *inhibitory receptive field* (IRF). Neurons with complex receptive fields usually give no response to diffuse, unstructured light stimuli projected into their receptive fields. Figure 5–33 illustrates the responses of two neurons in the visual cortex with complex receptive fields.

Many cortical neurons with complex receptive fields are much more strongly activated by *moved stimulus patterns* than by motionless patterns. Moreover, some of these visual-cortex neurons sensitive to motion require a specific *direction of motion* of the stimulus pattern. For example, a stimulus pattern with optimal spatial structure may have an excitatory effect only if it is moved through the ERF from left to right, whereas movement in the opposite direction does not activate the cell. Movement and direction sensitivity of cortical visual neurons no doubt reflect an adaptation to the fact that the image of the stationary environment is always shifting on the retina, with a continual movement of the eyes and body (see p. 190ff.). The "cerebral picture" of the stationary visual world must be derived during the brief fixation periods from retinal patterns that change with each eye movement.

Neurons of the visual cortex with complex receptive fields, as a rule, have a receptive field for each eye. These nerve cells, then, can be excited *monocularly,* by either eye alone. With *binocular* stimulation by the same patterns, the general result is greater activation *(binocular summation).* The receptive fields of a binocularly activated cortical nerve cell, imaged on regions of the left and right retinas, have only approximate geometric correspondence (see p. 169). The departures of these sites from the exactly corresponding retinal areas varies in different neurons. This disparity is such that a stimulus pattern provided binocularly is optimally activating when it is somewhat outside the horopter. This neuronal response is interpreted as a neurophysiologic correlate of binocular depth perception, discussed more extensively on pp. 167–170.

Structure and function of areas of the visual cortex. The nerve cells of the primary visual cortex, as in most regions of the cerebral cortex (neocortex), are arranged in six distinct cytoarchitectonic layers parallel to the cortical surface. In some of these, sublayers can be discerned (Fig. 5–34). The afferent axons from the lateral geniculate body end chiefly in Layer IV of the *primary visual cortex* (Area 17 or V1). Some of the neurons within this layer are excited from only one eye and inhibited by illumination of the other eye. This interaction presumably represents one of the neuronal components of binocular rivalry. But most of the other nerve cells in the visual cortex are excited by light stimuli to one eye as well as to the other (neurobiological basis of binocular fusion).

The nerve cells in Area V1 are organized not only within layers parallel to the surface but also in "columns" perpendicular to it. The receptive fields of the nerve cells in a vertical column are all in the same region of the retina (or of the field of

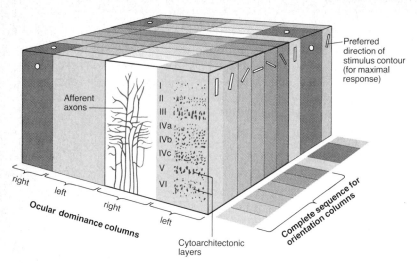

Fig. 5–34. Diagram of the "horizontal cytoarchitectonic layers" (I–VI), the "vertical" ocular-dominance columns, and the orientation columns in the visual cortex (Area 17, or V1) of the rhesus monkey [schematically redrawn from HUBEL and WIESEL (1977) and LIVINGSTON and HUBEL (1984)]. Within the ocular-dominance columns, the orientation columns are repeated in sequence; only one complete sequence is shown. Between the columns containing nerve cells that respond preferentially to contours having certain orientations within their receptive fields, there are larger regions, also columnar, containing nerve cells with no orientation preference for stimulus contours. These nerve cells respond to diffuse light; one of their functions is color-specific signal transmission. The receptive fields are concentrically organized

view). A distinction is made between *ocular-dominance columns,* within which excitation from one eye is always stronger than from the other, and *orientation columns.* The orientation columns are substructures within the ocular-dominance columns (Fig. 5–34). When cortical neurons are tested with contours oriented in various directions, to see which produces the greatest excitation, one finds a progressive change in optimal orientation across adjacent columns. Between the orientation columns are larger regions within which the receptive fields of the nerve cells have no detectable orientation-specificity. These nerve cells, however, are very often color-specific. This functional cytoarchitecture of Area V1 indicates a spatial distribution of signal processing according to the different qualities of vision (color, orientation of contours).

Visual regions of the cerebral cortex other than Area V1. Systematic microelectrode exploration of the occipital, occipitoparietal, and temporal parts of the cerebral cortex of the rhesus monkey in recent years has shown that visual signal processing occurs in extensive regions of the cerebrum (Fig. 5–35). This finding is consistent with clinical observations in humans. Adjacent to the anterior edge of the primary visual cortex (V1) are large visual areas with a regular, "retinotopic" representation of the retina similar to that in Area V1. Some of the nerve cells in these areas (V2, V3 and V4) respond very selectively to certain stimulus features

A   B

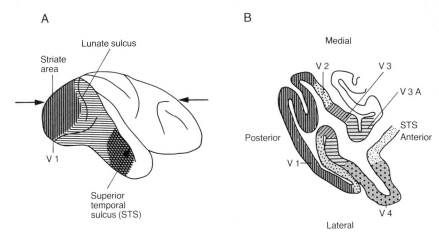

Fig. 5–35. A The distribution of the visual areas in the cerebral cortex of a rhesus monkey. Area V1 (or 17) occupies a large part of the outer occipital surface. The horizontally hatched region comprises the parts of the visual cortical areas V2, V3, V4 and STS that are visible on the surface. In these visual areas there is a regular retinocortical projection ("retinotopic" representation), which is not present in the visual regions of the inferior temporal gyrus (cross-hatching). The latter contain nerve cells responsive only to very complex visual stimuli. For example, in the depths of the superior temporal sulcus, near the tip of the pointer, there are cells that respond preferentially to faces or face-like configurations. *B* Horizontal cross section through the occipital cortex of the rhesus monkey at the level of the arrow in *(A)*. The various cortical areas are identified by different symbols. Modified from S. ZEKI, Nature *274,* 423–428 (1978)]. STS: cortex region in the vicinity of the superior temporal sulcus

— contours or movement (V2), particular color signals (V4), or movement including motion along the "Z axis" (i. e., toward or away from the head; STS region). Nerve cells in the part of the inferior temporal gyrus that is doubly shaded in Figure 5–35 respond to considerably more complex visual patterns. In these regions there is no retinotopic organization. A region deep in the superior temporal sulcus contains nerve cells responsive only to faces or stimulus configurations that resemble faces.

Neuronal bases of form perception. The formal properties of a shape that is seen — its contours, corners and interruptions of contour — are each detected by different classes of nerve cells in the primary (V1) and secondary (V2) visual cortex. These cortical visual neurons have "complex" receptive fields and respond preferentially to interrupted contours in certain orientations, to edges, and to corners, especially when these stimuli are moved in a certain direction. The movement-sensitivity of many visual neurons is presumably an adaptation to the necessity of "reconstructing", by neuronal means, a picture of the stationary world from a sequence of optical images of this world that are shifted on the retina. Altogether at least 15 classes of neurons, each optimally activated by a different stimulus feature, have been found in the primary and secondary visual cortices; these are distributed in each case over the entire cortical projection region of the visual field. By recording in succession from a great many different nerve cells in the visual cortex, one can reconstruct the spatial pattern of excitation that exists at one instant in the neurons of a single cortical class, exposed to a particular visual stimulus pattern. Figure 5–36 illustrates a simplified attempt at such reconstruction. The spatial patterns of excitation in the various neuron classes reflect various features of the stimulus pattern. Because the projection of the retina onto the visual cortex is nonlinear, the spatial distribution of excitation in the many thousand nerve cells of a neuron class is not as simple as Figure 5–36 implies. This diagram is meant simply to make clear the simultaneous, multiple representations of a single visual image that can occur in patterns of excitation of different neuron classes of the visual cortex. It may also give the reader an impression of the complexity of processing that confronts the neurophysiologist studying single nerve cells in the mammalian visual cortex. The neuronal mechanisms extracting form from the multiple representations of visual information in cortical excitation patterns are still entirely obscure. But from observations of patients in whom visual

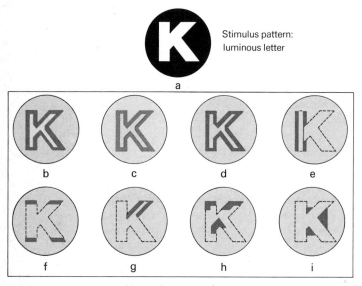

Stimulus pattern:
luminous letter

a

Neuronal representations

Fig. 5–36. Diagram of the processes of excitation elicited by a luminous letter *K* in various neuronal layers of the retina and the central visual system. (a) The image of the letter on the retina and the spatial pattern of excitation in the receptor layer of the retina. (b and c) Pattern of excitation in the output layer of the retina (the ganglion cells). In (b) through (i) the excitation is indicated by *red bars.* (b) "On"-center neurons. (c) "Off"-center neurons. (d) Pattern of excitation in the neuronal layers of the lateral geniculate body and some of the neurons of the visual cortex. The contours of the luminous letter produce excitation in the nerve cells. (e–i) Pattern of excitation in various neuronal layers of different nerve-cell classes in the primary, secondary, and tertiary visual cortices of the brain. The nerve cells here are excited only by contours with particular orientations, angles, or interruptions of outline. The illustration greatly simplifies the neurobiological relationships; the spatial distribution of excitation in the various nerve-cell layers of the cortex is not linearly related to the extent of the stimulus pattern

form and object perception is impaired (those with *visual agnosia*), it is known that these functions require not only the visual projection fields of the occipital cerebral cortex, but also the higher association regions in the parietal cortex.

Q 5.13. Which of the following statements apply to the receptor potentials of single cones in the vertebrate retina?
a) Under illumination a depolarizing receptor potential is formed.
b) Under illumination a hyperpolarizing receptor potential is formed.
c) Under illumination the membrane potential of the receptor does not change.
d) The receptor potential has nothing to do with ion movements through the membrane.
e) There is a linear relationship between the amplitude of the receptor potential and the stimulus intensity.
f) There is an approximately logarithmic relationship over 2–3 $\log_{10}$ units between the amplitude of the receptor and the stimulus intensity.

Q 5.14. Which of the following statements apply to rhodopsin (R)?
a) R consists of opsin and retinene.
b) R consists of γ-globulin and vitamin A.
c) R is identical with the visual pigment in the cones.
d) The concentration of R increases in the rods during dark adaptation.
e) The concentration of R decreases in the rods during dark adaptation.
f) A solution of R looks red, but becomes colorless after illumination.

Q 5.15. Complete the following sentences correctly: The "on"-center neurons of the retina (ganglion cells) respond to illumination of the RF center with (activation/inhibition), whereas darkening of the RF center leads to (activation/inhibition). Illumination of the RF periphery of the "on"-center neurons elicits (activation/inhibition), and darkening elicits (activation/inhibition). RF center and RF periphery are therefore function-ally . . . . organized. As the mean intensity of light falling on the retina is increased, the diameter of the RF center becomes (larger/smaller).

Q 5.16. Which of the following are correct?
The receptive fields of ganglion cells in the mammalian retina:
a) Are smaller in the foveal region than in the periphery of the retina
b) Are equal in size, on the average, over the whole retina
c) Can be subdivided into a functionally distinct center and surround, in light-adapted conditions
d) Are found only in neurons of the fovea
e) Are in some cases antagonistically organized with regard to spectral sensitivity
f) Are no larger than the receptive fields of a single photoreceptor

Q 5.17. Knowing the organization of the receptive fields of the nerve cells in the visual cortex, we can understand why the following properties of visual stimulus patterns are particularly important in form perception:
a) Mean luminance
b) Contours
c) Interruptions in outline
d) Colors
e) The fact that the image of the environment is reversed on the retina

5.4 Eye Movements and Sensorimotor Integration in Vision

In the preceding discussions of the various aspects of vision, the crucial role of *eye movements* in perception of the visual environment has not been taken properly into account. To understand the significance of sensorimotor integration during visual perception, one must know of the neuronal mechanisms by which eye movements are controlled. These, then, will be the first topic.

The human eye is moved by *six external eye muscles* (Fig. 5–37; cf. textbooks of anatomy). These muscles can operate in coordination according to quite different programs. Because the eye occupies its orbit like a ball in a socket, it can be moved to a wide range of angles — a prerequisite for the various programs directing the gaze. With respect to the coordinates of the head, the eye can make *horizontal, vertical, or rotational* (in the frontoparallel plane) movements. The latter are restricted to 5°–10°, whereas vertical and horizontal movements can move the visual axis (see p. 148) almost to the edges of the orbit. When vertical and horizontal movements are combined the eye moves diagonally, in directions that can be set at will by appropriate activation of the external eye muscles.

Conjugate eye movements; vergence. When a human with normal binocular vision glances about, his eyes move in such a well-coordinated way that the object being

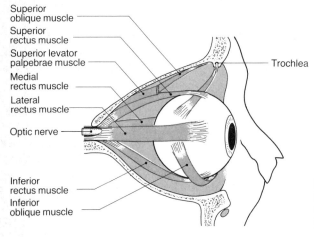

Superior oblique muscle
Superior rectus muscle
Superior levator palpebrae muscle
Medial rectus muscle
Lateral rectus muscle
Optic nerve
Inferior rectus muscle
Inferior oblique muscle
Trochlea

Fig. 5–37. Arrangement of the external eye muscles and of the eye in the orbit (diagrammatic)

fixated at any time (more precisely, a point on the object) is imaged in the *center of the fovea* of each eye. Closer observation of the movements of the two eyes shows that two "programs" can be distinguished. First, the eyes can be moved together upward, downward, to the left, or to the right. The two eyes move in the same direction with respect to the coordinates of the head. These binocular eye movements are called *conjugate eye movements.*

On the other hand, if the subject looks alternately at close and more distant objects, the two eyes carry out approximately mirror-image movements with respect to the head coordinates. During such *vergence movements,* the angle between the visual axes of the eyes changes. When a distant point is fixated, the visual axes are nearly parallel. If the gaze is then shifted to a nearby point, the visual axes converge *(convergence movements).* During subsequent refixation of a distant object the axes of the two eyes move apart, by *divergence movements,* until they are again nearly parallel. Vergence and conjugate movements can occur together — for example, when the gaze is shifted from a far-away object on the right to a nearby object on the left.

Rotational movements of the eyes in the frontoparallel plane are also binocularly coordinated. A slight "compensatory rolling" of the eyes occurs, for example, when the head is tilted to the side (see p. 232).

Dynamics of eye movement. When you look about casually, your eyes move from one fixation point to the next in quick flicks *(saccades).* The amplitude of the saccades can be only a few minutes of arc *(microsaccades)* or many degrees; large saccades, for instance, accompany a change of fixation point from the right to the left half of the visual field. The duration of the saccades varies between about 10 and 80 ms. The larger saccades normally occur along with supplementary head movements. Between the saccades are *fixation periods* lasting ordinarily between 150 and 400 ms.

When one is paying attention to a *moving object,* the eyes follow it with slow *pursuit movements* if its velocity is not too great. At speeds less than about 50°/s the angular velocity of the eyes corresponds approximately to that of the moving object. The function of the slow tracking movements is to keep the images of the moving object in the middle of the foveas — at the position where visual acuity is greatest. If the angular velocity of the moving object is greater than about 50°/s, the eyes do not keep up with the object; in such cases, when the object is not imaged at a fixed point on the retina by means of smooth pursuit gaze movements, correcting saccades are also employed in object tracking.

Pursuit movements, saccades, and fixation periods are various forms of eye control dependent on various "programs" in the oculomotor system of the brain stem. During fairly long periods of voluntary fixation (0.5–2 s in duration) slow, low-amplitude "drifts" of the fixation point occur. Even during the "best" fixation there is a superimposed *"microtremor"* of the eyes, movements of very small amplitude (1–3 min of arc) with dominant frequency components between 20 and 150 Hz.

The eye movements of binocular fixation. During conjugate and vergence movements, the oculomotor systems controlling movement of the two eyes are subordinated to a neuronal program coordinating the simultaneous movement. When this gaze control system fails to bring the visual axes of the two eyes to the same point, "squinting" or *strabismus* results, and the images formed on the foveas of the two eyes differ (see p. 168). As was discussed in Section 5.2, disturbing *double vision* can then occur. The gaze control mechanisms govern the relationship between excitation and inhibition in the oculomotor motoneurons of the brain stem and these, in turn, determine the relative contraction of the external eye muscles.

Figure 5–38 is a highly schematic diagram of the neuronal system by which horizontal eye movements are accomplished. The "centers" for binocular gaze control are in the region of the pontine and mesencephalic *reticular formation* of the brain stem, in the *superior colliculi* and in the *pretectal region.* Microelectrode recordings from the brain stem reticular formation have revealed that horizontal eye movements are controlled by the prepontine reticular formation (PPRF), and vertical eye movements by the mesencephalic reticular formation (MRF).

The *brain-stem centers controlling binocular movements* are themselves controlled by inputs from the visual cortex and the "frontal eye field" of the cerebral cortex. These neuronal connections are important with respect to the correlations between visual stimulus patterns and the scanning movements of the eyes (as discussed below) and to the guidance of pursuit movements. The nerve cells in the *superior colliculi* and the *pretectal region* receive both indirect visual afferents, via the cortex, and direct visual afferents from the eye by way of collaterals from some of the axons in the optic nerve (Fig. 5–31).

Figure 5–38 also indicates the connections of the *organs of equilibrium* (the labyrinths) to the brain-stem centers for monocular and binocular movement. These connections are primarily concerned with the reflex change in eye position elicited by change of the position of the head. But as a rule, in the waking human, the *oculomotor reflexes* elicited by excitation of the labyrinths are obscured by other neural commands controlling eye movements. Labyrinthine oculomotor reflexes are important chiefly in "holding" a fixation point when the head is moved suddenly. But the receptors in the labyrinth can be artificially or pathologically excited to such an extent that *vestibular excitation* becomes the sole determinant of eye movement. Under such conditions *vestibular nystagmus* and the associated *dizziness* (vertigo), discussed on p. 235, appear.

Precise control of the extent of eye movements — particularly in the case of slow pursuit movements, though the precision of the saccades is also affected to some degree — requires that the *cerebellum* be intact. In the cerebellum, the flocculus and paraflocculus in particular, vestibular and visual signals are processed in conjunction with signals reflecting eye and head position. The result of this analysis is passed on to the brain-stem centers controlling binocular movement, by way of cerebellar efferents.

Everyday experience tells us that eye movements can be indicators of the "internal psychological state". Attentiveness, tiredness, interest, fear, and indif-

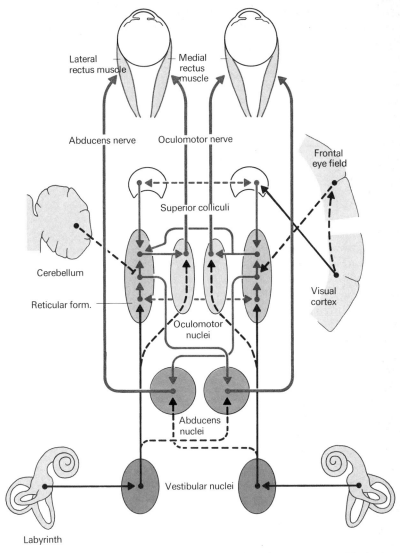

Fig. 5–38. Diagram of the subcortical centers for control of horizontal eye movements. For further explanation see text

ference can all change the frequency and amplitude of the saccades. This influence of the emotions upon eye movements is presumably mediated by the "nonspecific" neuron systems of the reticular formation, which in turn are affected by the "limbic system" (cf. **Fundamentals of Neurophysiology,** Chap. 8).

A simple and frequently used method of **measuring eye movements,** and one which is helpful in diagnosis, is **electrooculography.** This takes advantage of the

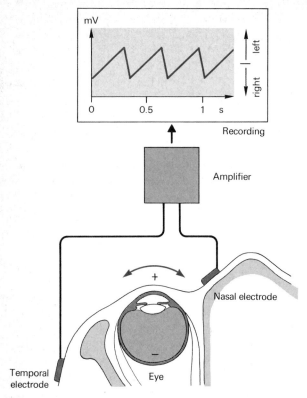

Fig. 5–39. Diagram showing the electrode positions for electrooculography and the recorded electrooculogram of optokinetic nystagmus

fact that there is a voltage difference between the cornea and retina of each eye — the **corneoretinal standing potential.** That is, the eye is an electrical dipole, the cornea being positive with respect to the retina (Fig. 5–39). The recording electrodes are attached with an adhesive paste to the skin over the bony rim of the eye socket, above and below the eye as well as nasal and temporal to it. When the anterior pole of the eye moves toward one of the electrodes, a voltage difference is created between the corresponding electrode pair, because the eye movement changes the direction of the axis of the electrical dipole. The voltage recorded by each pair of electrodes is approximately proportional to the displacement of the eye in the orbit. The electrooculogram can thus monitor the position of an eye relative to the coordinates of the head.

Eye movements and visual perception; nystagmus. First consider just horizontal eye movements. Figure 5–40 shows an electrooculogram recorded while a subject read texts differing in degree of difficulty. In this recording, movement of the eyes to the right causes an upward deflection of the trace, while movement to the left

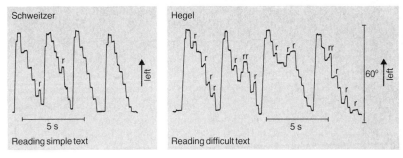

Fig. 5–40. Eye movements during reading of two texts varying in difficulty. The lines are sampled by 5 to 7 saccades, each followed by a period of fixation. In addition to the large backward saccades at the ends of the lines, there are smaller reverse saccades (r) during the lines, depending on the difficulty of the text; the reader does not ordinarily notice them. Texts: Albert Schweitzer, „Aus meiner Kindheit und Jugendzeit"; G. F. HEGEL, „Einführung in die Philosophie". Modified from GHAZARIAN and GRÜSSER (1977)]

deflects the trace downward. It is evident that during "uniform" reading, "silently" or aloud, the eyes move in quick *saccades,* with brief periods of *fixation between the saccades.* When the fixation point reaches the end of a line, it jumps to the beginning of the next line in a *single* saccade. Depending on their amplitude, saccades last between 10 and 80 ms; the average angular velocity of the eye during the saccades is between 50°/s and 600°/s. Unconscious backward saccades occur more often when the text is hard to understand.

A cyclic alternation between saccades and slow pursuit movements can occur while watching a moved stimulus pattern. When you look at the scenery through the side window of a moving automobile or train, your eyes alternate between conjugate slow horizontal movements and rapid saccades. During the slow *pursuit movements* the image of the fixated object is kept in the region of the fovea. That is, the tracking movement follows the relative movement of the object. This alternation between saccades and slow pursuit movements is called *nystagmus.* The example just described is *optokinetic nystagmus* ("railroad nystagmus"), so called because the nystagmus is elicited by moved optical stimulus patterns.

Optokinetic nystagmus can conveniently be induced in a subject reading the numbers of a measuring tape of the kind used in sewing, which is moved horizontally or vertically by the experimenter. By convention, the *direction of nystagmus* is considered to be that of the *rapid phase* (the saccades). Thus if the tape moves to the right, from the subject's point of view, a "left optokinetic nystagmus" results — slow tracking movements to the right are followed by saccades to the left that reset the eye's position and allow it to pick up a new fixation point. A stimulus commonly used for more precise analysis of optokinetic nystagmus is a pattern of horizontally or vertically moved light and dark stripes, projected on the inside of a hemicylinder.

Eye movements during normal viewing. When we casually observe a well-structured environment, saccades and periods of fixation alternate. The eye movements may be in any direction. A two-dimensional record of the sequential fixation positions of a subject examining a complex visual pattern is shown in Figure 5–41. Clearly, the eye movements tend to be determined by the contours, interruptions of contour, or places where two contours meet in the visual pattern. If the pattern is a human face, the eyes and mouth are fixated particularly often, and the right side of the face is preferred. Thus binocular fixation is controlled not only by the structure of the stimulus pattern, but also by the *significance* of its components. When a visual stimulus pattern is examined for some time, it is roughly reproduced, as a "movement image", in the record of the scanning movements of the eyes. The frequency of fixation characterizes the "conspicuousness" of certain substructures in the pattern. Psychologists involved in advertising have taken advantage of this finding, using measurement of eye movement to determine which visual structures in pictorial advertisements most "catch the eye", with the aim of increasing the effectiveness of the display.

Saccades shift the fixation point within the field of view; during the brief intervening fixation periods the visual signal is detected. During the rapid saccadic movement of the image over the retina, it is not perceived. There are various reasons for this. If the fixation point moves across a highly structured pattern during a saccade, the temporal fluctuations of intensity at each spot on the retina are usually far above the flicker fusion frequency (see p. 162). Thus the signal at the retina during a saccade corresponds quite closely to a brief "gray stimulus". A second factor, however, appears to be an active central inhibitory mechanism, whereby motion perception is suppressed during the saccades. In interpreting this phenomenon one must assume that the higher visual levels receive some feedback signals from the brain stem or cortical centers controlling eye movements. You can observe the inhibition of movement perception in yourself by the following simple experiment. Look at your eye in a mirror, and shift your gaze back and forth between the inside and outside edges of the orbits. You will probably detect no

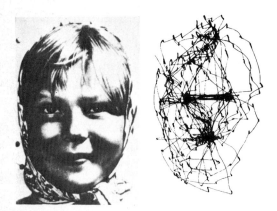

Fig. 5–41. Two-dimensional charting of the eye movements during viewing of a face. A subject looked at the photograph on the left for several minutes. Modified from Yarbus (1965)

movement of your eye. Now repeat this experiment with a second subject, watching the movements of one of his eyes in the mirror while he looks back and forth between his orbital edges. You will see his eye movements quite distinctly.

Coordination of eye movements and visual perception is mediated primarily by the connections between the visual cortex and the brain-stem regions governing binocular fixation. In Section 5.3 it was mentioned that some of the nerve cells in the visual cortex have *complex* receptive fields. For nerve cells in the secondary and tertiary visual cortices the most effective stimuli are *contours, interruptions of contour, and junctions of contour.* It seems highly likely, then, that these nerve cells control the scanning movements of the eyes, by way of their connections to the subcortical gaze control centers, in particular the superior colliculi. That scanning movements are also dependent on higher associative regions of the brain, however, is indicated by the relationship between eye movements and text during reading. When one reads, visual information is received only during the fixation periods. Preferred fixation points are the beginning of a line and the beginning of a word, the latter especially in the case of capitalized words. A long word may be fixated at several points. However, the probability of fixation is determined not only by this *physical structure* of the text, but by the *meaning* of the words it contains. Within a fairly long text, the same sequence of words can acquire different "fixation loci" when its meaning changes with the context. This observation implies that during reading the sensory speech area in the upper temporal gyrus of the cortex (Wernicke's region) also influences the movements of the eyes.

The triggering of eye movements by moving stimuli in the peripheral visual field. When a moving object appears suddenly in the periphery of the visual field, it induces a "reflex" saccade which may be accompanied by a head movement. Saccade and head movement are coordinated in such a way that the image of the "new" object is brought to the fovea centralis. This reflex is controlled by *movement-sensitive* neurons in the visual cortex and the superior colliculi. On the whole, the "conspicuousness" of moving objects in the visual-field periphery is greater than in the fovea. These reflex saccades are associated with a *redirection of attention* to the new object. The mechanism just described amounts to a biologically plausible *adaptation,* of value to early mammals and prehistoric man. The enhanced movement-sensitivity in the periphery of the visual field, and the reflex shifting of attention and direction of gaze, facilitate the recognition of a suddenly appearing moving visual stimulus — prey or predator, for example. Coincidentally, enhanced peripheral sensitivity is most useful under modern traffic conditions; it helps a driver or pedestrian to react appropriately to the unexpected appearance of a car at the edge of his field of view. Even today, then, a phylogenetically ancient mechanism continues to increase the probability of survival.

Q 5.18. Saccades are:
   a) Flicks of the eyes
   b) Slow tracking movements of the eyes

c) Rotational oscillations of the eyes
d) None of the above is correct.

Q 5.19. Which of the following records of electrical activity gives a measure of eye movement?
a) Electrocardiogram
b) Electroretinogram
c) Electrooculogram
d) Electroencephalogram
e) Electronystagmogram

Q 5.20. When a person looks at a picture the eye movements are:
a) Statistically random
b) Dependent on the colors in the picture
c) Dependent on the contours and their interruptions
d) Usually coordinated in the two eyes
e) Independent in the two eyes, but dependent on certain properties of the picture

Q 5.21. When you look at the scenery through the side window of a train moving at a steady speed, your eyes perform:
a) Jerky convergence movements
b) Optokinetic nystagmus
c) Labyrinth-induced movements
d) Irregular movements independent of the direction of movement of the train
e) None of the above is correct.

6 Physiology of Hearing

R. Klinke

The sense of hearing is fundamental in human life; hearing and speech together offer the most important means of communication among people, and are the basis of complex social interactions. It is not surprising, then, that loss of hearing can result in severe behavioral disturbance.

Men must have known since their early history that the ear is involved in the process of hearing. But it was not until the 17th century that the system of cavities buried in the mass of bone at the base of the skull was first suspected as the seat of audition. This system, the labyrinth, was eventually shown to be the organ of hearing, at the beginning of the 19th century. In the second half of that century a number of scientists turned their attention to the physiology of hearing and the problems of physical acoustics. The contributions of HELMHOLTZ are particularly notable, and his name is often heard even today. Nevertheless, many problems remained; some of them have been solved in this century, but many fundamental aspects of auditory physiology are still unclarified.

6.1 Anatomy of the Ear

An understanding of the physiology of audition requires some familiarity with the structure of the receptive apparatus. A brief review is given below, but this is not intended to be comprehensive. It is strongly suggested that the reader refers in addition to textbooks of anatomy.

The organ of hearing consists of the outer, middle, and inner ear (Fig 6–1). The *meatus,* the passage joining the first two of these, is closed at its inner end by the *eardrum,* or *tympanum.* This is thin membrane which has, in the healthy state, a mother-of-pearl sheen that provides the physician with a valuable diagnostic criterion. Behind the eardrum is the air-filled *cavity of the middle ear.* This space is connected to the pharynx (the throat) by a narrow passage called the Eustachian tube; when one swallows there is some exchange of air between throat and middle ear. Changes in external air pressure, like those experienced in air travel, cause an unpleasant feeling of "pressure in the ears". This is due to stretching of the eardrum because of the pressure difference between the atmosphere and the middle-ear cavity. Swallowing, which opens the Eustachian tubes, permits equilibration of pressures on the two sides of the eardrum.

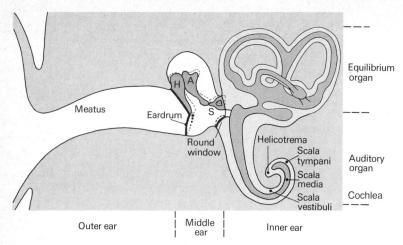

Fig. 6–1. Diagram of the outer, middle, and inner ear, greatly simplified. *H*, hammer; *A*, anvil; *S*, stirrup. The **dashed outlines** near *H*, *A*, and *S* show the extreme positions to which they can be driven as the eardrum oscillates

There are three little bones, the **ossicles,** in the middle ear; these are called the **hammer, anvil,** and **stirrup** (or the Latin equivalents, malleus, incus, and stapes). They are connected flexibly so as to form a structure like a chain. One of the processes of the hammer is fused to the eardrum. When the eardrum is moved by vibration in the air it transmits this motion to the chain of ossicles. The stirrup actually does resemble a stirrup, with its foot plate set into an opening in the bone called the **oval window.** The foot plate of the stirrup marks the boundary between the middle ear cavity and the third part of the auditory organ, the **inner ear.** The ossicular chain thus forms a bridge from eardrum to oval window — from the air to the inner ear. It is over this path that sound energy reaches the inner ear, which (as we shall now see) houses the sensory cells.

The **inner ear** lies within the temporal bone; it is in direct communication with the organ of equilibrium (cf. Fig. 6–1). The two organs together are called the labyrinth. Because of its shape, the inner ear is also called the **cochlea** (from the Latin for "snail" — it is shown partially uncurled in the drawing). We shall return to the equilibrium organ in the next chapter. The cochlea comprises three tubular canals running parallel to one another; these are coiled together to form a helical structure. Figure 6–2 shows a section through the axis of the helix, so that the canals wound around it are cut at several places. These canals are called the **scala vestibuli, scala media** or **cochlear duct,** and **scala tympani.** The human cochlea has about two and a half such helical turns. Its general arrangement can be seen in Figure 6–1; this simplified drawing shows only ca. one turn of the helix. The foot plate of the stapes at the oval window adjoins the scala vestibuli, which is filled (like the other canals) with fluid. Scala vestibuli and scala tympani contain the so-called **perilymph,** whereas the cochlear duct contains **endolymph.** The two fluids

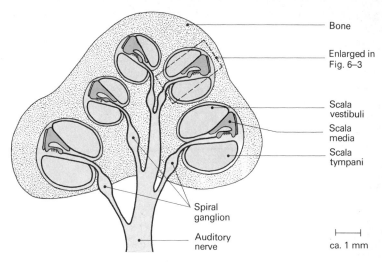

Bone

Enlarged in
Fig. 6–3

Scala
vestibuli

Scala
media

Scala
tympani

Spiral
ganglion

Auditory
nerve

ca. 1 mm

Fig. 6–2. Highly schematic section through the human cochlea, cutting several times through the helically coiled canals. The region within the ***dashed box*** is shown in more detail in Fig. 6–3

differ in chemical composition. The perilymph contains much Na^+, about the same concentration as the extracellular fluid, while the endolymph is rich in potassium, as is intracellular fluid. Scala vestibuli and scala tympani join at the ***helicotrema,*** the tip of the helix. At the base of the cochlea the two canals are separated from the middle ear cavity by rather similar structures. The oval window to the scala vestibuli is closed off by the stapes, with an ***annular ligament*** sealing the edges of the opening, while in the ***round window*** at the end of the scala tympani is a fine membrane, separating it from the middle ear cavity so that no perilymph can leak out into the middle ear.

Part of Figure 6–2 is shown in more detail in Figure 6–3. Here it can be seen that the boundary between scala vestibuli and cochlear duct is formed by a membrane called the ***vestibular*** (or ***Reissner's***) ***membrane.*** The boundary between cochlear duct and scala tympani is the ***basilar membrane,*** which bears the actual sensory apparatus, the ***organ of Corti.*** Within the organ of Corti, embedded in supporting cells, are the receptor cells. These are called ***hair cells*** because of their submicroscopic hairlike processes, the ***stereocilia. Inner*** and ***outer*** hair cells can be distinguished. The outer hair cells are arranged in three rows, whereas there is only one row of inner hair cells. Thus there are considerably more outer than inner hair cells.

Above the organ of Corti is a gelatinous mass, the ***tectorial membrane.*** This membrane is attached to the inner side of the cochlea, near the axis of the helix. It also touches the cilia of the hair cells, making relatively firm contact. This is certain at least in the case of the outer hair cells. Along the outer side of the cochlear duct is a region where blood vessels are concentrated, the ***stria vascularis.*** This structure plays a major role with regard to the energy requirements of the cochlea; in

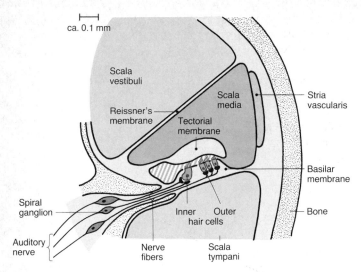

Fig. 6–3. Diagram of a cross section through one turn of the cochlea. The organ of Corti, on the basilar membrane, contains the receptor cells (hair cells). These are covered by the tectorial membrane

addition to its other functions, it maintains the high K$^+$ concentration of the endolymph.

The receptor cells in the organ of Corti are secondary sensory cells — that is, they do not have axons. The fibers which transmit excitation centrally from this organ have cell bodies in the ***spiral ganglion,*** which lies in the cochlea, coiled about its axis along with the canals (Fig. 6–2).

The nerve cells in this ganglion are ***bipolar cells.*** That is, they have two processes, one of which runs to the periphery, to the hair cells of the organ of Corti, while the other passes to the CNS in the ***auditory nerve.*** Inner and outer hair cells are innervated differently. Each ***inner hair cell*** synapses with many afferent nerve fibers, each of which probably makes contact with that hair cell alone. By contrast, the nerve fibers serving the ***outer hair cells*** are highly branched, each receiving synaptic input from many outer hair cells. Thus even though there are more outer hair cells, the majority of the fibers in the auditory nerve (the cochlear branch of the vestibulocochlear nerve) come from the inner hair cells.

Q 6.1.   Arrange the following structures in order from the air to the inner ear.
a) Hammer
b) Eardrum
c) Stapes
d) Anvil

Q 6.2.   Scala vestibuli and cochlear duct:
a) Are joined at the helicotrema

b) Are joined at the oval window
c) Are joined at the round window
d) Are not connected

Q 6.3. The organ of Corti is on:
a) The vestibular (Reissner's) membrane
b) The tectorial membrane
c) The basilar membrane
d) The tympanic membrane
e) The stria vascularis

Q 6.4. The stria vascularis plays a major role in:
a) Energy supply to the inner ear
b) Compensating movements of the stapes
c) Maintaining the ionic milieu in the endolymph
d) The production of perilymph
e) The resorption of perilymph

Q 6.5. The endolymph is rich in:
a) K^+
b) Na^+
and therefore resembles:
c) Intracellular fluid
d) Extracellular fluid
The situation in the perilymph is:
e) The same
f) Opposite

6.2 Human Auditory Performance

Physical properties of sound stimuli. An oscillating body, such as a tuning fork or the membrane of a loudspeaker, sets the surrounding air in oscillation by accelerating the air molecules in its immediate vicinity. These in turn transmit energy to the more distant surroundings so that there, too, the air molecules oscillate. These disturbances therefore spread out from the source in waves, with a velocity (in air) of ca. 340 m/s. This phenomenon is called *sound,* though to be precise one should say "airborne sound".

In water, for example, sound is propagated at a speed more than four times that in air. Oscillations are propagated by similar physical interactions within solid bodies (as in earthquakes, for example) but most biologists tend to distinguish the many forms of such "vibrations" from airborne "sound". Figure 6–4 illustrates the spatial distribution of pressure in a simple sound wave at a single instant of time; zones of increased pressure (greater density of air molecules) alternate with zones

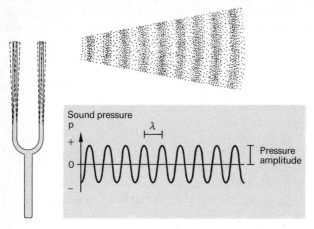

Fig. 6–4. Diagram of the state of part of the sound field around an oscillating tuning fork, at a single instant of time

of reduced pressure. A short time later, this entire series of waves would be seen displaced somewhat to the right. Thus it is this waveform and the energy associated with it that is propagated over long distances, not the air molecules. The motion of the latter is actually forward and backward (in accordance with the locally changing pressure gradients) along the direction of propagation; this is the reason sound waves are referred to as **longitudinal** waves (as opposed to the transverse waves that propagate along a string or a water surface).

The amplitude of the periodic pressure fluctuations (Fig. 6–4) is called the **sound pressure;** it can be measured with a microphone and used to describe the sound. Like any pressure, sound pressure has units of newtons per square meter. The range of sound pressures affecting the auditory system is so great, however, that it is more convenient, in fact a universal practice in acoustics, to use a logarithmic scale, the so-called **sound pressure level.** This is set up by adopting the arbitrary reference pressure level $p_0 = 2 \cdot 10^{-5}$ N/m^2 (which is near the threshold for hearing). The sound pressure level (L) of a given sound pressure p is then defined by the equation

$$L = 20 \log_{10} \frac{p}{p_0} \tag{6–1}$$

and the resulting units of L are called decibels (dB). Thus for a pressure level p equal to p_0, $L = 0$ dB. The "20" has a simple explanation: the log of ratio of sound power was originally called a "bel" (in honor of Alexander Graham Bell), in which there are of course 10 dB; but a decibel scale reflecting pressure is of more interest. Power is proportional to the pressure amplitude squared, and $\log p^2 = 2 \log p$; thus, $2 \cdot 10 = 20$.

As a sample calculation, to determine the sound pressure level of a tone with sound pressure $p = 2 \cdot 10^{-2}$ N/m² we proceed as follows:

$$\frac{p}{p_0} = \frac{2 \cdot 10^{-2}}{2 \cdot 10^{-5}} = 10^3$$

$$L = 20 \cdot \log_{10}(10^3) = 20 \cdot 3 = 60 \text{ dB}$$

That is, a sound pressure of $2 \cdot 10^{-2}$ N/m² corresponds to a sound pressure level of 60 dB. The left ordinate of Figure 6–6 gives values of sound pressure and the corresponding sound pressure levels.

Because other quantities — for example, voltages — are also sometimes expressed on a similar decibel scale, sound pressure levels (SPL) are often given as *decibels SPL.* This notation specifies that the numbers were obtained by the above definition, with reference pressure $p_0 = 2 \cdot 10^{-5}$ N/m².

A second parameter of sound, the frequency, is expressed in cycles per second, or *hertz* (in honor of the 19th-century German physicist H. R. HERTZ; abbreviated Hz). Since the velocity of propagation is determined by the medium, higher-frequency sounds have shorter wavelengths (cf. Fig. 6–4). In fact, frequency f, sound velocity c, and wavelength λ (lambda) are related as follows:

$$c = f \cdot \lambda \tag{6–2}$$

A sound characterized by only one frequency (for example, 2000 Hz) is called a *tone* (Fig. 6–5A). In everyday life, however, pure tones practically never exist. Ordinary sounds, from the most musical to the most noisy, almost always contain many frequencies. The sounds we consider musical comprise a limited number of frequencies, in general a fundamental tone with several harmonics (Fig. 6–5B). The fundamental determines the "repeat period" of the complex sound-pressure fluctuations (*T* in Fig. 6–5B). Harmonics are overtones at frequencies which are integral multiples of the fundamental frequency. Nearly pure tones can be obtained from various devices, but the "tones" produced by musical instruments contain harmonics. The different instruments vary in the number and relative

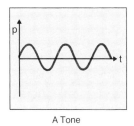

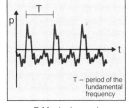

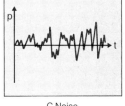

A Tone   B Musical sound   C Noise

Fig. 6–5. Plots of sound pressure versus time, for a pure tone (A), a musical sound (B), and noise (C).

intensity of the overtones accompanying a single fundamental. Some instruments cannot produce certain overtones; for example, the sound produced by closed organ pipes include only the odd harmonics, the frequencies f_0, $3f_0$, $5f_0$ and so on. It is such peculiarities of frequency spectrum that give rise to the variety of sounds in an orchestra. If a sound includes very many frequencies, it is "noisy", and if all frequencies are present at equal intensities the sound is called *white noise.* Other noises have different frequency spectra, but it is characteristic of all such sounds that records of the temporal variations in sound pressure reveal no obvious periodicity (Fig. 6–5C).

The occurrence of sound and the subjective sensation of hearing. Everyday experience shows that there are limits to our auditory abilities. That is, a certain sound pressure must be exceeded if a sound is to be perceptible to the human ear. The sound pressure at which a tone is just audible is called the *auditory threshold.* Its magnitude depends upon the frequency of the test tone. The bottom curve in Figure 6–6 shows the variation of auditory threshold with frequency, and indicates that the ear is most sensitive in the range 2000–5000 Hz. At these frequencies the threshold is exceeded at remarkably low sound pressure. At higher and lower frequencies, higher sound pressures are required.

As sound pressure is increased above the threshold level a tone is perceived as becoming steadily louder, regardless of its frequency. A clear distinction must be

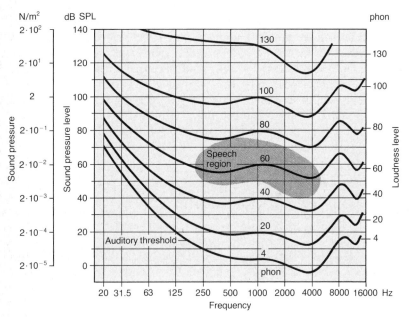

Fig. 6–6. Curves of equal loudness level. On the left ordinate the equivalent values of sound pressure and sound pressure level are given. The *red shading* represents the range of frequencies and intensity required for comprehension of ordinary speech

made between the (physical) *sound pressure* or *sound pressure level* (measured in N/m² or dB SPL, respectively) and the (subjectively experienced) *loudness*. The relationship between the two can be described quantitatively. An experimental subject can not only say when a tone becomes audible (crosses the auditory threshold) but can also report when two tones at the same frequency sound *equally loud.* Such an experiment is done by presenting the subject with a reference tone at 1000 Hz to be compared with a test tone, the frequency of which is varied in successive trials. With each pair of tones, the subject adjusts a potentiometer so as to change the sound pressure of the reference tone until the two sound equally loud. The sound pressure of the reference tone at this setting, in decibels SPL, gives the loudness level of the test tone in *phon* (e. g., if the reference tone is set at 70 dB SPL, the loudness level of the test tone is 70 phon). Because it is used as the standard, a 1000-Hz tone necessarily has identical decibel and phon values. In a typical experiment, a healthy subject will perceive a 4000-Hz tone at 70 dB SPL as being as loud as a 1000-Hz tone at 80 dB SPL; in this case the loudness level of the 4000-Hz tone is 80 phon. When phon values are plotted for test frequencies over the whole audible range, an *equal-loudness contour* (or *isophone*) is obtained. A set of equal-loudness contours is shown in Figure 6–6; these represent averages from the reports of a large number of healthy subjects, with the test tones set at a different sound pressure level for each curve. All tones, regardless of frequency, that lie on one of these curves are regarded as equally loud. The auditory threshold is also given by an isophone; all tones on this curve are equally loud — just barely perceptible. The average auditory threshold of healthy humans is 4 phon.

If sound pressure is increased sufficiently a subject eventually experiences pain in the ear. This occurs at about 130 phon, the *pain threshold.* Such high sound pressures can actually damage the ear if the duration of exposure is long enough. Indeed, sounds of very long duration can cause trauma even at sound pressures well below the pain threshold (cf. p. 208).

In a second type of experiment, the subject is asked to say when a test tone sounds *n* times (for instance, two or four times) as loud as a 1000-Hz reference tone at 40 dB SPL. When measured in this way, the loudness of the tone is expressed in *sones.* A tone judged four times as loud as a 1000-Hz, 40 dB reference tone has a loudness of 4 sones; the loudness of a test tone half as loud as the reference is 0.5 sones, and so on. In setting up the sone scale, then, the subject is required to make a higher-level discrimination than with the phon scale, for which it was necessary only to determine equivalence. Nevertheless, a reproducible relationship between the two scales is found. Above 40 phon the sensation of loudness follows a simple power function of the sound pressure, with exponent 0.3; a 10-phon increase causes a doubling of the perceived loudness. Below 40 phon this relationship does not hold; loudness is doubled by a smaller increase in sound pressure.

Evaluation of noise; measurement of hearing ability. The sone scale is very relevant to the evaluation of severity of noise disturbances. However, since it can be determined only by the judgments of experimental subjects or sophisticated equipment, estimation of loudness by this means is laborious and in general impracticable. The phon scale is also defined in terms of human judgments and cannot be measured directly. However, it is possible to design a sound-pressure meter that does not respond equally to all frequencies, but rather weights them in the same way as the human ear. The greatest sensitivity of such a measuring instrument is in the middle frequency range (cf. the threshold curve of Fig. 6–6), and it is less sensitive at higher and lower frequencies. Readings from such a device are designated by *dB (A),* the A denoting a certain filter curve. They correspond *approximately* to phon values — that is, to the loudness level. Because these meters are easy to operate they are used in noise evaluation even though some inaccuracy is involved. For example, the noise of an idling car motor may amount to about 75 dB (A). It is worth noting that prolonged exposure (for example, throughout 8-h working days) to more than 90 dB (A) over the course of years causes hearing impairment.

Whereas the scale of sound pressure level is physically defined, the *loudness-level scale* described above is based on subjective judgments of "equality". How accurate are the reports of subjects in these tests? This question can be answered by determining how small a difference in loudness can be detected. It turns out that equal loudness can be judged quite accurately. In the near-threshold range two tones at the same frequency are perceived to be of different loudness when their sound pressures differ by 3–5 dB (the *difference threshold*). The higher the sound pressure, the smaller the difference threshold. At 40 dB SPL, the difference threshold is only about 1 dB.

As is clear in Figure 6–6, the *audibility of a tone* depends not only on the sound pressure but also on the frequency. An adult can hear sounds with frequencies in the range 20–16,000 Hz (16 kHz). Frequencies above 16 kHz are called *ultrasonic,* while those below 20 Hz are *infrasonic.* All events audible to us, then, are associated with sounds between 20 Hz and 16 kHz, and between 4 and 130 phon — the area between the top and bottom curves in Figure 6–6. The red area in the middle of the diagram represents the range of frequencies and intensities required for the understanding of conversational speech (the spectral composition of the human voice under various conditions of course covers a broader area).

Patients who are "hard of hearing" have elevated auditory thresholds; that is, in order to perceive sound they require higher sound pressures than a normal person. The clinical determination of auditory threshold is called *audiometry.* Various tones are presented to the patient through earphones, a procedure which tests the response to airborne sounds (cf. p. 212). The clinician begins with tones of an intensity certain to be subthreshold, and slowly increases the sound pressure until the patient reports hearing a tone. The sound pressure at that point is entered on a diagram. If the threshold of a patient is some dB above the normal threshold, the diagnosis is a corresponding *hearing loss.* The diagram of threshold deviations vs. frequency, in which all the data from such a test are entered, is called an *audiogram* (Fig. 6–7). Standard audiogram forms are available, with preprinted coordinates and the normal threshold represented by a straight line labelled "0 dB". The standard notation differs from that of Figure 6–6 in that thresholds

HEARING RECORD

NAME .... INITIAL TEST DATE ....

ADDRESS .... TESTED BY ....

AGE .... SEX ....

AUDIOGRAM

HOSP. OR CLINIC ....

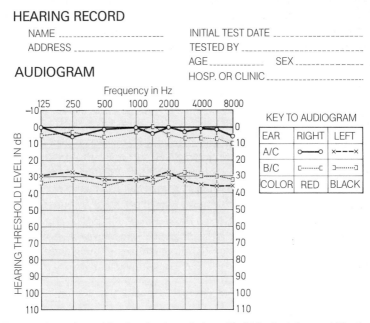

Fig. 6–7. Audiogram of a patient with a hearing loss of about 30 dB in the left ear. A/C, air conduction; B/C, bone conduction

higher than normal are plotted downward, so that the difference in decibels is represented graphically as a "loss". These relative figures should not be confused with the actual sound pressure level (identified as decibels SPL). For a discussion of evoked response audiometry see p. 222.

Loss of hearing in the high-frequency range is a routine accompaniment of old age. This phenomenon is called ***presbycusis.***

The human auditory system is of course also capable of judging ***pitch,*** which is a correlate of the frequency of a tone. In musical terms, an increase in pitch by an octave is accomplished by doubling the frequency of a tone: $f_1 = 2 f_0$. The organization of the tone scale in terms of octaves is a fundamental aspect of occidental music, and reflects the basic physics of most musical instruments. Psychophysical measurements of "pitch", however, reveal systematic departures from the physical situation. If the experimenter presents a reference tone higher than 2 kHz and asks the subject to select a frequency that seems to be twice as high in pitch, the selected tone tends to differ in frequency by more than a physical octave. Nevertheless, the physical octave remains the standard for tuning musical instruments. The octave is subdivided into 12 steps, which in equal-tempered tuning differ successively by the factor $\sqrt[12]{2}$; however, such tuning need not be followed in all cases, so that some instruments may depart slightly from this standard.

The human ability to discriminate pitch is remarkably good. In the optimal range, around 1000 Hz, we can distinguish frequencies that differ by only 0.3%, or about 3 Hz. This value is called the *frequency-discrimination threshold.* One can also assign a pitch to a musical sound that is not a pure tone; the perceived pitch is that of a pure tone at the fundamental frequency of the sound.

Auditory orientation in space. Another important function of the auditory system is its contribution to spatial orientation. Everyday experience shows us that the *direction of a sound source* can be estimated fairly accurately. Binaural hearing (with both ears functional) is a prerequisite. This ability rests on the physical properties of sound waves and the fact that one ear is usually somewhat farther from the sound source than the other, and oriented differently to it. Because sound is propagated with a finite velocity, it arrives at the more distant ear *later,* and is lower in *intensity* at that position. Figure 6–8 shows how the difference in propagation time can be computed. The difference in path length Δl is $d \cdot \sin \alpha$, where d is the distance between the two ears and α is the angle between the sound source and the median plane of the head. The difference of arrival times Δt is then expressed by

$$\Delta t = \frac{\Delta l}{c} \tag{6–3}$$

where c is the speed of sound.

With $\alpha = 30°$ and a distance $d = 0.17$ m between the ears, the delay is

$$\Delta t = \frac{0.085}{340} = 2.5 \cdot 10^{-4} \text{ s.}$$

But the auditory system can detect much smaller interaural delays. Delays as short as $3 \cdot 10^{-5}$ (or half this, under optimal conditions) can certainly be detected; this delay corresponds to an angle of about 3° between sound source and midline.

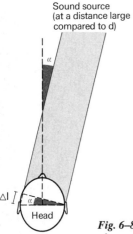

Sound source
(at a distance large
compared to d)

Head

Δl

d

Fig. 6–8. Geometric relationships used to calculate the delay in incidence of sound at the two ears; see text

That differences in both ***propagation time and intensity*** do in fact affect the perceived direction of sounds can be demonstrated experimentally. The subject of such a psychophysical experiment wears earphones, so that time of stimulation and intensity can be independently varied. It turns out that a delay in the presentation of a sound at one ear can be compensated by raising the intensity at that ear, and conversely. Comparable results have been obtained in recordings from single nerve cells in the lateral and medial nuclei of the ***superior olive.*** These nuclei are the chief site of ***neuronal processing*** of the signals from the two ears with respect to spatial orientation. The results of these analyses are transmitted to higher centers; at the highest level, in the auditory cortex, there are cells that can be activated solely by sound arriving at a certain angle with respect to the head (cf. p. 221).

But the mechanisms described so far do not explain why direction can be discriminated regardless of whether the ***sound source is in front*** of the listener or ***behind*** him. Figure 6–8 could be extended to show that the difference in delay and intensity at the two ears may remain unchanged with a source behind the head. Some accessory mechanism is required, and this is the ***pinna*** — the external ear. Because of its shape, sounds originating in front of the subject are perceived as quite distinct from identical sounds coming from behind. This fact can be turned to advantage in tape-recording music. With a model of a head in which microphones are mounted in the positions of the eardrums, excellent stereophonic recordings can be made.

Q 6.6. A singer's high C, in the physical sense, is:
  a) A pure tone
  b) A note with fundamental and harmonics
  c) A noise

Q 6.7. The sound pressure that measures 20 dB SPL is doubled. The resulting sound pressure level is:
  a) 22 dB
  b) 26 dB
  c) 40 dB
  d) All the above are false

Q 6.8. Isophones are:
  a) Curves of equal sound pressure
  b) Curves of equal sound pressure level
  c) Curves of equal loudness level
  d) Curves of equal loudness

Q 6.9. The points below the zero line in the clinical audiogram represent:
  a) The threshold sound pressure, at which the patient first reports the sensation of sound
  b) The sound pressure level of the auditory threshold of the patient
  c) The hearing loss in dB

Q 6.10. Localization of a sound source is possible if:
  a) It is in front of the head or a little to the side, otherwise not
  b) It is in front of, behind, or to the side of the head
  c) It is less than 30° off the line pointing straight ahead
  d) Both eyes and ears are employed, otherwise not

6.3 Functions of the Middle and the Inner Ears

The last section presented some of the capabilities of the auditory system as a whole. In this section and the one that follow we shall consider the way this performance is achieved.

Role of the middle ear. As stated in Section 6.1, the eardrum responds to sound and relays its energy of oscillation along the chain of ossicles to the inner ear, or more precisely to the perilymph of the scala vestibuli. Sound conducted along this pathway is said to be *airborne.* But a sensation of sound is also produced if an oscillating body — for example, a tuning fork — is placed in direct contact with the skull. In this case it is primarily the bones of the skull that are vibrated, so that there is *bone conduction* of the sound. In everyday life bone conduction plays a role only in the hearing of one's own voice. Otherwise all airborne sound reaches the inner ear via the eardrum and ossicles; the once-popular hypothesis that high frequencies travel to the inner ear by bone conduction has failed to be confirmed in experiments. Nevertheless, clinical tests of bone conduction are of considerable diagnostic value, as we shall see below.

Airborne sound must be transmitted from the air to the fluid filling the inner ear. Normally, when sound waves encounter a transition from air to liquid, most of the sound energy is reflected at the interface. In the case of the ear such reflection would obviously be counterproductive. The complicated mechanism of the eardrum-ossicle apparatus is Nature's "invention" to reduce such losses by reflection. In engineering terms, the apparatus *matches the acoustical impedance* of the air to the inner ear. As a result, losses by reflection are considerably reduced and more sound energy reaches the inner ear. The mechanism is in principle analogous to the coating of photographic objective lenses, which also serves to reduce reflection, at the air-glass interfaces. Impedance matching in the middle ear is brought about chiefly by two factors. First, the area of the eardrum is considerably greater than that of the stapedial foot plate. With transmission of a given force via the ossicles, the area difference itself accounts for an amplification of pressure at the oval window as compared with that at the eardrum. Second, the arms of the ossicular chain are so arranged that their lever action brings about a small pressure amplification.

The system thus resembles a *transformer* in its operation, though other factors are involved. The mechanism as a whole accounts for an improvement of auditory performance by about 15–20 dB.

It is important to note the construction of the ossicular chain. The distribution of mass in the ossicles is such that internally generated, bone-conducted sound (e. g. by footsteps) does not stimulate the inner ear.

Fine muscles, the so-called *middle ear muscles,* are attached to the hammer and stirrup. These give reflex contractions to sound stimuli, which impede sound transmission; but apparently they offer no appreciable protection from injury by intense sound. Nothing more is known about the function of these middle-ear reflexes.

Sound reception in the inner ear. Place theory. When sound strikes the ear, the *stapes* transmits energy to the *perilymph of the scala vestibuli* (cf. Fig. 6–1). The stapes oscillates back and forth, driving the perilymph with it. Because the fluids in the inner ear are nearly incompressible, a corresponding movement must occur elsewhere, at the *round window.* When the stapes moves inward the membrane over the round window is pushed outward, and conversely. During these movements of the stapes there are simultaneous displacements of the nearby, basal parts of the cochlear duct involving the *basilar and vestibular membranes.* This region oscillates in time with the stapes, toward the scala tympani and the scala vestibuli in alternation. For simplicity in the following discussion, we shall consider the cochlear duct as a whole — the scala media, filled with endolymph, and its bounding vestibular and basilar membranes. The initial displacement of the base of the cochlear duct, described above, starts a wave travelling along the duct from the basal end to the helicotrema, rather as a wave can be sent along a rope held horizontally. The shape of this wave at two instants of time is shown in Figure 6–9, with the duct represented as a simple line. Maintained tones cause the stapes to go into maintained oscillation, and such *travelling waves* pass continually along the endolymph-filled duct.

Rather than attempt a physically precise description of the wave mechanics here, we shall resort to a simplified description of the situation, as revealed by the experiments of VON BEKESY several decades ago. During exposure to sound, the

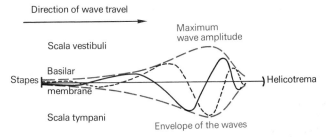

Fig. 6–9. Travelling waves along the cochlear duct, which is represented simply by a line in the diagram. The stapes end of the cochlea is at the *left* and the helicotrema, at the *right* of the diagram. The two wave formations shown *(solid and dashed curves)* occur at different instants of time. The *red curve* shows the envelope of all the wave formations, indicating the extreme displacements due to the waves, at each point along the cochlea

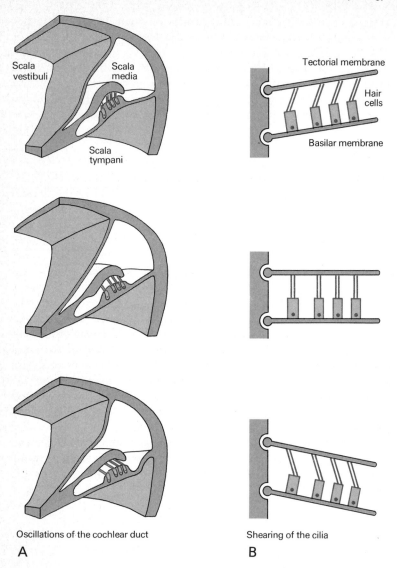

Oscillations of the cochlear duct

A

Shearing of the cilia

B

Fig. 6–10. A Three-dimensional diagram of the oscillation of the cochlear duct. ***B*** Shearing of the cilia as the basilar membrane oscillates

basilar membrane swings up and down as shown in the exaggerated three-dimensional drawing of Figure 6–10. Actually, the amplitudes are very small — about 10^{-10} m in the threshold range. Because the ***stiffness of the basilar membrane*** decreases from the stapes to the helicotrema, ***velocity of propagation*** of the waves becomes gradually smaller toward the helicotrema and the waves at first increase in amplitude. But further on, because of certain physical peculiarities

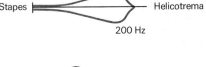

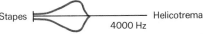

Fig. 6–11. Maximal amplitudes of oscillation
of the basilar membrane during exposure
to tones of different frequency; frequency-to-
place mapping

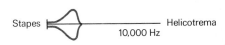

of the fluid-filled canals, the waves are damped and eventually disappear altogether, in general before they have reached the helicotrema. Somewhere between the site of origin of a wave at the stapes and the point where it terminates, therefore, there is a point of maximum deflection. This maximum occurs at a different location for each frequency, shifting toward the *stapes region* as frequency is *raised* and lying more in the *vicinity of the helicotrema* with *low* frequencies (cf. Fig. 6–11). Th existence of these *points of maximum displacement* thus maps each frequency in a sound stimulus onto a particular place in the cochlear duct. The sensory cells are primarily excited at the site of the maximum, so that each frequency excites different sensory cells. This, in brief, constitutes the *place theory of hearing.*

Stimulus reception by the hair cells. As Figure 6–10 shows, sound causes the cochlear duct to swing alternately toward the scala vestibuli and the scala tympani. One effect of this complex motion is a *displacement of the basilar and tectorial membranes* relative to one another. This is illustrated by the highly schematic Figure 6–10B. Because the *cilia of the hair cells* are in contact with the tectorial membrane, the displacement exerts a *shearing force* on them so that they are bent. This *shear of the cilia* constitutes the adequate stimulus of the hair cells.

Before the *process of transduction* (transformation of the stimulus into a neuronal signal) by the hair cell can be described, a few other facts must be introduced. If a microelectrode is used to measure the potentials in the inner ear, with the scala vestibuli as the reference site, the cochlear duct exhibits a strong positive potential ($\sim +80$ mV; Fig. 6–12). With respect to the same reference level, the stria vascularis and the organ of Corti exhibit negative potentials. The positive endocochlear potential is maintained by chemical processes in the stria vascularis. All these potentials are observable in the *absence of sound,* so they are called *standing* (i. e., steady) *potentials.*

When *sound strikes the ear,* additional potentials appear — the so-called cochlear microphonic potentials and the action potentials of the auditory nerve. The term *microphonic potential* comes from the fact that this potential (which can

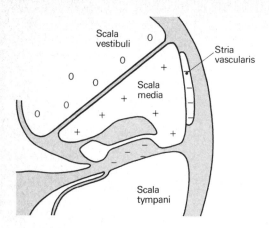

*Fig. 6–12.*Standing potentials in the inner ear, as discussed in the text

be recorded, for example, at the round window) behaves like the output voltage of a microphone — that is, it reproduces closely the *fluctuations in sound pressure.* The microphonic potential follows the stimulus 1. with essentially no latency; 2. it has no refractory period or 3. measurable threshold, and 4. it is not fatiguable. In all four respects it differs from most biological potentials, and in particular from action potentials. Probably the microphonic potential represents the extracellularly recordable *sum of the receptor potentials* of all the excited hair cells. It is thought that the acoustic stimulus produces a synchronized change in the electrical resistance of the membrane of the receptor cell, as a result of shearing of the cilia. Because there is a steep potential gradient (associated with the standing potentials) between the endolymph space and the interior of the receptor cell, amounting to some 150 mV, changes in membrane conductance are accompanied by a rapid influx or efflux of ions, which in turn produce the receptor potential in the hair cell. This is the mechanism ordinarily called the *battery hypothesis.* Further, it is thought that the receptor potential of each individual hair cell causes a *release of transmitter* at its basal pole. This substance then elicits excitation of the afferent nerve fibers.

The *action potentials* in the fibers of the auditory nerve, accordingly, signal excitation of the hair cells to the CNS. These action potentials can be recorded with microelectrodes. Their properties will be described in the next section.

It ist not clear yet why two types of hair cells are necessary for the function of the cochlea.

When the ear is presented with a click (a very brief pressure pulse), the fibers in the auditory nerve are excited synchronously and a compound action potential can be recorded; that is, the action potentials of the individual Fibers are discharged at nearly the same time and therefore summate. Figure 6–13 shows both the *cochlear microphonic potential* (CM) and the *compound action potential* (CAP) of the auditory nerve in response to a click. When a prolonged sound is given, the individual fibers in the auditory nerve do not discharge in synchrony, and a compound action potential is not observed.

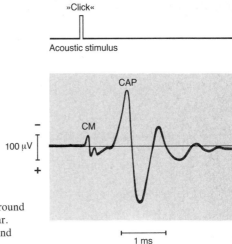

»Click«

Acoustic stimulus

Fig. 6–13. The potentials recorded at the round window when a click is presented to the ear. *CM*, cochlear microphonic; *CAP*, compound action potential

Middle-ear and inner-ear deafness. It was noted above that the bones of the skull can be set into oscillation directly — for example, by contact with an oscillating tuning fork. With such strong stimuli, the vibrating bone can excite the inner ear. This ***bone conduction*** is important in clinical examinations, for the following reason. Hearing impairments can be subdivided roughly into two kinds: 1. ***disturbances of conduction,*** in which the ***middle ear*** fails, for various reasons, to transmit adequate sound energy to the inner ear, and 2. inner-ear deafness, in which the middle ear is intact but there is damage in the ***cochlea,*** to the hair cells or to the afferent nerve fibers. Audiometric tests should examine not only the responses to ***airborne sound*** (as described on p. 208), but also the efficacy of ***bone conduction.*** The examiner places a vibrator on the mastoid process, the bony knob behind the external ear, on the side of interest. It is evident that when impaired hearing is due to ***inner-ear damage*** the auditory theshold to both airborne and bone-conducted sound is expected to be increased — the receptor process itself is affected. But in the case of ***middle-ear deafness*** the conduction of airborne sound is impaired while the inner ear remains functional, so that the threshold to bone-conducted sound is unchanged. The audiogram of Figure 6–7 reflects inner-ear damage; the patient's theshold to both bone-conducted and air-conducted sound is elevated.

There is a very simple procedure to determine whether a patient with hearing difficulty on one side only has suffered damage to the middle or inner ear. It is called ***Weber's test.*** The stem of an oscillating tuning fork (256 Hz is the most useful frequency) is pressed against the midline of the skull. If it is the inner ear that is damaged the patient reports hearing the tone on an unaffected side. But if the fault lies in conduction through the middle ear, the patient claims to hear the tone on the damaged side; in clinical terms, the tone is said to be "lateralized to the affected side".

Q 6.11. The eardrum-ossicle apparatus:
  a) Serves exclusively to bridge the space separating the eardrum from the oval window
  b) Reduces loss due to reflection at the transition of the sound from the air to the inner ear
  c) Because of its linked-lever construction prevents damage of the inner ear by sound
  d) Is a phylogenetic relict, evolved from the gill arches and with no particular significance in mammals

Q 6.12. The term "travelling wave" as used with respect to sound reception refers to the notion:
  a) That standing waves are produced in the cochlea by sound
  b) That a wave passes from the helicotrema to the stapes, forming a frequency-dependent maximum between the two
  c) That a wave passes from stapes to helicotrema, forming a frequency-dependent maximum between the two
  d) That sound spreads through the air in the form of waves

Q 6.13. The place theory says:
  a) That a sound stimulus excites only the hair cells at a single site on the basilar membrane
  b) That each frequency component of a sound excites the hair cells at a particular site on the basilar membrane
  c) That the fibers of the auditory nerve all arise at a single site, the spiral ganglion

6.4 The Auditory Nerve and the Higher Stations of the Auditory Pathway

Conditions under which auditory nerve fibers are stimulated. Each fiber in the auditory nerve comes from a narrowly circumscribed region of the cochlea or from a single inner hair cell. Because particular places in the cochlea are associated with particular frequencies, each nerve fiber can be optimally excited by a sound of a certain frequency. This frequency is called the *characteristic frequency* of the fiber. A fiber in the auditory nerve, then, is excited most readily when the ear is stimulated by sound at the characteristic frequency of that fiber (Fig. 6–14). Pure tones of very low intensity will excite specific single fibers in the nerve. If the ear is stimulated with tones at frequencies other than the characteristic frequency of a fiber under study, the fiber can be activated only if the intensity is raised sufficiently. This property of "tuning" is illustrated in Figure 6–15, a graph showing for each frequency the sound pressure required to produce a just-threshold response in each of two fibers differing in characteristic frequency ($\sim$ 3000 and 4600 Hz). The shaded area above each curve indicates the range of frequencies and intensities over which the fiber is responsive. Such curves are called *"tuning*

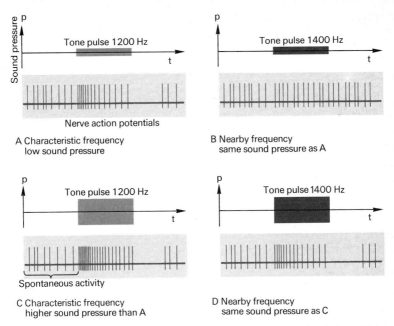

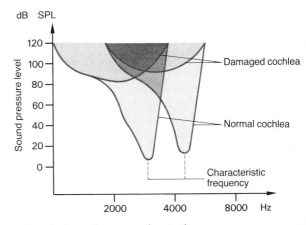

Fig. 6–14. Discharges of a single fiber in the auditory nerve in response to stimulation with its characteristic frequency and a nearby frequency, at two different intensities

Fig. 6–15. Tuning curves of two fibers in the auditory nerve (see text)

curves. "When the sound pressure is low, the nerve fibers are very selective — i. e., tuned to narrow frequency bands. If a sound stimulus contains several frequencies, all the corresponding groups of nerve fibers are activated. The *duration* of a stimulus is coded by the duration of activation, and its *intensity* by the degree of activation. As sound pressure level is increased, not only are the fibers concerned *more strongly excited* (their discharge rate is increased), but additional fibers (having nearby characteristic frequencies) are *recruited.* Recruitment is also illustrated in Figure 6–15: when the parameters of the sound stimulus lie in the doubly shaded overlap area, both fibers are excited. When the inner ear is damaged (by exposure to noise, for example), the fibers become less sensitive (one becomes hard of hearing) and the frequency selectivity is lost. As a result, complex sounds such as speech can no longer be so accurately analyzed. Speech then becomes harder to understand.

In summary, we can say that at the level of the primary afferent fibers a sound stimulus is analyzed into its frequency components. At higher stations on the auditory pathway, the nature of the processing is quite different.

Anatomy of the auditory pathway. Figure 6–16 is a much simplified diagram of the most prominent parts of the auditory pathway. For clarity, only the paths from the left ear are shown. The arrow tips indicate relay points, where the neurons synapse with higher-order ones; the diagram does not distinguish between inhibitory and excitatory synapses. The primary afferent fibers run to the *cochlear nucleus,* which is subdivided into a *ventral* and a *dorsal* part. From the ventral part a ventral tract proceeds to the *olivary complexes,* both ipsilateral and contralateral. Thus the nerve cells in each olivary complex receive inputs from both ears. Here is the lowest level in the brain at which an opportunity exists for comparison of the acoustic inputs to the two ears — an interaction already mentioned in Section 6–2 in connection with the sensation of directionality of sound. The *dorsal cochlear nucleus* sends out a dorsal tract. These fibers cross to the opposite side and there synapse with neurons in the *nucleus of the lateral lemniscus.* Some of the ascending fibers of the olivary-complex cells project to the same side, and some cross to the opposite side. Above the lateral lemniscus the auditory tract proceeds by way of two relay stations, the *inferior colliculus* and the *medial geniculate body,* to its final destination, the *primary auditory cortex* in the temporal lobe. The tract thus consists of sequences of at least five or six neurons. In fact there are still other relay points not shown in the diagram of Figure 6–16, so that even longer chains are possible. Moreover, many collaterals are sent out from the auditory pathway. Finally, the auditory system contains not only afferent, centripetal fibers which pass from ear to cerebral cortex, but also an efferent, centrifugal system (running in the opposite direction) which has been omitted in Figure 6–16; the function of this efferent system is not entirely clear.

Response criteria of central auditory neurons. Neurons in the auditory nerve can be excited by quite simple stimuli, such as pure tones, but the neurons at higher levels of the auditory pathway ordinarily require more complex sounds. Although cells in the *ventral cochlear nucleus* behave like those in the auditory nerve, those in the *dorsal cochlear nucleus* show distinctly different responses. Under certain conditions these neurons are *inhibited* by auditory input. The inhibition is brought about by extensive *reciprocal connections* among the neurons.

Recordings from cells at still higher levels often reveal no response at all to pure tones. These cells respond to *complex patterns of sound* such as amplitude- or

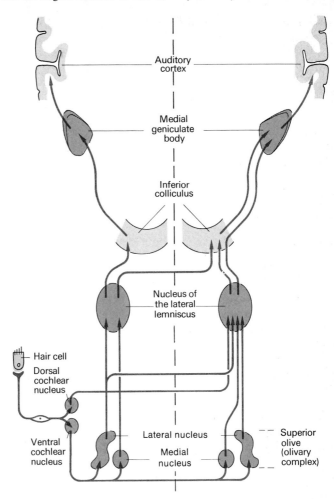

Fig. 6–16. Highly simplified diagram of the auditory pathway, as discussed in the text

frequency-modulated sounds — sounds with continuously changing intensity or frequency. Other neurons respond only to the onset, or only to the termination, of a sound stimulus, and so on. A common finding is that a cell is activated at some frequencies and inhibited at others. As a rule of thumb, we can say that *the higher the level of a neuron in the auditory pathway, the more complicated the sound patterns required to excite it.* It was once thought that the *frequency selectivity* of neurons responding to pure tones would be enhanced at higher levels, but this is not the case. Higher-level neurons are not appreciably more sharply tuned than those in the auditory nerve; in fact, many cells in the *auditory cortex* can be activated over a very broad band of frequencies.

The *sounds encountered in ordinary life* are very rarely pure tones. They usually have a variety of components, as in the complex stimuli mentioned above. This is particularly true of *speech,* which presents a continuously changing pattern; some elements are very brief, and simultaneous amplitude and frequency modulation is the rule. Evidently the neurons in the higher parts of the auditory pathway are specialized to extract specific characteristics of such complex sounds — for example, the change of frequency within a spoken word — and thus identify certain constellations of stimuli. Cells responding to such particular constellations are the auditory analogs of the complex or hypercomplex neurons of the visual cortex (cf. p. 183). In both modalities, such cells extract certain features of a stimulus, contributing to the process of *pattern recognition.*

Another way the neuronal processing of a sound stimulus can be monitored is via the potentials recorded by electrodes on the scalp, with the skull intact. These potentials represent the summed activity of many neurons but are much attenuated, so that electronic computers are needed to analyze them. Such measurements form the basis of so-called evoked response audiometry (ERA), a method currently being tried as a diagnostic aid regarding the origins of hearing impairment, at the level of the cochlea or higher, and other neurological diseases.

Adaptation in the auditory system. The phenomenon of adaptation is common to all sensory systems, and the auditory system is no exception. It is a property of both the peripheral receptors and the central neurons. *Adaptation* to a given sound level results in an *increase in auditory threshold,* but it does not follow that it is undesirable or useless. Adaptation to certain intensities and frequencies can actually *lower the difference threshold,* enhancing discrimination of different sound pressure levels. For example, the 4000-Hz tone in Figure 6–6 at 33 dB SPL has a loudness level of 40 phon, and same tone at 52 dB SPL has a loudness level of 60 phon. In this part of the graph, then, an increase of 19 dB in sound pressure is required to achieve a difference in loudness level of 20 phon. If, however, the ear is adapted by long exposure to 4000 Hz, the isophones in this region shift upward; in particular, those for lower loudness levels move further than those for higher levels. As a result, a 20-phon difference in loudness level requires a change of less than 19 dB SPL — for example, 14 dB. To put it another way: *A given difference in sound pressure level causes a greater difference in loudness level in the adapted state.* The subjective difference becomes greater, so that the discrimination threshold is lowered.

The discussion so far may have left the impression that the sensation of *pitch* rests entirely upon the frequency-dependent localization of displacement in the cochlea as postulated by the *place theory,* or on the tuning of the auditory-nerve fibers, to their characteristic frequencies (cf. p. 218). However, not all psychophysical observations concerning pitch sensations can be explained by the place theory alone. For example, if the ear is stimulated by a sequence of brief pulses of pressure (clicks) at intervals of 5 ms, subjects perceive a pitch of 200 Hz as expected. However, if the sound is first filtered so that only frequencies above a certain value (say, 800 Hz) are passed, the frequency 200 Hz is no longer present in the resulting stimulus. Nevertheless, the subjective pitch is still reported as 200 Hz. No convincing explanation of this phenomenon has yet been offered, but it cannot be explained by the place theory alone. The brain presumably "reconstructs" an impression of pitch from the periodic features of the stimulus (e.g., a pressure pulse every 5 ms), performing "periodicity analysis".

Q 6.14. Let us assume that a sound activates fibers of the auditory nerve having several different characteristic frequencies — about 800 Hz, 1600 Hz, and 3200 Hz. Fibers with characteristic frequencies between these values are not activated. The reason for this can be:
a) That the sound contains several frequencies
b) That the sound intensity is very high
c) That the nerve fibers in the auditory nerve have spontaneous activity
d) a and b explain the observation equally well.

Q 6.15. The following are among the relay stations in the auditory pathway:
a) Cochlear nucleus
b) Reticular formation
c) Superior colliculus
d) Medial geniculate body
e) Lateral geniculate body
f) Auditory cortex
g) Superior olive
h) Lentiform nucleus

Q 6.16. Primary afferent fibers in the auditory nerve can be excited:
a) By any sound stimulus as long as it is suprathreshold
b) Only by pure tones
c) Only by complex sounds such as frequency- or amplitude-modulated tones
d) Only by the onset or termination of a sound ("on" and "off" neurons)

7 Physiology of the Sense of Equilibrium

R. Klinke

7.1 Anatomy and Physiology of the Peripheral Organ

Receptors of the equilibrium organ, and the stimuli that excite them. Within the temporal bone, next to the cochlea, is the vestibular organ — a transducer intimately involved in the maintenance of equilibrium. The relative orientation of these parts of the labyrinth was shown in Figure 6–1 (cf. also Fig. 7–5). The vestibular organ is phylogenetically related to the ear, particularly with respect to the *receptors* of the two systems. In both cases, the receptors are *hair cells.* The adequate stimulus of the hair cells in the organ of Corti, as described in Chapter 6, is shearing of the cilia. This is also true in the vestibular organ, but here the shearing forces arise in a different way. First we shall consider how the receptor cells of the equilibrium organ are stimulated, before describing the macroscopic structure of the organ. Figure 7–1 illustrates the operation of this mechanism in one kind of sensory subunit of the vestibular organ, the *macula.* The cilia of the hair cells project into a gelatinous mass in which small granules of high specific gravity are embedded. The mass and its contents together are called the *otolith membrane.* There is a stepwise gradation in length of the cilia, the largest (called the *kinocilium*) being differently constructed than the rest. This differentiation distinguishes these hair cells from those of the cochlea, which lack a kinocilium and have only *stereocilia.*

The upper drawing in Figure 7–1 shows the *macula* at rest. If the head is tilted to one side or the other, the force of gravity slightly displaces the otolith membrane as shown in the two lower drawings. As it moves this small distance with respect to the sensory epithelium, it bends the cilia. This bending constitutes the stimulus to the receptors. The afferent nerve communicates this state to the CNS as follows: The fibers are active (the *resting activity*) even in the neutral position. If the cilia are bent in one direction, the discharge rate is increased, and if they bend to the other side it is reduced. Increased activation of the afferent nerve fiber occurs when the shearing force in the bundle of cilia is in the direction of the kinocilium; inhibition occurs in the opposite direction (Fig. 7–2). The main effective stimulus of the macula, then, is *gravity.* The force of gravity is a special case of *linear (translational) acceleration.* The maculae also respond to all other forms of translational acceleration — for example, that associated with the starting up or braking of a car. Under such conditions the otolith membrane shifts over the underlying sensory epithelium, just as a movable object slides forward when the brakes of a car are suddenly applied.

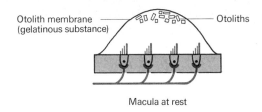

Macula at rest

Tilt   Tilt

Fig. 7–1. Diagram of a macula organ during tilting of the head (the adequate stimulus of the organ) in two directions

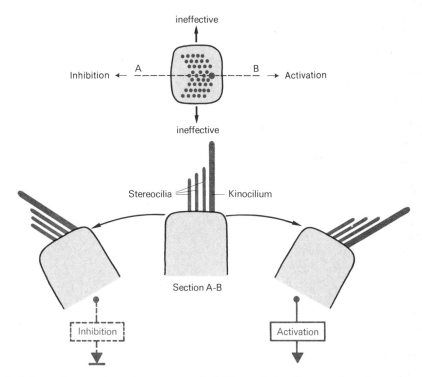

Fig. 7–2. Upper diagram shows the arrangement of cilia on a hair cell as seen from above; the *lower* is a section through the cell tilted in different directions. Shear toward the kinocilium activates the afferent fiber, while shear in the opposite direction reduces its discharge rate. Shear perpendicular to this direction has no effect

Structure and function of the statolith organs and semicircular canals. Two maculae (also called *statolith organs*) are present on each side, the macula of the *utricle* and that of the *saccule* (cf. Fig. 7–5). Both of these are fixed with respect to the skull. In the utricle the macula is approximately horizontal when the body is upright (as in the upper drawing of Fig. 7–1), and that in the saccule is vertical. When the head is tilted, the organs are displaced to angles between horizontal and vertical, as in the lower drawings of Figure 7–1. For every possible orientation of the skull, the effect of gravity is to move the otolith membranes into particular positions with respect to the sensory epithelium. As a result, there is a quite specific constellation of excitation in the associated afferent nerve fibers. Central neuronal evaluation of this pattern of excitation from the vestibular system provides *information about the position of the skull in space.*

Each vestibular organ includes another distinct sensory system, the *semicircular canals.* The receptors in the semicircular canals respond to *rotational acceleration* rather than linear. The principle of their construction is shown in Figure 7–3. At one site in each of the closed, circular, fluid-filled canals is an enlargement, the *ampulla.* Within this a gelatinous membrane, the *cupula,* projects into the fluid; its *specific gravity* is exactly that of the surrounding *endolymph,* and because of this the cupula (unlike the otolith membrane) does not move with respect to the canal during linear acceleration. But rotational acceleration does affect the cupula, because of the inertia of the endolymph. If the skull, initially at rest, is turned, the endolymph at first tends not to move; since the cupula is attached to the wall of the canal, it is pulled in a direction opposite to the direction of rotation (right-hand drawing in Fig. 7–3). The cilia of the receptor cells extend into the cupula, so that when the cupula is distorted there is a shearing force on the cilia. As in the maculae, this shear is the adequate stimulus of the receptor. The afferent nerve

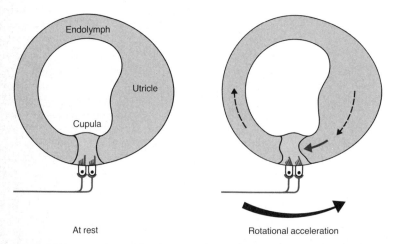

At rest   Rotational acceleration

Fig. 7–3. Diagram of a semicircular canal, showing the cupula within the ampulla. On the *right* is shown the imposed position of the cupula during angular acceleration

fibers, like those from the macula organs, exhibit **resting activity** in the absence of shear of the cilia. Bending of the cupula in one direction causes an **increase in the discharge rate,** and bending in the other direction causes a **decrease** (see Figs. 7–6 and 7–7). In the horizontal semicircular canal the fibers are excited when the cupula is displaced toward the utricle (cf. Fig. 7–5). This happens in the left canal when rotation of the head is toward the left.

    Rotational accelerations can have components about all three independent axes. The head can be 1. turned about its vertical axis, 2. inclined forward or backward, and 3. tilted to either side. A single semicircular canal cannot represent accelerations about all these axes and all their possible combinations. The nervous system requires at least **three semicircular canals,** one for each axis of rotation. A glance at Figures 7–4 and 7–5 will show that we do in fact have three canals on each side, arranged roughly **perpendicular to one another.** Their orientation in the skull is approximately as shown in Figure 7–4. On each side there is a **horizontal,** an **anterior vertical,** and a **posterior vertical** semicircular canal. The vestibular organ on each side thus comprises *five* subunits, *two* maculae (in utricle and saccule) and *three* semicircular canals. The shapes of the canals are not perfect circles. As shown in Figures 7–4 and 7–5, they are joined over parts of their courses. Finally, it should be mentioned that the so-called horizontal semicircular canal is not precisely horizontal when the head is in the normal position; its anterior margin is raised slightly, so that the plane in which the canal lies forms an angle of about 30° with the horizontal.

    The canals, the utricle, and the saccule consist of fine membranes that form closed tubes (hence the term **membranous labyrinth**). The system is filled with

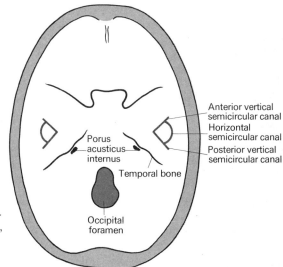

Fig. 7–4. Orientation of the semi-circular canals in the human skull, as seen by an observer looking down from above at the base of the skull

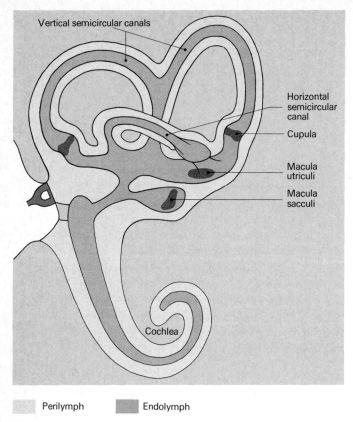

Perilymph   Endolymph

Fig. 7–5. Diagram of the labyrinth, showing continuity of the lymph spaces in vestibular organ and cochlea

endolymph, and this endolymph space is in communication with that of the cochlea. Moreover, the membranous labyrinth is surrounded by perilymph, which again is continuous with that of the organ of Corti. The system of cavities in the bone which contains both cochlea and vestibular organs (cf. Fig. 6–1) is called the *bony labyrinth.*

Behavior of the cupula during brief and prolonged rotation. Certain properties of cupular mechanics are of special interest. Figure 7–6 represents graphically the angular acceleration accompanying a brief rotation of the head from one position to another, along with the angular velocity, the calculated degree of deflection of the cupula in the horizontal semicircular canal, and the experimentally determined activity of one of the primary afferents from this ampulla. Clearly, the deflection of the cupula and the activity of afferent nerve fibers reflect the angular velocity and not the angular acceleration, even though the forces causing deflection of the cupula are forces of acceleration. The role of acceleration is more prominent in the

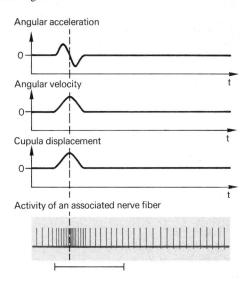

Case 1: brief movement (e. g. turning of the head)

Fig. 7–6. Movement of the cupula and the response of an afferent nerve fiber during a brief rotation. The effective acceleration and the angular velocity are also indicated

experiment of Figure 7–7, which represents *prolonged* uniform rotation on a turntable. The animal is accelerated at first, until a certain angular velocity has been reached. This velocity is then maintained for a considerable period. The figure shows that during the acceleration phase the cupula is deflected from its resting position, and during the steady rotation it slowly returns to the resting position. The reason for this is that friction between the endolymph and the canal wall causes the lymph slowly to catch up with and eventually to follow the rotational motion of the body; once it has caught up there is no difference between the rotational motion of the body and that of the endolymph. Under these conditions no forces exist to deflect the elastic cupula. The neuronal activity increases or decreases according to the amount and direction of cupula displacement. When movement is stopped, all these phenomena are reversed. The cupula is deflected in the opposite direction, and after the body is at rest it slowly (over 10–30 s) returns to its resting position as the rotation of the lymph slows as well.

The *differences in behavior of the cupula* associated with the *duration of rotation,* such that after a brief rotation it returns immediately to the resting position, are due to mechanical properties of the cupula-endolymph system that will not be discussed here. But it is important to bear in mind that the forces causing deflection of the cupula are *accelerations.* It should also be clear that the semicircular canals have evolved to signal the *short* rotational movements that occur in everyday life, and that the turntable situation is an unphysiologic stimulus.

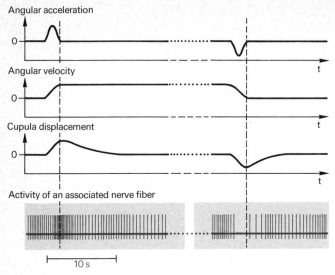

Angular acceleration

Angular velocity

Cupula displacement

Activity of an associated nerve fiber

10 s

Case 2: prolonged movement (e.g., on a turntable)

Fig. 7–7. Movement of the cupula and the response of an afferent nerve fiber during maintained rotation. The accelerations (positive at onset, negative at termination of rotation) and angular velocity are also indicated

Q 7.1. The following are elements of the vestibular organ:
a) Macula of the utricle
b) Macula of the saccule
c) Macula lutea
d) Anterior vertical semicircular canal
e) Posterior vertical semicircular canal
f) Horizontal semicircular canal
g) Scala vestibuli

Q 7.2. The adequate stimulus to the semicircular canal is:
a) Translational acceleration
b) Rotational acceleration
c) Rotational velocity
d) Oscillation of the stapes

7.2 Central Nervous Basis of the Sense of Equilibrium

Central connections of the receptors of the vestibular organ. The receptors in the vestibular organ, like those in the cochlea, are secondary sense cells. The associated afferent nerve fibers originate in the *vestibular ganglion* (ganglion of Scarpa); this is situated in the temporal bone near the vestibular organ. The fibers project into the region of the **vestibular nuclei** (cf. Fig. 7–8), in the medulla oblongata. This is the first station in which the discharge rates of the vestibular-nerve fibers are evaluated. There are four different nuclei on each side. If the vestibular organ is to participate in maintaining the balance of the body, there must be central connections between its afferents and the motor centers that can mediate the necessary regulation. Outputs from the vestibular nuclei are sent:

a) Along the **vestibulospinal tract,** and ultimately influence the motoneurons to the extensor muscles
b) Directly to the **motoneurons of the cervical cord**
c) To the **eye-muscle nuclei** (cf. Fig. 5–38)
d) To the **cerebellum**
e) To the **vestibular nuclei** on the opposite side, so that the inputs from the two sides can be processed together
f) To the **reticular formation**
g) By way of the **thalamus** to the posterior central gyrus of the **cortex,** which is involved in the conscious processing of vestibular inputs
h) To the **hypothalamus;** these fibers play a role in bringing about motion sickness (cf. p. 235).

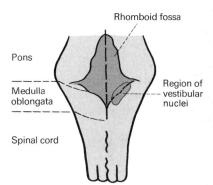

Rhomboid fossa

Pons

Medulla oblongata

Region of vestibular nuclei

Spinal cord

Fig. 7–8. Position of the vestibular nuclei in the medulla oblongata

Because the heads of the higher vertebrates are moveable with respect to their bodies, signals from the **vestibular receptors** alone cannot give an unambiguous picture of the position of the body in space (Fig. 7–9). There must be additional information about the position of the head with respect to the body. This is provided by the receptors of the cervical joints and musculature (muscle spindles, Golgi receptors), which are linked to the vestibular nuclei via central neurons (cf. Sec. 2.2).

Static and statokinetic reflexes. Vestibular nystagmus. Balance is maintained by reflexes, without conscious intervention. Although conscious analysis of spatial impressions is possible, one cannot perform efficient regulatory tasks without the built-in reflexes for their execution. For example, it is impossible to learn to fly an airplane "blind" (e. g., in the fog) on the basis of one's conscious spatial sensations;

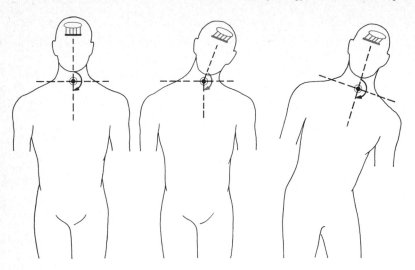

Fig. 7–9. Diagram of the macula organs and neck receptors in different positions of the body (see text)

instruments must provide the information required. The reflexes elicited by the vestibular organ can be subdivided into two groups, the so-called *static and statokinetic reflexes.* The static reflexes maintain equilibrium when one is standing quietly, sitting and in some cases lying down, in all the various positions. The *macula organs* are responsible for these *static reflexes.* That is, signals from receptors in the macula organs affect central nervous circuits so as to excite those muscle groups that must be active in order to keep the body in balance in the desired position. *Compensatory rolling of the eyes,* which can be particularly well observed in cats (cf. Fig. 7–10) but which also occurs in humans, is also a static reflex. It ensures that horizontal and vertical lines are imaged on the retina in the same way. Neck receptors, of course, are also involved in this reflex. *Statokinetic* reflexes, on the other hand, occur during movements and are movements themselves. Among them is the reflex turning elicited in a free fall. For example, a

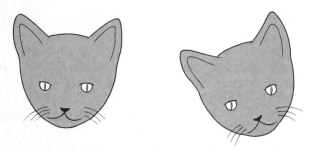

Fig. 7–10. Compensatory rolling of the eyes, by which the pupils are kept aligned with the vertical

cat always lands on its feet, regardless of the position from which it began to fall. Statokinetic reflexes can be elicited by the *macula organs* and/or the *semicircular canals.* Another statokinetic reflex is the *lifting response.* This amounts to an appropriate reaction to free fall, in which extensor tonus is increased when the animal is moved downward and vice versa.

A particularly striking statokinetic reflex is *vestibular nystagmus* (Fig. 7–11). Its vestibular origin can be demonstrated by rotating the subject in a completely dark room, so that no visual stimulation is possible. The vestibular stimulation causes eye movement in a direction opposite to that of rotation of the body, so that the direction of gaze is preserved. The neuronal connections involved, from the vestibular nuclei to the oculomotor nuclei, are shown in Figure 5–38. This *compensatory eye movement* is of course effective only over a certain rotation. Before the eyes reach the limit of their range of lateral movement, there is a *rapid* movement in the direction of rotation — the eyes snap ahead and fixate on a new spot. This rapid phase is followed by another *slow* movement, again compensating for the rotation.

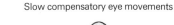

Slow compensatory eye movements

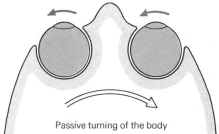

Passive turning of the body

Fig. 7–11. Direction of eye movement during vestibular nystagmus

When the head or body is *rotated about the vertical axis* only the horizontal semicircular canals, for practical purposes, are affected. A deflection of the cupulae in the two horizontal canals, then, produces a *horizontal nystagmus.* The direction of the two (fast and slow) components of the nystagmus depends on the direction of rotation (and hence of cupular bending). The *direction of the nystagmus* is, by convention, described clinically as that of the *rapid phase.* That is, in a "right nystagmus" the rapid phase is to the right. This terminology is compatible with that for *optokinetic nystagmus* (cf. p. 195).

If a subject is passively rotated, one initial effect is stimulation of the vestibular apparatus and another is a relative displacement of the visual environment. Each of these alone elicits nystagmus (vestibular nystagmus and optokinetic nystagmus). The two supplement one another. One of the most important functions of the semicircular canals, then, is to provide extra insurance that when the head is moved the eyes will move in the opposite direction. Further details of static and statokinetic reflexes are given in Chapter 6.4 of *Fundamentals of Neurophysiology.*

Clinical significance of nystagmus. Nystagmography is a useful tool for testing the function of the vestibular apparatus; the response most often measured is *postrotatory* nystagmus. The subject sits on a rotating chair and is rotated at a uniform velocity for a considerable time. The movement is then suddenly stopped. Figure 7–7 showed how the cupula is affected by this event; interruption of prolonged rotation causes it to be deflected, in a direction opposed to that in which it was bent when the rotation began. Deflection of the cupula elicits nystagmus regardless of the cause (acceleration or deceleration), and the resulting nystagmus in this case is called postrotatory nystagmus. The expected direction of this nystagmus can easily be worked out. The inertia of the endolymph bends the cupula in the direction in which it had been rotating, and this is interpreted as rotational acceleration in the opposite direction. Interruption of uniform rotation to the left, then, produces postrotatory nystagmus to the right — a pattern of eye movements shown in the recording of Figure 7–12.

Note, however, that during tests of postrotatory nystagmus *visual fixation must be prevented.* Otherwise nystagmus might be suppressed by the dominance of the visual system over the vestibular. For this reason the patient wears glasses with very strong convex lenses and a built-in light source (Frenzel's spectacles). These make the patient myopic and unable to fixate, while allowing the examining physician to follow easily the movement of the eyes. During clinical tests for the presence of *spontaneous nystagmus* it is also essential that visual fixation be eliminated with similar apparatus.

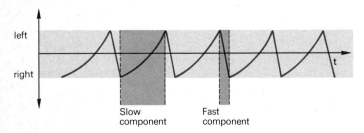

Fig. 7–12. Nystagmogram

Another diagnostic procedure involving vestibular nystagmus is *thermal stimulation* of the horizontal semicircular canal. An advantage in this case is that the right and left horizontal canals can be tested separately in order to detect differences in sensitivity on the two sides. In patients with certain diseases, this test may also reveal that one of the semicircular canals has become completely nonfunctional. The procedure is to tilt the head of the patient back about 60°, so that the horizontal canal is vertical. Now the *external meatus* of the ear is rinsed with cold or warm water. The outer edge of the horizontal semicircular canal is very close to the meatus, and there is sufficient heat transfer to cool or warm it. The effect is diagrammed in Figure 7–13; the warmed endolymph becomes lighter and

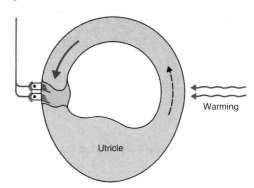

Fig. 7–13. Deflection of the cupula during caloric stimulation of a semicircular canal

therefore rises, causing a flow of endolymph around the canal and a deflection of the cupula; the result is **caloric nystagmus.** The application of warm water produces nystagmus toward the treated side; obviously, the nystagmus in response to rinsing with cold water will be in the opposite direction. The sensation of turning experienced by the subject during caloric nystagmus corresponds in direction to the rapid phase of the eye movement.

The central connections underlying vestibular nystagmus are such that the slow phase is elicited by the vestibular system, whereas the rapid return of the eye is triggered by the reticular formation.

A final point of interest with regard to the production of caloric nystagmus by endolymph flow is that this mechanism can operate only in the earth's field of gravity; it is only under the influence of gravity that density differences in the endolymph can induce flow. However, experiments during space flights have shown that caloric nystagmus can also be elicited in zero-gravity conditions. This implication is that the discharge rates in the vestibular nerve are also directly affected by the thermal stimulus.

Because of the link between vestibular system and **hypothalamus,** strong **excitation of the vestibular apparatus** is often associated with unpleasant sensations — dizziness, nausea, sweating, and the like. Such symptoms are called **kinetosis** (motion sickness). Kinetosis is particularly likely to result when the organ is subjected to constellations of stimuli to which it is not accustomed (as happens, for example, at sea). Coriolis accelerations are particularly effective in eliciting kinetosis, as are any discrepancies between visual sensations and the signals from the vestibular organs. (One is more susceptible to seasickness in the cabin of a boat than on deck, where the horizon provides a reliable point of reference.)

Acute interruption of labyrinthine function leads to nausea, vomiting, profuse sweating and nystagmus toward the intact side. There is also a tendency for the patient to fall toward the affected side. **Chronic** loss of a labyrinth can be compensated relatively well, as long as the patient can orient visually. In the dark, however, the deficit becomes very noticeable.

Q 7.3.   When the body is in a resting position information about its position in space is available from the follwing sense organs:
a) Eyes
b) Neck receptors
c) Macula organs
d) Semicircular canal organs
e) Organ of Corti

Q 7.4.   About how long does it take for the cupulae to return to their resting position after a prolonged uniform rotation has been stopped?
a) 100 ms
b) At most 1 s
c) 10–30 s
d) Usually more than 1 min

Q 7.5.   Acute damage to the labyrinth gives the following symptoms:
a) Nausea
b) Vomiting
c) Sweating
d) Nystagmus toward the intact side
e) Nystagmus toward the damaged side
f) Anxiety states
g) None of the above symptoms, all of which appear only when the damage is chronic

8 Physiology of Taste

H. Altner

The organs subserving the sense of taste are located in the region of the oral cavity, in particular on the tongue. In discussing the sense of taste it seems useful to turn first to the structure of these organs and their connections with the CNS. We shall see that the receptor organs, the *taste buds,* are mounted on *papillae* (folds in the skin of the tongue) of three different forms. The taste buds and the sense cells they contain, however, cannot be grouped into particular morphologic types. Of the basic dimensions of the taste sensation, two — quality and intensity — will be discussed in detail (Sec. 8.1). There are four *basic sensations:* sweet, sour, salty, and bitter. In the second section (8.2) it is shown that the ability to discriminate these categories may well be derived from the specificity of receptor molecules. But there are no quality-specific receptor types; quality and concentration are apparently encoded by the graded response of large numbers of receptors.

8.1 Morphology of the Organs of Taste; Subjective Taste Physiology

Orientation and structure of the taste buds. The surface of the human tongue is covered with a mucous membrane, folded at many points to form little peglike projections called *papillae.* Figure 8–1 is a diagram of the distribution of the three types of papillae – vallate, foliate, and fungiform — over the tongue's surface.

The three types differ in their distribution. Only the *fungiform papillae* are scattered over the entire surface. The *vallate papillae,* of which there are only 7–12 in humans, appear from above to be round structures 1–3 mm in diameter; they are restricted to a zone across the back of the tongue near its base. The third type, the *foliate papillae,* are arranged as closely packed folds along the back edges of the tongue. They are well developed in children, but are very much less prominent and numerous in adults.

The *filiform papillae,* which cover the remaining surface of the tongue, are not shown in Figure 8–1 because they bear no taste buds. The term "bud" refers to the shape of these organs (drawn in red in Fig. 8–2). Their location on the papillae varies; in the case of vallate and foliate papillae, there are many taste buds in the side walls but none on top. In the fungiform papillae, the taste buds are limited to the surface of the "cap" of the "mushroom", which may be as much as 1 mm in diameter.

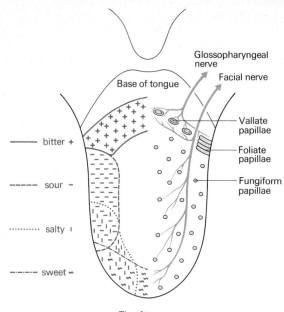

Fig. 8–1. Diagram summarizing the distribution of gustatory papillae, their innervation, and the regions of maximum sensitivity to the different qualities, on the human tongue. The dense array of fungiform paillae on the edges and tip of the tongue has been omitted for clarity. Sensitivity to "salty" is greatest in the anterolateral third of the tongue; that to "sour" may extend beyond the indicated area, to the base of the tongue

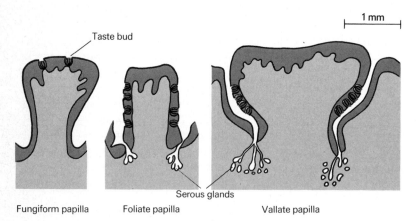

Fig. 8–2. Position of the taste buds *(red)* on the three types of gustatory papillae

A single taste bud is about 70 μm high, with a diameter of about 40 μm. A human has about 2,000 taste buds, roughly half of which are on the vallate papillae. Each taste bud contains 40–60 individual cells.

Embedded in the connective tissue below the vallate and foliate papillae are serous glands with ducts opening in the depressions between papilla and wall or between neighboring papillae (Fig. 8–2); their secretion serves to wash away particles of food and microorganisms. In addition, the presence of this secretion lowers the concentration of stimulus substance in the vicinity of the taste buds.

Within the taste buds, three types of cells can be distinguished: **sensory cells, supporting cells, and basal cells** (Fig. 8–3). Water-soluble substances that reach the surface of the tongue can diffuse through a pore into a fluid-filled space over the taste bud; here they contact the membranes of the microvilli that form the outer ends of the sensory cells. The taste receptors are secondary sensory cells, without axons to conduct impulses centrally. Their responses are transmitted by afferent fibers that form synapses near the bases of the sensory cells. In Figure 8–3 only 2 fibers are shown, but actually about 50 fibers enter and branch within each taste bud.

The **life span of the sensory cells** in the taste buds is short; there is a continual **exchange of sensory cells.** On the average, a sensory cell is replaced by its successor after only 10 days. The shedding of the cells can be monitored by marking the cell

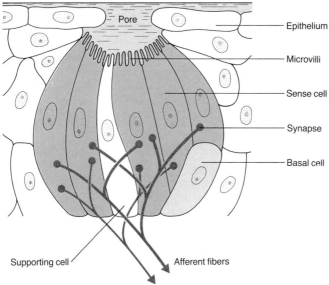

Fig. 8–3. Structure and innervation of a taste bud. The elements of the taste organ, the sensory, supporting, and basal cells, are arranged rather like the leaves in a bud. The whole structure is set below the epithelial surface, so that the microvilli of the sensory cells project into a fluid-filled space above them. Only two afferent fibers are shown (in **red**); actually about 50 fibers enter and branch within a single taste bud

nuclei with radioactive ^{3}H-thymidine and checking the number of marked nuclei that remain after some time has passed. The lost cells are replaced by new sensory cells derived from **basal cells.** During the changeover, the synapses between the afferent fibers and the old cells must be disrupted and new synapses formed. This kind of reorganization raises a number of interesting questions, particularly in view of the fact that the sensory cells differ in their sensitivity to various stimuli. For example, an exchange of sensory cells might result in a **change in the taste profile,** the characteristic pattern of responses in the afferent fibers which will be discussed in the next section.

Central connections. The afferent fibers signalling the responses of the aggregate of taste buds are divided between two cranial nerves, the *facial nerve* (VII) and the **glossopharyngeal nerve** (IX). This subdivision generally matches the areas of the tongue served by the fibers (Fig. 8–1). Thus the fibers from the vallate and foliate papillae run predominantly in the glossopharyngeal nerve, while those from the fungiform papillae in the front part of the tongue enter the **chorda tympani,** a branch of the facial nerve. Children have additional taste organs, in the epithelium of the soft palate and in the back wall of the throat, as far as the larynx; these are innervated chiefly by the **vagus nerve** (X).

In the brain, the taste fibers on each side join to form the **solitary tract.** This tract ends in the medulla oblongata, in the **nucleus of the solitary tract,** where the afferent fibers synapse with second-order neurons. The axons of the latter neurons proceed to the **ventral thalamus** as part of the medial lemniscus. A third set of neurons communicates between this region and the cerebral cortex. The cortical taste fields are in the lateral region of the **postcentral gyrus.**

The basic taste sensations. Under natural conditions — for example, during eating — the mouth region is exposed to complex stimuli comprising several modalities. Because the mouth cavity is in open communication with the nasal cavity, odor substances can diffuse up to the odor receptor in the nose and give rise to other sensations. Furthermore, there are thermoreceptors, mechanoreceptors and pain fibers in the mucous membranes of mouth and tongue, and these may also be stimulated. What is usually called a "taste" is actually a multimodal sensation, in which sensations of odor, heat or cold, pressure, and perhaps even pain are superimposed on the real gustatory sensations.

In the case of odors, it is difficult to arrange the many different stimuli in groups of related substances that can be regarded as odor qualities. By contrast, there are four quite distinct **basic taste sensations: sweet, sour, salty, and bitter.**

Apart from these basic qualities, two **accessory qualities — alkaline and metallic** — can be distinguished. The sensation alkaline (or soapy) is produced by stimulation with potash (potassium carbonate). And some metals and metal salts have a specific "metallic" taste.

Table 8–1 lists certain substances in each of the basic categories. It is apparent in the table that **H^+ ions** are the factor determining a **sour** taste. But as far as the other three qualities are concerned, it is practically impossible to predict which quality any particular substance will have on the basis of its physical and chemical properties. Substances that taste similar can differ widely in chemical structure, whereas even optical isomers can have quite different tastes; certain amino acids taste sweet in the D form and bitter in the L form. It is clear that the stimuli acting under natural conditions are complex, comprising several qualities, so that most taste sensations are mixed.

Table 8–1. Examples of substances in the four basic taste categories

Sweet	Sour	Salty	Bitter
Glucose	Hydrochloric acid	Table salt	Quinine sulfate
Saccharose	Acetic acid	Ammonium chloride	Nicotine
Saccharin	Citric acid	Magnesium chloride	Caffeine
D-leucine	Tartaric acid	Sodium fluoride	L-leucine
Beryllium chloride			Magnesium sulfate

The *detection thesholds* are at different concentrations for the various qualities. The threshold concentration for quinine sulfate (8 μmol/liter, or 0.006 g/liter) is a good example of the fact that substances with a *bitter* taste are detected at very low concentrations. The detection threshold for saccharine is 23 μmol/liter (0.0055 g/liter), for grape sugar 0.08 mol/liter, and for cane sugar 0.01 mol/liter (14.41 g/liter and 3.42 g/liter, respectively). These data are characteristic, and indicate that the thresholds for mono- and disaccharides are considerably higher than those for synthetic sweeteners. The thresholds for acetic acid (0.18 mol/liter, or 0.108 g/liter) and table salt (0.01 mol/liter, or 0.585 g/liter) exemplify the general rule that thresholds for *sour* and *salty* substances are of about the same order of magnitude as those for the saccharides mentioned above. The thresholds for acids reflect approximately the degree of dissociation. Comparison of the thresholds for grape and cane sugar implies that a solution of grape sugar must be more concentrated than a cane-sugar solution that tastes equally sweet. An experimental test of solutions at various suprathreshold concentrations confirms this prediction.

But the usefulness of such precise threshold data is limited, because there is considerable individual variability in the thresholds for most substances. It would be more realistic to speak in terms of *threshold ranges.*

Intensity of sensations. The simple comparison of different test solutions indicates that the intensity of a taste sensation depends upon the *concentration* of the substance concerned. In threshold determinations, it turns out that the effect of diluting a solution of stimulus substance can be compensated by stimulating a larger *area on the surface of the tongue* — that is, by stimulating a larger number of receptors. This effect can probably be attributed to spatial facilitation. There is a corresponding relationship between *concentration and duration* of a stimulus, in the threshold region. These findings can be summarized in the expressions $C \cdot A^n = k$ and $t \cdot C^n = k$, where C is the concentration of the substance in solution, A is the area of the stimulated part of the tongue and t is the time during which the stimulus acts. k is a constant for each substance tested; the exponents n are also specific to the stimulus substance. These expressions do not include all the parameters affecting the intensity of a taste sensation; the *temperature* of the stimulus solution also plays a role. Moreover, it should be kept in mind that the sense of taste exhibits a definite *adaptation* — during long exposure to a stimulus the intensity of the sensation decreases. Still another factor is the secretion of the serous glands, which dilutes the stimulus substance at the taste buds and thus can change the intensity of sensation.

Tests of series of dilutions of salt solutions in the near-threshold range, in many cases, show that the sensation can change in quality as a function of concentration. Solutions of table salt of 0.02–0.03 mol/liter taste sweet, whereas concentrations of 0.04 mol/liter or more taste salty. This *shift in quality* is perhaps understandable in view of the fact that the taste fibers exhibit a broad spectrum of sensitivities within each quality (cf. Sec. 8.2).

As Figure 8–1 shows, the different *regions of the human tongue vary in sensitivity* to the four basic qualities. The tip of the tongue is particularly sensitive to sweet substances, and the middle parts of the outer edges are most responsive to sour stimuli. Salty stimuli are most effective in an area on the edge of the tongue that partially overlaps these two regions. Bitter substances affect most strongly the receptors near the base of the tongue, in the region of the vallate papillae. Therefore *damage to the glossopharyngeal nerve* reduces the ability to detect bitter substances, whereas after a block of conduction in the *facial nerve* only bitter substances can be detected.

Like other sensory systems, the taste system is influenced by hormones. *Glucocorticoids* affect one's ability to discriminate taste qualities.

Functional disturbances. The condition in which the thresholds for taste perception are above the normal range is called *hypogeusia.* In *ageusia* there is no taste sensation at all; saturated solutions of salt or sugar cannot be distinguished from water. The perception of bitter substances is most often affected. *Dysgeusia* is a distortion of taste such that sensations — usually unpleasant — are experienced that do not correspond to the stimulus, or without any stimulus. It is observed in various disease states, especially carcinomas. Because the distorted taste affects choice of food and the amount consumed, it can influence the general condition of a patient. In some cases of dysgeusia the administration of *zinc* has proved helpful.

Q 8.1.   The afferent fibers from the taste buds are:
a) The axons of the gustatory sense cells
b) Unbranched fibers ending in synapses on the gustatory sense cells

    c) Branched fibers ending in synapses on the gustatory sense cells
    d) Sensory fibers ending on the surface of the epithelium between the gustatory sense cells.

Q 8.2. List from memory the names of the nerves from the taste organs, and two higher stations in the taste pathway.

Q 8.3. Match the following substances with the associated taste quality:
1. Caffeine, 2. magnesium chloride, 3. citric acid, 4. glucose, 5. nicotine, 6. tartaric acid, and 7. quinine sulfate
    a) Sweet
    b) Sour
    c) Salty
    d) Bitter

Q 8.4. How concentrated, in relative terms, must a solution of cane sugar be in order to taste just as sweet as 1. a grape-sugar solution? 2. a saccharine solution?
    a) More and less concentrated, respectively
    b) More concentrated in both cases
    c) Less and more concentrated, respectively
    d) Less concentrated in both cases

Q 8.5. To which taste qualities do 1. the tip of the tongue and, 2. the area just ahead of the base of the tongue respond most strongly?
    a) Sweet stimuli
    b) Sour stimuli
    c) Salty stimuli
    d) Bitter stimuli

8.2 Objective Taste Physiology

In this section we shall discuss the likely possibility that the ability to **discriminate taste qualities** depends on the **specificity of receptor molecules** in the membranes of the sensory cells. It might seem surprising that such a mechanism would be reflected only diffusely or not at all in the specificity of response of the individual sensory cell and afferent fiber. How can quality and concentration then be coded? This question can be answered by taking into account the constellation of responses of large numbers of cells or fibers. Therefore we shall first describe these, and in conclusion discuss briefly the biological significance of the sense of taste.

    Microelectrodes can be used to record the activity of both single taste sensory cells and afferent fibers. Such recordings show that neither the receptors themselves nor the fibers leading to the CNS give quality-specific responses; as a rule,

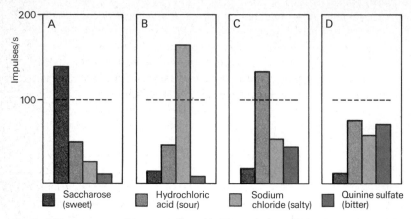

Fig. 8–4. The responses of four taste fibers (A–D) to solutions of stimulus substances of different qualities. The typical patterns of differing excitation are called taste profiles

stimuli in more than one category are effective. Figure 8–4 shows the change in discharge rate of four afferent fibers (A–D) during stimulation with substances representing the four basic qualities. It is evident that each fiber responds to stimuli of several categories, but there are distinctions if one considers the various gradations of sensitivity. That is, stimulation with a solution of a substance at a certain concentration activates the various fibers by different amounts. The pattern of excitation typical of each single fiber, in response to a range of substances, is called its *taste profile.* The most nearly quality-specific fibers are those that respond with an increased discharge rate to sugar solutions. Comparative studies have shown that possession of such relatively specific fibers is particularly characteristic of monkeys.

Recordings from the individual sensory cells have shown that they, too, respond with a *graded relative specificity.* The responses of the fibers from these cells, to this extent, reflect those of the cells. But the afferent fibers branch within the taste buds (cf. Fig. 8–3), so that each fiber receives excitation from a number of sensory cells differing — one must assume — in specificity. Moreover, it has been found that sensory cells in different papillae synapse with collaterals from a single afferent fiber. That is, the taste fibers receive input from sensors distributed over fairly large areas of the tongue. These areas are called receptive fields (Fig. 8–5). The receptive-field situation is complicated by the fact that individual sensory cells can be innervated by several different fibers.

To summarize, the graded relative specificity of the taste fibers results from, 1. the graded relative specificity of the sensory cells and, 2. the branching of the taste fibers to form receptive fields. The discharge rate of a single afferent fiber (cf. Fig. 8–4) changes, therefore, depending both on the quality of a stimulus and on its concentration. The extent to which the stimulated area covers the receptive field of the fiber is of course also an important factor. The clear implication, with respect to the coding of a stimulus situation, is that the activity of a single fiber cannot provide

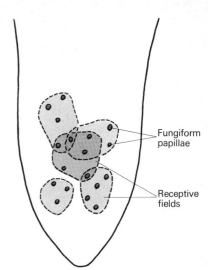

Fungiform
papillae

Receptive
fields

Fig. 8–5. Receptive fields on the rat
tongue. The individual afferent fibers
respond to stimuli over extensive regions,
which may exhibit multiple overlap; each
region includes several fungiform papillae

unambiguous information about quality or concentration. Only a **comparison** of
the level of excitation in several fibers can reveal characteristic activity patterns
that tell something about the quality of the stimulus. Given that the quality is
known, the frequency of impulses in each individual fiber would serve to measure
the concentration of the stimulus substance. The distinguishing aspects of a
stimulus substance, then, are coded in such a way that a complex but characteristic
pattern of excitation is generated by the simultaneous but different responses of a
large number of neurons.

The primary process. If a taste receptor is to be excited, there must be an
interaction between molecules of the stimulating substance and specially differentiated places in the membrane of the sensory cell where **receptor molecules** are
located. This interaction is called the primary process; it is thought to begin with
adsorption of the stimulus molecule. When this happens the receptor, probably a
protein molecule, is assumed to change its structure. This **conformational change**
of the receptor molecule could in turn lead to a local **permeability change** in the cell
membrane. Such a cellular "amplifier mechanism" could account for the generation of a receptor potential.

   Evidence of the **existence of specific receptor molecules** includes the observation
that certain plant substances and drugs, such as cocaine and gymnemic acid
(derived from the Indian plant *Gymnema sylvestre*), selectively block the sensation
of taste of certain qualities. Gymnemic acid evidently combines with the receptor
molecules for sweet substances, since application of this agent renders such
substances tasteless. The primary process in the membranes of taste sensory cells
has not yet been adequately explained, but a working hypothesis is that it
resembles that at cholinergic synapses, where particular molecules change the
permeability at special membrane sites.

Role of the sense of taste. The taste buds on the tongue respond to stimuli within or directly in front of the mouth. In other words, the sense of taste is involved in *short-distance orientation,* in all the higher vertebrates. Among fish, on the other hand, the sense of taste can also contribute to *long-distance orientation.* In water, taste substances can move, by diffusion and convection, from quite distant sources to the taste buds, which may even be distributed over the entire body surface of a fish.

In addition to its role in short-distance orientation, the human sense of taste has the important function of triggering a number of *reflexes.* For example, the rinsing of the tongue by release of secretion from the serous glands is controlled by a reflex that is under the influence of the taste buds. The secretion of saliva is also triggered reflexly by appropriate stimulation of the taste receptors. Indeed, the composition of saliva varies according to the pattern of stimuli acting on the sensory cells, and the secretion of gastric juices is also affected by taste stimuli. Finally, the sense of taste has been shown to be involved in eliciting vomiting.

Q 8.6. How does a given afferent fiber from the taste buds respond to taste substances?
a) Equally strongly to substances of the same quality.
b) To different degrees, though the substances are of the same quality
c) Equally strongly to substances of different quality
d) To different degrees when the substances are of different quality

Q 8.7. What is the basis of the graded specificity of single taste fibers?
a) The lack of absolute specificity among the sensory cells
b) The branching of the fibers and the existence of receptive fields
c) The overlapping of the receptive fields

Q 8.8. Which of the following responses can be triggered reflexly by the excitation of taste receptors?
a) Coughing
b) Serous-gland secretion
c) Secretion of saliva
d) The flow of tears
e) Choking

The suggested reading list for this chapter appears with that for chapter 9 on p. 275.

9 Physiology of Olfaction

H. Altner

The human nose is capable of discriminating thousands of different odor sub-stances, but this achievement is modest compared with the performance of other organisms. This relative lack of olfactory ability, combined with the dominant importance of our other sense organs, may well be one reason why people have had little interest in research on the olfactory system. Another is the difficulty of experiments on the sense of smell — with humans, certainly, but also with other animals. As a consequence, neither subjective nor objective criteria have permit-ted clear definition of odor qualities; there is little order in the bewildering variety of adequate olfactory stimuli. On the other hand, as this chapter will show, the olfactory pathway in mammals is well known. Structural and physiologic analysis has revealed a number of interesting properties of the system — for example, that the signals sent to the brain are under efferent control. Much has also been learned about the significance of the sense of smell in autonomic regulatory and emotional attitudes.

9.1 The Olfactory Mucosa; Peripheral Mechanisms of Olfactory Reception

The first subject of this section is the morphology of the olfactory organ and the cells it comprises. We shall then turn to the variety of stimulus substances; these cannot be classified as to quality, on the basis either of the sensations they elicit or of the responses of individual sensory cells.

Location and cellular organization of the olfactory epithelium. The nasal cavity is divided into two spaces, left and right, by a partition called the nasal septum. The surface area of each space is enlarged by folding to form ridges, the conchae, which project into the interior from the outside walls. As Figure 9–1 shows, in the adult human three conchae are arranged one above the other on each side. The entire nasal cavity is lined with a mucous membrane, but the olfactory sensory cells are restricted to a small area, the olfactory region (shown in red in Fig. 9–1). The olfactory region covers the whole of the upper concha and forms islands on the middle concha. There is also olfactory epithelium on the adjacent parts of the septum. The respiratory region — the part of the nasal mucosa that lacks olfactory cells — is a ciliated epithelium made up of two layers of cells, among them the goblet cells which produce the mucus.

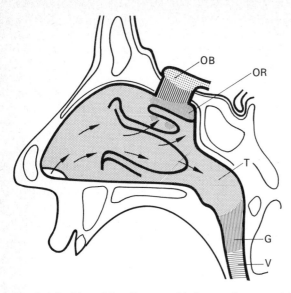

Fig. 9–1. Position of the olfactory epithelium, and pattern of air flow, in the human nose as seen from the side. The olfactory region *(OR, red)* is restricted to the upper and middle conchae. The axons of the sensory cells here form the fila olfactoria *(black)*, which run to the olfactory bulb *(OB)*. The regions from which fibers pass to the trigeminal *(T)*, glossopharyngeal *(G)* and vagus *(V)* nerves are also indicated

In the human fetus, the mucosa on the septum contains closed tubules that appear to lead nowhere. These are rudiments of the vomeronasal (Jacobson's) organ, an olfactory organ that plays an accessory, and in some cases important, role in many amphibians, reptiles, and mammals. It no longer exists in humans.

Figure 9–2 shows the structure of the *olfactory mucosa,* a several-layered epithelium with two predominant cell types, the olfactory cells and the supporting cells. As in the taste buds (cf. Chap. 8), basal cells are also present; these can develop into olfactory cells, and are thus immature sensory cells. The olfactory cells (unlike gustatory sensory cells) are primary sensory cells, sending out axons from the basal pole. These fibers form thick bundles beneath the sensory epithelium; these (also called *fila olfactoria*) run to the olfactory bulb.

At their apical poles the olfactory cells bear modified cilia, enclosed by the layer of mucus that covers the olfactory epithelium. The molecules of an odor substance must diffuse through part of this mucus layer before they reach the most peripheral part of the olfactory cells, the membranes of the cilia. The mucus is derived from three sources: 1. Bowman's glands, 2. the goblet cells of the respiratory region, and 3. the supporting cells of the olfactory epithelium, which thus serve a dual function. The kinocilia of cells in the respiratory region act to control the flow of mucus.

Odor sensations are not mediated exclusively by the sensory cells in the olfactory region. The respiratory region includes, in addition to the cell elements already, mentioned, free endings of sensory fibers of the fifth cranial nerve, the trigeminal;

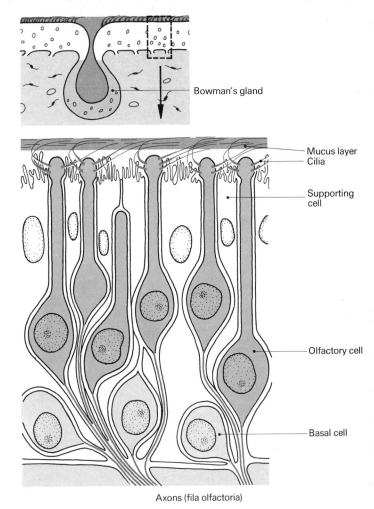

Bowman's gland

Mucus layer
Cilia

Supporting
cell

Olfactory cell

Basal cell

Axons (fila olfactoria)

Fig. 9–2. Elements of the olfactory epithelium. *Above,* mucous membrane in the olfactory region; *below,* the cells of which the olfactory mucosa is composed

these also respond to odor substances. Thus even if the fila olfactoria are completely transected, as may happen in an accident, the sense of smell is to some extent preserved.

Odor qualities. Everyday experience demonstrates that we can disciminate thousands of different substances by their smell. But in contrast to the situation in gustatory physiology, subjective experiments on olfaction have not succeeded in providing a clear distinction between odor qualities. There is something arbitrary about each attempt to impose such an organization. But for practical considerations a series of qualities has been defined, a list of *odor classes* or *primary odors.*

Some of these are listed below, each with two examples of chemically pure odor substances in that category:

Flowery: α-ionone, β-phenylethyl alcohol
Etheric: 1,2-dichlorethane, benzylacetate
Musky: Ring ketones (C_{15-17}) such as civetone and musk ketone
Camphorous: 1,8-cineole, camphor
Sweaty: Isovalerianic acid, butyric acid
Rotten: Hydrogen sulfide, ethyl mercaptan
Pungent: Formic acid, acetic acid

Just these few examples make it clear that chemically similar substances can fall into different odor classes, and that members of a single class can differ considerably in chemical structure. The naturally occuring scents that have given their names to the primary classes (for example, the perfume of flowers, the smell of sweat, and the odor of rotting meat) are as a rule *odor mixtures* in which certain components predominate.

Of the population in Europe 0.1%–1% has been shown to have specific "odor blindness". The symptom of such *partial anosmia,* which in some cases may be inherited, is that a small number of substances that smell similar (e. g., certain musky odors) cannot be detected. The existence of partial anosmias is evidence that a delimitation of odor qualities is possible to a certain extent.

Coding. As with taste sensations (cf. Chap. 8), the primary process underlying the sense of smell is poorly understood, though again it is thought that the molecules of an odor substance interact with specialized molecules in the membrane of the olfactory cell, the receptor molecules. The large number of effective odor substances alone makes it unlikely that the sensory membrane contains a particular receptor molecule for each odor substance. Presumably several *related odor substances* react with a *common receptor molecule.* Evidence for the existence of receptor molecules that can interact with more than one odor substance is given by the phenomenon of partial anosmia mentioned above. Nevertheless, the separate stimuli must somehow be coded, to account for the known recognition of the individual odors.

The way the parameters of the stimulus, in particular the nature and concentration of the odor substance, are coded should be most readily discernible from recordings of the responses of single receptor cells. Such recordings have shown that the olfactory cells exhibit *characteristic response spectra.* Each single cell is excited, to different degrees, by many substances, but the relative sensitivity to various effective substances (at given concentrations) varies from one cell to another. Evidently stimuli to the olfactory cells, like those to the taste buds (cf. Chap. 8), are coded in such a way that at a given concentration each odor substance elicits a particular pattern of excitation involving many sensory cells. That is, the relative level of excitation of a great number of receptors contains the information about the nature of the substance. As concentration increases, in most cases the frequency of impulses increases, though some odor substances inhibit the spontaneous activity of the sensory cells.

The olfactory sensory cells of insects, usually located on bristle-like projections of the cuticular exoskeleton, are much more accessible to electrophysiologic procedures than are vertebrate olfactory cells. Here the results differ from those obtained with vertebrates, in that receptors have been found with highly specific responses to certain odor substances. Another intriguing finding, from experiments with the silkworm moth, is that a conducted action potential can be elicited if only a single molecule of the attractant substance produced by the female strikes the membrane of a male sensory cell. There is no reason to suppose that the situation is fundamentally different in the olfactory cells of humans and the other vertebrates.

Q 9.1. (A) How many conchae are there in each chamber of the nasal cavity, and (B) on which of them is the olfactory region located?

A. a) Three or four   B. a) On all of them
    b) Three   b) On the top one
    c) More than three   c) On the bottom one
    d) Two   d) On the two upper ones
    e) One or two   e) On the two lower ones

Q 9.2. Which of the following cell types are to be found in the olfactory region of the nasal mucosa?
a) Olfactory cells
b) Goblet cells
c) Supporting cells
d) Basal cells

Q 9.3. List from memory the names of four odor classes.

Q 9.4. What is meant by the term "partial anosmia"?
a) Destruction of the olfactory region
b) An inability to smell a small number of related odors
c) A general increase in the threshold to odor stimuli
d) A reduced sensitivity to musky smells

Q 9.5. How are odor substances coded in the response of the sensory cells?
a) By the response of quality-specific sensory cells
b) By the response of substance-specific sensory cells
c) By the formation of specific patterns of excitation over a large population of sensory cells

9.2 Subjective Olfactory Physiology; Central Connections

We shall first discuss the finding that a distinction can be made between the threshold for detection of an odor and that for its recognition. Then it will be shown that the strength of such sensations increases relatively slowly as the intensity of the stimuli is raised. Analysis of the olfactory pathway has revealed that efferent control of the excitatory input is exerted near the periphery. Moreover, the olfactory sense by no means serves only in orientation; it also affects the course of vegetative processes and may well influence emotional attitudes.

Detection threshold and recognition threshold. At low concentrations of odor substance, just sufficient to elicit the sensation of smelling "something", people as a rule cannot say what the odor is. They simply perceive that there is an odor. Only at higher concentrations does the smell of the substance become recognizable, so that the odor can be specifically identified. It is useful, therefore, to think in terms of a *detection threshold* and a *recognition threshold.*

The human nose is very sensitive to many substances. Butyric acid, which is in the class of sweaty smells, is detected at a concentration as low as $2.4 \cdot 10^{12}$ molecules/liter of air — equivalent to a dilution of the pure substance by a factor of 10^{10}. The detection threshold for butyl mercaptan, a substance with an unpleasant rotten garlicky smell, is 10^{10} molecules/liter air (dilution $2.7 \cdot 10^{12}$).

If one knows the detection threshold for a substance and the number of receptors, one can calculate the corresponding number of molecules of odor substance per olfactory cell per inspiration (or "sniff"). Such a calculation for butyl mercaptan gives a result of at most eight molecules per cell per sniff at threshold.

Considerably lower thresholds have been measured for animals other than man. The astonishing olfactory acuity of dogs is widely known. Eels are actually capable of detecting beta-phenylethyl alcohol at a dilution of $1 : 2.86 \cdot 10^{18}$, which is equivalent to putting one ml of this substance into a lake with 58 times the volume of Lake Constance.

The intensity of sensation. When suprathreshold stimuli are given, the sensation becomes stronger as the concentration of the odor substance is increased. The relationship is describable by Stevens' power law — sensation is proportional to $(C - C_0)^n$ (cf. p. 17). When plotted on double logarithmic coordinates such data fall on a straight line, the slope of which is a measure of the rate of increase in strength of sensation as concentration is increased (Fig. 9–3). The exponent n, which reflects the slope, is 0.5–0.6 in the case of olfaction. This is a rather small slope in comparison to that of some other sensory modalities; in other words, olfactory sensations change relatively slowly with changes of the stimulus.

If stimuli are maintained for long periods the intensity of the sensation falls off — *adaptation* occurs. With prolonged high-intensity stimuli adaptation may even be complete, so that the sensation disappears entirely. Adaptation can be measured by the increase in threshold observed after a period of stimulation.

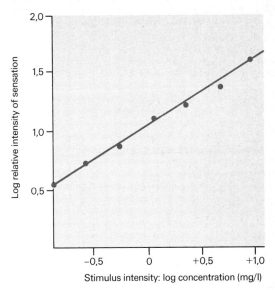

Fig. 9–3. Dependence of the strength of an odor sensation upon the concentration of the substance (in this case, pentanol). The slope of the line is small as compared with that for other sensory modalities

Stimulation of trigeminal fibers. The fibers of the trigeminal nerve are said to respond preferentially to pungent or burnt odors. But in experiments on animals these fibers respond as well to substances that do not smell at all acrid to humans. Observations of patients with unilateral destruction of this nerve also suggest that the trigeminal component makes a more general contribution to odor sensations.

Central connections. In the preceding section it was mentioned that the bundled axons of the olfactory cells, the *fila olfactoria,* run to the olfactory bulb. On the way they pass through the cribriform plate of the ethmoid bone. Figure 9–4 shows that the cellular elements in the olfactory bulb are arranged in layers. Proceeding centripetally, these layers are, 1. the layer of the fila olfactoria, 2. the layer of the glomeruli, 3. the outer plexiform layer, 4. the layer of the mitral-cell somata, and 5. the layer of the granule cells. The conspicuously large mitral cells represent the second-order neurons of the olfactory pathway. They send out one main dendrite, on the distal branches of which are the synapses with the fibers from the olfactory cells. The dendritic branches of the mitral cells, together with the endings of fibers that terminate there, form spherical masses, the glomeruli.

About 1,000 afferent fibers converge on each mitral cell. Axons of olfactory cells also end at and form synapses with the periglomerular cells, which provide lateral communication among the glomeruli.

The axons of the mitral cells constitute the olfactory tract. This tract, either directly or by way of its connections with other tracts, transmits olfactory signals to many regions of the brain. Among these are the olfactory bulb on the other side,

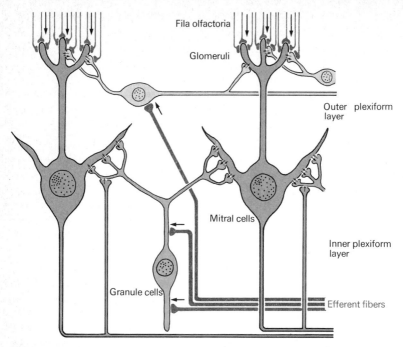

Fig. 9–4. Diagram of the layers in the olfactory bulb, showing the connections among the cells. The cells between the glomeruli, the periglomerular cells, can transmit lateral influences between mitral cells; both periglomerular and granule cells mediate efferent control. The fila olfactoria and efferent fibers are shown in **red.** At the dendrodendritic synapses, **red arrows** symbolize inhibition and **black arrows,** excitation

the prepiriform area and the piriform lobe, the hippocampal formation, and via the amygdaloid complex, the autonomic nuclei of the hypothalamus.

The output of excitatory signals from the olfactory bulb is under efferent control, applied at a peripheral level. In Figure 9–4 the centrifugal fibers are shown in red. These axons terminate at granule cells and periglomerular cells, and are thus in a position to modify excitatory inputs from the fila olfactoria at the level of the mitral cells. The schematic representation in Figure 9–4 is a much simplified survey of the complicated connections within the olfactory bulb. It does show, however, that dendrodendritic contacts are made between mitral and granule cells as well as between mitral and periglomerular cells. Such contacts mediate information flow in both directions — from the mitral cells to the periglomerular and granule cells, and conversely, from these to the mitral cells. Figure 9–4 also indicates the possibility of lateral interactions among the mitral cells, by way of the periglomerular cells.

As mentioned above, excitatory signals from the olfactory organ are transmitted to the autonomic nuclei of the hypothalamus. The function of this connection has not yet been adequately studied. It is certain that in various mammals activity in these pathways influences phenomena associated with reproduction. An important finding in this respect is that sensory cells and neurons in the olfactory pathway are influenced by *steroid hormones.* In rodents estradiol, testosterone and aldosterone act at various levels in the system. One result may well be to enhance responsiveness to *pheromones,* odor substances produced by a sexual partner which are perceived mainly by way of the vomeronasal organ.

But the full *significance of the sense of smell* in mammals goes beyond both this participation in the control of reproduction and its obvious role in the search for food. For example, odor substances serve as signals in the social relationship of groups and individuals. The group to which an animal belongs can be communicated by an *odor signal,* just as the occupant of a territory can label its boundaries with scent marks. Among humans the sense of smell has lost in importance in comparison with other senses, but its significance still tends to be underestimated. Emotions, for example, may be affected more widely then we realize; a familiar perfume can evoke a strong mood. The abovementioned connections between the olfactory organ and the limbic system might account for such effects. But these relationships have received little attention; better known is the fact that some unpleasant odors can elicit protective reflexes in humans, including sneezing and choking. And substances with a sharp smell, such as ammonia, can cause a reflex interruption of breathing.

Functional disturbances. In cases of *hyposmia* the threshold for detection and/or recognition is raised; in *anosmia* no odor sensations can be elicited. A person with *dysosmia* experiences unpleasant sensations of smell abnormally, either in response to an inappropriate odor substance (cacosmia) or in the absence of an olfactory stimulus (phantosmia). Such disturbances of olfaction can have various causes; for example, they may accompany allergic rhinitis or result from head trauma. Some partial anosmias are innate.

Q 9.6. Which is associated with higher concentrations, a) the detection threshold or b) the recognition threshold?

Q 9.7. Which of the following indicates the degree of adaptation of the sense of smell?
a) An increased sensitivity to odor substances
b) A rise in the detection threshold
c) A lowering of the recognition threshold

Q 9.8. Which of the following elements exerts efferent control in the olfactory bulb?
a) Fila olfactoria
b) Centrifugal fibers in the olfactory tract
c) Granule cells
d) Periglomerular cells

10 Thirst and Hunger: General Sensations

R. F. Schmidt

The feeling of thirst we experience when we have not drunk enough fluids, and our feelings of hunger when we have not eaten recently, cannot be ascribed to a particular sense organ or part of the body. For this reason they are called "general sensations". Other examples of general sensations are tiredness, shortness of breath, and sexual appetite. From the viewpoint of sensory physiology, a characteristic they all share is that they can be elicited by one or more *adequate stimuli originating within the body itself,* rather than in its environment. These stimuli are detected by receptors, some of which are still unknown, and thus produce the associated general sensations (Fig. 10–1A). For example, we shall explain below that a "concentrating" of the body fluid due to lack of water is sensed by osmoreceptors, the result being a sensation or feeling of thirst (Fig. 10–1B). One can also imagine that during the course of the day waste materials accumulate in the blood, and that these are responsible for a feeling of tiredness (cf. Sec. 9.2 in *Fundamentals of Neurophysiology*), or that certain hormones elicit feelings of sexual desire, or favor the occurrence of such feelings, when their concentration in the body is high enough.

The stimuli adequate to elicit general sensations also elicit activities directed toward reducing the intensity of such sensations or eliminating them. That is, the stimuli for general sensations induce *drives,* motivational states that "drive" the organism to provide whatever is felt to be lacking. Although such drives are controlled by sensations, they may also occur independently (Fig. 10–1A). A lack of water in the body leads not only to a sensation of thirst but also to a search for water which, if successful, removes the deficiency (Fig. 10–1B). In the broadest terms, *the satisfaction of a drive eliminates the releaser of the general sensation.*

The drives associated with general sensations serve to *ensure survival* of the individual or species. As a rule, therefore, they must be satisfied. They are inborn and need not be learned. But during a lifetime they are modified by numerous influences, especially at the more advanced phylogenetic levels. These influences act at various points in the overall process. A description of drives and their modification is outside the framework of this book; here we shall treat only the aspects of thirst and hunger related to sensory physiology, as examples of the category of general sensations.

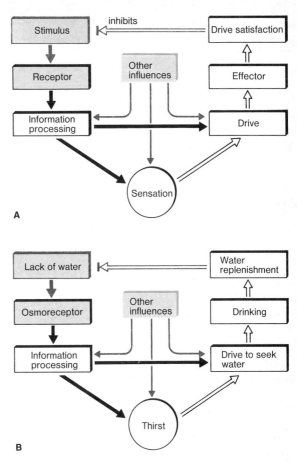

Fig. 10–1 A,B. Diagramm of the relationship between general sensations and drives. *A* General representation of the way the sensations and drives are interrelated. *B* Production of a feeling of thirst and activation of the drive to find water during water deficiency. Other receptors in addition to the osmoreceptors are responsible for producing the sensation of thirst (cf. Fig. 10–2). The *vertical red bars* at the tips of the *top arrows* indicate that satisfaction of the drive (the provision of water in *B*) leads to elimination of the stimulus (water deficiency in *B*)

10.1 Thirst

Conditions under which a sensation of thirst appears. The adult human body consists of about 70%–75% water by weight (without taking the fat deposits into account). This high water content of the body is *maintained within very narrow limits.* Normally it fluctuates by only about ± 0.22% of the weight of the body, so that in a 70 kg man the variation is around ± 150 ml. If the body loses water amounting to more than 0.5% of its weight (about 350 ml, for a person weighing

70 kg) thirst results. There are four physiological ways in which the body can lose water: by producing urine, by sweating, as water vapor in the exhaled air, and (usually to a limited extent) in the feces. This water must be replaced if the vital, delicate equilibrium among the many dissolved substances is not to be upset. As the *water-balance data* in Table 10–1 show, a person in a temperate climate eating ordinary food obtains water chiefly by drinking, but also as a component of his solid food, and to a lesser degree as a product of the oxidative decomposition of that food in his body. The totals reflect the daily turnover of water in an adult, which amounts to about 3%–4% of the body weight.

Table 10–1. Daily water balance in the adult (from MUNTWYLER, 1973)

Water uptake	ml	Water loss	ml
Drinking	1200	Urine	1400
In solid food	900	Lungs and skin	900
Water from oxidation	300	Feces	100
Totals:	2400		2400

Another factor affecting the sensation of thirst is the division of the body's water into *two compartments* with different properties. About two thirds of the body fluid is in the cells, the *intracellular space,* and the remaining third is in the *extracellular space.* About three quarters of the extracellular water occupies the gaps between the cells, the interstitial space, and the rest is in the *vascular system,* forming the aqueous phase of the blood plasma (the blood minus the corpuscles). The extracellular and intracellular fluids are separated by the cell membrane and are of different composition, particularly regarding the cations and anions. For present purposes, the important difference is that the *extracellular fluid contains large quantities of Na^+,* whereas the *intracellular fluid is rich in K^+* but poor in Na^+ (for further details see Table 2–1, p. 23, in *Fundamentals of Neurophysiology,* 3rd Ed.). The blood plasma and the interstitial fluid are in communication through the walls of the capillaries; they differ negligibly in salt content, but the protein content of the plasma is considerably higher than that of the interstitial fluid.

The cell membranes separating intracellular and extracellular spaces are readily permeable to water, but their permeability to salts is considerably less. We shall assume in this discussion, for simplicity, that the membranes are impermeable to salts. The net *diffusion of water* through such semipermeable membranes (i.e., permeable only to water) is always *in the direction of the space with the higher salt concentration* (i.e., lower "water concentration"). If the salt concentration in the two spaces is the same, water diffuses through the cell membrane equally in both directions, so that there is no net displacement of water. But if water is removed from one of the spaces, so that the salt concentration there rises, water moves in from the other space until the concentration is again equal in both. (This process is called *osmosis,* and the hydrostatic pressure difference which would just counteract the net tendency of water to diffuse across a semipermeable membrane between two fluid spaces differing in salt concentration is the *osmotic pressure.* A salt solution with the same osmotic pressure as normal body fluid is called an *isotonic* solution. Correspondingly, *hypertonic* and *hypotonic* designate salt solutions more or less concentrated, respectively, than normal body fluid). For example, if water is withdrawn from the plasma owing to urine production in the kidney, water diffuses from the interstitial space into the plasma and from the cells into the interstitial space. On the other hand, if a cell in a sweat gland secretes sweat (i.e., loses water), water must diffuse from the interstitial space into the gland cell.

The physiologic water losses of the body (urine, sweat, moisture in the expired air) together cause *loss of water from both the extracellular and intracellular spaces.* There is a concomitant *increase in the salt concentration* in these solutions; they become hypertonic, though normally only slightly so. A further result is a *reduction in the secretion of saliva,* which gives rise to the feeling of dryness in mouth and throat so characteristic of thirst. If the appropriate receptors were present, then, reduced water in the body could be measured a) by the volume or osmotic pressure of the cells, b) by the volume or osmotic pressure of the extracellular space, or c) indirectly by the reduction in saliva secretion and the resulting dryness of the mucous membranes.

The adequate stimuli for the sensation of thirst. To decide which of the changes just mentioned might be responsible for producing the sensation of thirst, each factor must be studied experimentally *in isolation;* that is, the water or salt content of one space must be changed without affecting the other, or the rate of saliva secretion alone must be modified. Such experiments have been done on animals, the amount of water drunk serving as an indicator of the degree of experimentally induced thirst. The most important results of these experiments will be described in the following paragraphs.

Following intravenous infusion of a hypertonic NaCl solution, a dog drinks twice as much water as it does after intravenous infusion of an osmotically equivalent solution of urea. In the former case, because the cell membranes are impermeable to Na^+ ions, water leaves the cells. But the cell membranes are readily permeable to urea, so that when it is injected the concentrations in the intracellular and extracellular spaces equilibrate, with a distinctly smaller change in cell volume and tonicity (salt concentration) of the cells. This finding has been confirmed by repetition of the experiment, with many modifications, on a wide variety of mammals. The inference to be drawn is that *reduction of cell volume,* the salt content of the cells remaining constant (but not the concentration, which rises), *elicits thirst.*

If the amount of Na^+ in the extracellular space is experimentally reduced (for example, by a change in diet or by means of an artificial kidney), the extracellular space loses water; part is released from the body, and part diffuses into the cells. Under these conditions, even though there is an increase in cell volume, thirst is experienced. (The subject also feels a desire for table salt, but we shall not go into that here). Moreover, it is possible experimentally to reduce the volume of extracellular fluid without changing its NaCl concentration, so that there is no change in cell volume; in this case, too, thirst results. We can conclude that *decrease in volume of the extracellular fluid* also elicits thirst. Experiments have shown that the effects of the above two factors are additive; *simultaneous decrease* of cell volume and of the volume of extracellular fluid gives rise to particularly *intense thirst.*

The *dryness of the mouth* accompanying essentially all forms of thirst is caused, as mentioned above, by a *reduction in the secretion of saliva.* This phenomenon reflects the shortage of water. But contrary to earlier interpretations, it does not appear to be the cause but rather a *symptom* associated with the general feeling of thirst. This is demonstrated by the following findings. Moistening the mouth and throat surfaces does not eliminate the sensation of thirst, though it can relieve it somewhat. Nor can thirst be relieved or prevented by local anesthesia of the oral mucosa, or even by complete denervation of the mouth and throat region. Finally congenital absence of the salivary glands (in humans) or their surgical removal (from animals) has no appreciable effect on water consumption; the normal amount is drunk.

Receptors and central mechanisms. The neural structures chiefly responsible for regulating salt/water balance lie in the *diencephalon,* particularly in the *hypothalamus and its vicinity* (cf. *Fundamentals of Neurophysiology,* Sec. 8.8). This part of the brain is especially involved in the control and regulation of the vegetative functions of the body. Experiments have revealed the presence of *osmoreceptors* here, mostly in areas anterior to the hypothalamus. These are sensors that respond to *increase of the intracellular salt concentration when the cell loses water.* The injection of very small amounts (less than 0.2 ml) of hypertonic solutions of NaCl into certain parts of this region, for example, causes goats to begin drinking 30–60 s later, and to continue for 2–5 min, in the process consuming 2–8 liters of water. Electrical stimulation of the same neural structures also elicits prolonged drinking. When certain hypothalamic areas have been ablated surgically or coagulated, drinking can be reduced or eliminated even though body water is depleted. All these results indicate that *osmoreceptors in the diencephalon serve as sensors for the thirst induced by cellular water deficiency* (Fig. 10–2). Neuronal structures in the hypothalamus evidently play a crucial role in processing the information from these osmoreceptors.

As far as the *sensors underlying the thirst elicited by lack of water in the extracellular space* are concerned, we have only suggestions and indirect evidence. At present it appears that the *stretch receptors* in the walls of the large veins near the heart and the atria not only influence the circulation of the blood, but also participate in the regulation of water balance and arousal of thirst (Fig. 10–2). The hypothalamus is an important processing center for signals from the stretch receptors (by way of the vagus afferents). There is also evidence that in addition to the neural components, *hormonal factors* (in particular the renin/angiotensin

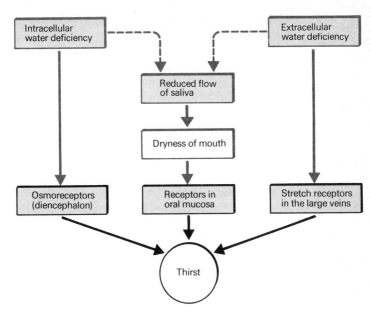

Fig. 10–2. Production of the sensation of thirst. The receptors involved are marked by the *gray shading.* Above them are *boxes* indicating their adequate stimuli. Dryness of the mouth is an indirect consequence of intracellular and extracellular lack of water

system) are involved in producing thirst. At present, however, we cannot say just how these factors act or how important they are.

The reduced flow of saliva and the resulting *dryness of the mouth* associated with water deficiency are signalled by *receptors in the mucous membranes of the mouth and throat.* Experiments on animals have shown that various kinds of receptors are present there — mechanoreceptors, cold and warm receptors, and perhaps water receptors. The extent to which each of these participates in eliciting this *peripheral component of thirst* is not known. If these receptors are stimulated when there is no general water deficiency in the body, as may happen as a result of speaking, smoking, breathing through the mouth, or eating very dry food, the *"false thirst"* they elicit can be satisfied by moistening the oral mucosa. In the case of genuine thirst, as mentioned above, moistening the throat may lessen but it will not quench the thirst sensation.

Thirst, then, is a *general sensation based on the integrated response of many receptor types,* some in the periphery and others in the CNS. These are summarized in Figure 10–2. The diencephalon, and the hypothalamus in particular, appear to play a dominant role in the integration of this multitude of afferent inputs. We do not know how accurately the results of experiments on animals can be applied to humans, nor do we know which central structures give rise to the sensation of thirst. But it can be assumed that the relationships diagrammed in Figure 10–2 are indicative of those operating in the human.

The *sensation of thirst does not adapt.* Again, animal experiments have corroborated this subjective experience. The amount of water consumed after intravenous injection of hypertonic saline solution was shown to be independent of the rate of infusion. That is, the thirst elicited by the injection of a specific amount of solution was the same whether the NaCl concentration rose very slowly or very rapidly. Because thirst does not adapt, the only way to alleviate the sensation is to consume water (cf. Fig. 10–1B).

Satiety. Between the moment drinking is begun and the time the water deficiency is relieved there is a considerable delay; the water in stomach and intestine must first be absorbed (that is, moved into the circulating blood), a process occurring primarily in the small intestine. But it is a common observation, and one repeatedly confirmed in animal experiments, that the feeling of thirst ceases (i. e., drinking is stopped) long before the water deficiency in the extracellular and intracellular spaces could have been compensated. That is to say, *postabsorptive satiety* is preceded by *preabsorptive satiety;* this obviously prevents the consumption of too much water, covering the period until the absorbed water can take effect (Fig. 10–3). Experiments on animals have shown that this preabsorptive mechanism operates with great precision, the amount of water drunk corresponding quite closely with that required in the long run.

The *receptors and underlying mechanisms of preabsorptive satiety* are not known. A dog with an esophageal fistula drinks about twice as much water as a

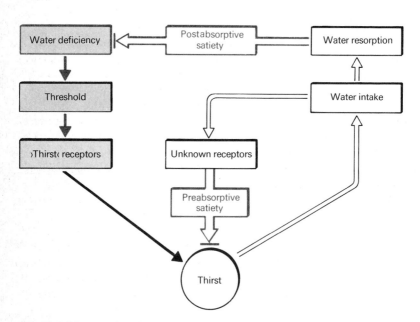

Fig. 10–3. Diagram of preabsorptive and absorptive satiety by water intake. The receptors shown in Fig. 10–2 are indicated here by the single box labeled "Thirst" receptors

normal dog with the same water deficit, and then stops drinking for 20–60 min. Therefore drinking itself, or the associated motor and sensory processes, causes a certain transient relief of thirst. Stretching of the stomach by the fluid consumed also appears to be important. Water poured directly into the stomachs of rats and other animals causes an equivalent reduction of the amount of water drunk. But the associated neural mechanisms remain unclear.

Once the deficit has actually been compensated *(postabsorptive satiety),* a certain time elapses before the sensation of thirst recurs, even though there is a steady (but slow) physiological loss of water. That is, there is a threshold for thirst. As was mentioned at the outset, this threshold is equivalent to a loss of about 0.5% of the body's weight in water. This *thirst threshold* confines the appearance of thirst to occasional intervals; without this, one would rather inefficiently spend a great deal of time drinking small amounts of water. In summary, then, the water content of the human body *fluctuates between a maximum following postabsorptive satiety and a minimum,* which in the ideal case is *a little below the thirst threshold.* But fluctuations in water content of the human body are often greater than this. One reason is that we often consume more water than necessary to compensate for the losses; another is that it is not always possible to satisfy our thirst as soon as it becomes noticeable.

Primary and secondary drinking. Drinking that results from an absolute or relative lack of water in one of the fluid spaces of the body is called *primary drinking,* while drinking with no apparent necessity for water replenishment is called *secondary drinking. Secondary drinking is in fact the usual way* that water is supplied! In general we (and other mammals) tend to consume the physiologically required water in advance. For example, fluid is drunk during and after eating — we seem to have learned to adjust the amount drunk to the kind of food eaten. If it is salty we drink more even in the absence of the sensation of thirst. Habits also appear to play a role, but our information about the mechanisms by which we estimate our water requirements in advance is very sparse. In any case, *primary drinking* is basically an *emergency response* seldom experienced by people leading well-regulated lives.

Clinical thirst. An increase in thirst during illness can be the consequence of *abnormally large water loss,* with the thirst mechanisms functioning normally. On the other hand it can indicate *disturbances of the thirst mechanisms* or of control of *salt/water balance.* Outstanding examples of the first case are the loss of water during continuous vomiting or severe diarrhea, as occurs in cholera. Another well-known example of the first case is diabetes insipidus, in which the lack of antidiuretic hormone, ADH, causes the body to excrete many liters of hypotonic urine per day. These patients suffer from unquenchable thirst, and their entire daily routine revolves about the constant need to drink. Further details of the many aspects of clinical thirst are available in textbooks of pathophysiology and clinical medicine.

Q 10.1. Body water is contained in two large spaces, the intracellular and the extracellular space. The ratio (intracellular volume) : (extracellular volume) is
a) 5 : 1
b) 2 : 1
c) 1 : 1
d) 1 : 3
e) 1 : 10

Q 10.2. The human body consists of about 70%–75% water by weight. The threshold for the appearance of a sensation of thirst is water loss amounting to how much of the body's weight?
a) 0.05%
b) 0.1%
c) 0.5%
d) 1.0%
e) 10.0%

Q 10.3. Which of the following factors participate(s) in generating a feeling of thirst
a) Increase of tonicity of the intracellular fluid
b) Lowering of tonicity of the intracellular fluid
c) Increase of cell volume
d) Decrease of the volume of the extracellular fluid
e) Lowering of the tonicity of the extracellular fluid

Q 10.4. Which receptors are involved in signalling water deficiency in the body?
a) Chemoreceptors in the carotid body
b) Osmoreceptors in the diencephalon
c) Stretch receptors in the stomach
d) Stretch receptors in the swallowing musculature
e) Stretch receptors in the large veins

Q 10.5. Which of the following forms of drinking is the more common in human fluid replenishment?
a) Primary drinking
b) Secondary drinking
c) Primary and secondary drinking are equally common

10.2 Hunger

The need to consume food. The energy balance of any animal is maintained in equilibrium if the energy content of the food corresponds to the energy used up by muscular work, chemical processes (growth, reorganization) and heat loss. Excess food intake causes deposition of fat and thus increase in weight, while lack of food leads first to mobilization and utilization of fat deposits and if prolonged impairs bodily function and eventually causes death.

Man and the other animals nomally adapt their food intake to changing needs, depending on the amount of work done, the climate, and the nutritional value of their food. This *short-term regulation of food intake* is superimposed on a *long-term regulation,* which makes up for temporary inadequacies in the diet and ensures a return to the normal body weight. For example, when animals are fattened by force-feeding and then return to normal conditions, they eat less than control animals. As the animals return to their original control weights, their food consumption slowly increases. Conversely, after a period of fasting the original body weight is regained by temporarily increased food consumption.

Lack of food causes *sensations of hunger,* and the associated feeding drive leads to food intake and eventually to *satiety* (cf. Fig.10–1A). What mechanisms are responsible for eliciting hunger and for the attainment of satiety? One may also ask whether short-term and long-term regulation of food intake are subserved by the same or different mechanisms. In spite of extensive research, these questions have not yet been fully answered. The gaps in our knowledge will become apparent in the discussion that follows.

One clear finding is that several factors are involved in the sensations of hunger and satiety. The relative importance of the various factors, however, is not at all clear, nor is it yet known whether all relevant factors have been discovered.

Factors eliciting hunger. Subjective experience indicates that *hunger* is a *general sensation* localized in (or projected to) the stomach region; it appears when the stomach is empty, and vanishes or gives way to a *feeling of satiety* once the stomach is filled with food. Some early students of the problem postulated that hunger is elicited by *contractions of the empty stomach.* According to these authors this idea is consistent with the finding that the stomach, in addition to the ordinary contractions by which food is processed and transported, also contracts when it is empty. Such contractions appeared to be closely correlated with the occurrence of hunger, so that they could contribute to the sensation. These contractions may possibly be signalled to the CNS by *mechanoreceptors in the stomach wall* (on the left in Fig. 10–4). But the effect of empty-stomach contractions on hunger should not be overestimated; when the stomachs of animals are experimentally denervated or removed altogether, their eating behavior is hardly affected. Thus such contractions may be one factor leading to the sensation of hunger, but it is a dispensable one.

A crucial role in eliciting hunger seems to be played by the glucose (grape or blood sugar) dissolved in the blood. This sugar is the most important source of energy for the cells of the body. The glucose level of the blood and the availability of glucose to the individual cells are controlled hormonally. It has been shown experimentally that a ***decreasing availability of glucose*** (not the blood-sugar level itself) is very well correlated with feelings of hunger and powerful contractions of the stomach. That is, the factor "availability of glucose" is a critical parameter in the development of hunger.

This ***"glucostatic" hypothesis*** is further supported by various experimental findings indicating that ***glucoreceptors*** probably exist in the diencephalon, liver, stomach, and small intestine. For example, when gold thioglucose (gold is a cell poison) is injected into mice many cells in the diencephalon, which apparently take up particularly large amounts of glucose, are destroyed; this damage severely disrupts feeding behavior. That is, the glucoreceptors ordinarily signal a reduced availability of glucose and hence tend to induce hunger (Fig. 10–4).

Another idea about the way hunger is elicited, for which there is less experimental evidence than for the glucostatic hypothesis, is the ***thermostatic hypothesis.*** This is based on the observation that warm-blooded animals consume food in amounts inversely proportional to the temperature of the environment. The colder their surroundings, the more food they eat and vice versa. The internal (central)

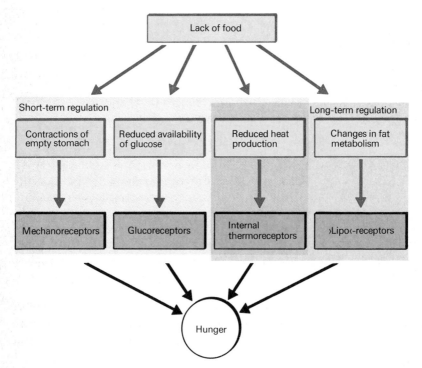

Fig. 10–4. Production of the sensation of hunger. The receptors involved are shown below their adequate stimuli. The factors and receptors involved in short-term and long-term regulation of food intake are grouped within the ***gray shaded areas***

thermoreceptors of the body (cf. Sec. 2.3) could thus serve as sensors in the process of integrating the overall energy balance. A *decline in total heat production* would cause the *internal thermoreceptors* to trigger the sensation of hunger (Fig. 10–4). It is possible to show experimentally that local cooling and warming in the diencephalon, the seat of the central thermoreceptors, can bring about changes in feeding behavior as predicted by this hypothesis; but other interpretations of the same results are not ruled out.

Excessive food intake leads to the deposition of fat in the body, and if food is insufficient the fat deposits are used up. Assuming the existence of *liporeceptors,* such departures from the ideal weight of the body could be monitored by way of the intermediate products of fat metabolism that appear during deposition or utilization; hunger or satiety signals could arise in this way (on the right in Fig. 10–4). There is some good experimental evidence for the *lipostatic hypothesis,* in particular the observation mentioned above that force-fed animals subsequently eat less than under control conditions, until their fat deposits are gone.

In this interpretation, the lipostatic hunger mechanism serves chiefly in *long-term regulation* of food intake, whereas the contractions of the empty stomach and the glucostatic mechanism are primarily involved in *short-term regulation.* The thermostatic mechanism possibly participates in both (cf. the gray shading in Fig. 10–4). With such a variety of physiological mechanisms subserving the feeling of hunger, even under the most complex conditions the sensation of hunger and the feeding drive ensure the consumption of food in appropriate amounts.

Satiety. As in the case of drinking, food consumption by man and other animals is usually stopped long before absorption of the food from the digestive tract has eliminated the energy deficit that originally led to hunger and feeding. All the processes that cause an organism to end its meal are together termed *satiety.* The feeling that one has had enough to eat, as everyone knows from his own experience, is something more than just the disappearance of hunger; among its unique aspects (some of which are associated with pleasure) is the distinct feeling of *fullness* if too much food has been eaten. The sensation of satiety gradually recedes as time passes after a meal and eventually, after a more or less long neutral period, gives way to renewed hunger. By analogy with the processes by which *thirst is quenched,* we can take as a premise that *satiety is initially preabsorptive,* that is, results from processes related to feeding itself, whereas the later absorption of nutrients produces a *postabsorptive satiety* and prevents the immediate recurrence of hunger. We shall now turn to the processes underlying these two kinds of satiety.

A number of factors are probably responsible for *preabsorptive satiety.* Animals with an esophageal fistula — through which the food swallowed leaves the body before reaching the stomach — eat for considerably longer periods than prior to the operation, and repeat their meals at shorter intervals. The stimulation of *olfactory receptors, gustatory receptors, and mechanoreceptors* of nose, mouth, throat, and esophagus that occurs during eating, and possibly the *act of chewing* itself, (on the left in Fig. 10–5) apparently contribute to preabsorptive satiety,

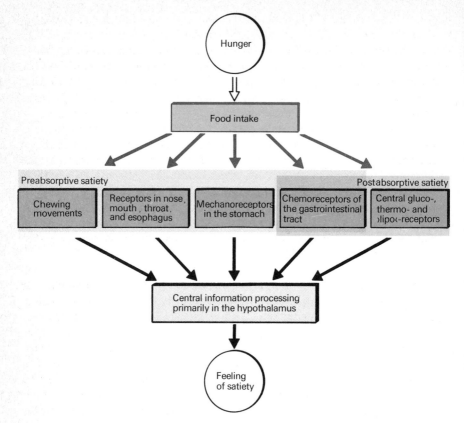

Fig. 10–5. Production of the sensation of satiety by food intake. The factors and receptors involved in preabsorptive and postabsorptive satiety are grouped within the **gray shaded areas.** Chewing movements can contribute to preabsorptive satiety via a direct central efference copy of the motor patterns of chewing, via the receptors activated during chewing (e. g., muscle spindles and tendon organs), or both

although the data at present available suggest that their influence on initiating and maintaining the sensation of satiety is slight. Another factor seems to be the **stretching of the stomach** by the food (middle of Fig. 10–5). If the stomach of an experimental animal is filled through a fistula before its mealtime, there is a reduction in the oral food intake. The **degree of compensation** is related not to the nutritional value of the food, but to the volume of the initial stomach contents and the time they were introduced. In the extreme case, oral food consumption can be inhibited completely for weeks if large amounts of food are put directly into the stomach shortly before the scheduled mealtimes. Stretching of the stomach (and perhaps of the adjacent intestine as well) is therefore certainly involved. Finally, **chemoreceptors** in the stomach and upper parts of the small intestine (Fig. 10–5) are apparently sensitive to the glucose and amino acid content of the food. The existence of appropriate "glucose" and "amino acid" receptors in the intestinal wall has been demonstrated electrophysiologically.

Postabsorptive satiety may also involve the digestive-tract **chemoreceptors** just mentioned, because they can signal the concentrations of utilizable nutrients still remaining in the tract. These are supplemented by all the enteroceptive sensory processes introduced during the discussion of short-term and long-term regulation of hunger. The *increased availability of glucose, increased heat production* as the food is processed, and the *changes in fat metabolism* affect the corresponding central receptors (on the right in Fig. 10–5); the effects are the reverse of those giving rise to hunger (red shading in Fig. 10–4). In this sense hunger and satiety are two sides of the same coin. The (short-term) sensation of hunger triggers eating and the feeling of (preabsorptive) satiety brings it to an end. But the amount of food eaten and the duration of the pauses between meals are also determined by the processes we have called "long-term regulation of food intake" and "postabsorptive satiety" — processes which, as we now realize, overlap more or less extensively (cf. Figs. 10–4 and 10–5).

Psychological factors involved in the regulation of food intake. In addition to the above *physiologic factors* a number of *psychological factors* are involved in the control of feeding behavior. For example, the time at which food is eaten and the amount consumed depend not only on the feeling of hunger, but also on the habitual mealtimes, the amount of food offered, its palatability, and so on. Other animals as well as humans regulate the amount eaten according to when the next mealtime is expected, and how much energy will probably be used in the meanwhile. This element of *planning in feeding behavior,* by which energy is supplied in advance, is analogous to "secondary drinking" (cf. p. 263), the ordinary pattern of water consumption.

Our desire for certain foods is called *appetite.* It can stem from the sensation of hunger or can appear independently (as when one sees or is offered something especially delicious). Appetite often has a somatic basis — for example, the craving for salty food when the body has lost salt — but it can also be independent of physical needs, reflecting innate or acquired individual preferences. Such acquired behavior, as well as rejection of certain foods, is often a matter of food availability and cultural standards, some of which have their roots in religious attitudes. Viewed in this light, the "palatability" of a dish — the predominant elements of which are its smell, taste, consistency, temperature, and the way it is prepared and served — depends very much on our *affective response* to it. Examples are numerous and easily found at regional, national, and international levels.

Practically everyone confronted with a tempting selection of food occasionally eats more than he requires. The *mechanisms of short-term regulation are overruled.* A subsequent reduction in food consumption should ensue, but not everyone in today's affluent societies behaves in this way. The reasons for failure of long-term regulation are, unfortunately, barely understood. Programs for the prevention and treatment of obesity are hard to design and often unsuccessful;

obesity, with all its associated dangers to health, seems to have reached epidemic proportions in many western countries.

In conclusion we must mention the relationship of food consumption to *neuroses and psychoses.* Increased eating, or the refusal of food, is often used as a substitute satisfaction, or protest, when the difficulty actually lies in the areas of other drives. The best known example is *anorexia nervosa,* a form of abstinence from eating most common in girls at puberty; this disturbance in development of the psyche can be so severe as to result in death by starvation.

Central mechanisms of hunger and satiety. The *hypothalamus,* a structure intimately involved in the control of autonomic functions (cf. the section on central mechanisms of thirst), also appears to be the chief central *processing and integrating structure for hunger and satiety.* Bilateral destruction of tissue in certain ventromedial regions of the hypothalamus causes extreme obesity in experimental animals, as a result of overeating. On the other hand, the destruction of more lateral areas can occasion refusal to eat and eventually death by starvation. These findings are paralleled by comparable results of local stimulation via electrodes implanted in the hypothalamus and of experiments with gold thioglucose. Thus for some time the attention of researchers was directed almost exclusively to the hypothalamus. As a result, the *role of other brain structures* in regulating food intake is very little known. It is certainly an oversimplification to say, on the basis of the experiments just mentioned, that the entire central information processing is localized in two hypothalamic "centers", one of which acts as a "satiety center" and the other as a "hunger center". According to this hypothesis destruction of the satiety center would result in disinhibition of the hunger center and hence compulsive eating, whereas if the hunger center were destroyed there would be a permanent sensation of satiety with rejection of all food. But the situation is clearly more complicated. For example, the anticipatory intake of food and liquid mentioned above clearly requires the participation of higher levels of the brain (limbic system, association cortex). Nor should it be overlooked that eating and drinking are complex motor acts that demand correspondingly extensive participation of the motor system.

Q 10.6. Which of the following processes probably participate(s) in producing a sensation of hunger?
   a) An increase in the intermediate products of the metabolic breakdown of fat deposits
   b) A decrease in heat production
   c) Vigorous contractions of the empty stomach
   d) Dryness in the mouth and throat region
   e) Increased availability of glucose

Q 10.7. Which of the following receptors are involved in short-term control of food intake, and which in long-term control? (Some overlap is possible).
   a) Internal thermoreceptors
   b) Mechanoreceptors in the stomach wall

    c) "Lipo"-receptors
    d) Glucoreceptors

Q 10.8. Which of the following receptors are involved in preabsorptive satiety, and which in postabsorptive satiety? (Some overlap is possible).
    a) Glucoreceptors in the diencephalon
    b) Mechanoreceptors in the stomach
    c) Amino-acid receptors in the gastrointestinal tract
    d) Olfactory and taste receptors
    e) Central thermo- and liporeceptors
    f) Glucoreceptors in the gastrointenstinal tract

11 Suggested Reading

The references listed below, mostly major textbooks, monographs and review articles, were chosen by the authors of the individual chapters. Additional references can be found in the corresponding chapters of *Human Physiology* (R.F. SCHMIDT and G. THEWS, eds.: Springer, Berlin — Heidelberg — New York, 1983).

References for Chapter 1

CARTRETTS, E. C., FRIEDMAN, M. P., (eds.): Handbook of Perception, Vol. 1+2. Academic Press New York and London (1974).

GROSSMAN, P.: A Textbook of Physiological Psychology. John Wiley & Sons, Inc. New York — London — Sidney, pp. 1–932, 1967.

HAMANN, W., IGGO, A., (eds.): Sensory receptor mechanisms. Singapore: World Scientific 1984

Handbook of Physiology. I The Nervous System. Vol. III Sensory Processes, Part 1. (Sect. ed. J.M. BROOKHART, V.B. MOUNTCASTLE). Bethesda, Md.: American Physiological Society 1984

Handbook of Sensory Physiology. Vol. 1: Principles of Receptor Physiology (ed. W.R. Loewenstein). Vol. IV: Olfaction (ed. L.M. Beidler). Vol. VII 4: Visual Psychophysics (eds. D. Jameson, L.M. Hurvich). Berlin — Heidelberg — New York: Springer 1971.

MARKS, L. E.: Sensory Processes. New York — London: Academic Press 1974

MILNER, P. M.: Physiological Psychology. Holt, Rinehart and Winston, London — New York — Sidney — Toronto, pp. 1–531, 1971.

RUCH, F. L., ZIMBARDO, P. G.: Psychology and Life, 9th Edition. Scott, Foresman and Company, Glenview — Illinois — London 1975.

STEVENS, S. S.: Psychophysics. New York — London — Sidney — Toronto: John Wiley 1975.

References for Chapter 2

CACIOPPO, J. T., PETTY, R. E. (eds.): Social Psychophysiology. New York — Guilford: 1983.

DE REUCK, A. V. S., KNIGHT, J. (eds.): Touch, Heat and Pain. London: Churchill 1969.

HAMANN, W., IGGO, A. (eds.): Sensory Receptor Mechanisms. Singapore: World Scientific 1984

HÖLZL, R., WHITEHEAD, W. E. (eds.): Psychophysiology of the Gastrointestinal Tract. New York: Plenum Press 1983

IGGO, A. (ed.): Handbook of Sensory Physiology, Vol. II: Somatosensory System. Berlin — Heidelberg — New York: Springer 1973

KENSHALO, D. R. (ed.): Sensory Functions of the Skin of Humans. New York: Plenum Press 1979

KORNHUBER, H. H., ASCHOFF, J. C. (eds.): Somato-Sensory Systems. Stuttgart: Thieme 1976.

ROWE, M., WILLIS, W. D. (eds.): Development, Organization and Processing in Somatosensory Pathways. New York: Alan R. Liss 1985

SCHMIDT, R.F., THEWS, G. (eds.): Human Physiology. Berlin — Heidelberg – New York: Springer 1983.

Schwartz, G.E., Shapiro, D. (eds.): Consciousness and Selfregulation. Vol. I: New York: Wiley 1976.
Sherrington, C.S.: The muscular sense. In: Schäfer's Textbook of Physiology, Vol. 2, 1002–1025. London, Edinburgh: Pentland 1900
Torebjörk, H.E., Schady, W., Ochoa, J.: Sensory correlates of somatic afferent fibre activation. Human Neurobiol. *3*, 15–20, 1984
Vallbo, A.B., Johansson, R.S.: Properties of cutaneous mechanoreceptors in the human hand related to touch sensation. Human Neurobiol. *3*, 3–14, 1984.
Zotterman, Y. (ed.): Sensory Functions of the Skin in Primates. Oxford: Pergamon Press 1976.

References for Chapter 3

Brodal, A.: Neurological Anatomy in Relation to Clinical Medicine. 3rd ed. New York — Oxford: Oxford University Press 1981
Darian-Smith, I.: Touch in primates. Ann. Rev. Psychol. *33*, 155 (1982)
Garner, V.R.: Uncertainty and Structure as Psychological Concepts. New York: John Wiley 1962.
Iggo, A. (ed.): Somatosensory System, Handbook of Sensory Physiology. Berlin — Heidelberg — New York: Springer 1973, Vol. II.
Kenshalo, D.R. (ed.): The Skin Senses. Springfield/III: Charles C. Thomas 1968.
Loewenstein, W.R. (ed.): Principles of Receptor Physiology. Handbook of Sensory Physiology. Berlin — Heidelberg — New York: Springer 1971, Vol. I.
Merzenich, M.M., Kaas, J.H.: Principles of organization of sensory-perceptual systems in mammals. Progress in Psychobiology and Physiological Psychology, Vol. 9, 1 (1980)
Milner, P.M.: Physiological Psychology. London — New York — Sidney — Toronto: Holt, Rinehart & Winston 1970.
Mountcastle, V.B. (ed.): Medical Physiology, 14th ed. St. Louis; Mosby 1980, Vol. I.
Penfield, W., Rasmussen, T.: The Cerebral Cortex of Man. New York: Macmillan 1950.
Ruch, T.C., Patton, H.D.: Physiology and Biophysics. Philadelphia—London: Saunders 1966.
Shannon, C.E., Weaver, W.: The Mathematical Theory of Communication. Urbana: The University of Illinois Press 1949.
Stein, R.B.: The information capacity of nerve cells using a frequency code. Biophys. J. *7*, 797 (1967)
Wiener, N.: Cybernetics, Cambridge/Mass.: MIT Press 1948.
Zimmermann, M.: Neurophysiology of nociception. In: International Review of Physiology, Neurophysiology II. Porter, R. (ed.) University Park Press, Baltimore 1976, Vol. X. pp. 179–221.
Zotterman, Y. (ed.): Sensory Function of the Skin in Primates. Oxford: Pergamon Press 1976.

References for Chapter 4

Bond, M.R.: Pain. Its Nature, Analysis and Treatment. Second Edition. Edinburgh: Churchill Livingstone 1984.
Bromm, B. (ed.): Pain Measurement in Man. Amsterdam: Elsevier 1984
Fordyce, W.E.: Behavioral Methods of Chronic Pain and Illness. Saint Louis: Mosby 1976
Kosterlitz, H.W., Terenius, L.Y. (eds.): Pain and Society. Weinheim: Verlag Chemie 1980
Lewis, Th.: Pain. London: Macmillan 1942. Facsimile edition 1981.
Livingston, W.K.: Pain Mechanisms. New York: Plenum Press 1943. Republication 1976.
Melzack, R., Wall, P.D.: The Challenge of Pain. New York: Basic Books 1983.
Schmidt, R.F., Thews, G. (eds.): Human Physiology, Berlin — Heidelberg — New York: Springer 1983
Wall, P.D., Melzack, R. (eds.): Textbook of Pain. London: Churchill Livingstone 1984

WILLIS, W. D.: Control of nociceptive transmission in the spinal cord. Progress in Sensory Physiology 3 Heidelberg: Springer 1982

WILLIS, W. D.: The Pain System. The neural basis of nociceptive transmission in the mammalian nervous system. Karger, Basel 1985.

References for Chapter 5

BAKER, R., BERTHOUZ, A. (eds.): Control of gaze by brain stem neurons. Amsterdam — New York: Elsevier 1977.

DESMEDT, J. E.: Visual Evoked Potentials in Man: New Developments. Oxford: Clarendon Press 1977.

FUCHS, A. F., BECKER, W. (eds.): Progress in Oculomotor Research. Amsterdam — New York — Oxford: Elsevier 1981.

GRAHAM, C. H. (ed.): Vision and Visual Perception. New York — London — Sidney.: J. Wiley 1965.

GRANIT, R.: Receptors and Sensory Perception. New Haven, Yale University Press 1955.

HELMHOLTZ, H. VON: Physiological Optics (transl. of 3rd edition). New York: Optical Society of America 1924.

HEIN, A., JEANNEROD, M. (eds.): Spatially Oriented Behavior. New York — Berlin — Heidelberg — Tokyo: Springer 1983.

HERING, E.: Outlines of a Theory of the Light Sense (engl. transl.). Cambridge Mass: Harvard Univ. Press 1964.

HOWARD, I. P.: Human Visual Orientation. Chichester – New York: John Wiley 1982.

JUNG, R. (ed.): Handbook of Sensory Physiology. Vols. VII/3a und 3b Berlin — Heidelberg — New York: Springer 1973.

MAFFEI, L. (ed.): Pathophysiology of the Visual System. Den Haag — Boston — London: Junk 1981.

ORBAN, G. A.: Neuronal Operations in the Visual Cortex. Berlin — Heidelberg — New York: Springer 1984.

SCHMIDT, R. F., THEWS, G. (eds.): Human Physiology. Berlin — Heidelberg — New York: Springer 1983.

WALLS, G. L.: The Vertebrate Eye and its Adaptive Radiation. New York — London: Hafner 1963.

WRIGHT, W. D.: The Measurement of Colour. 3. ed. London: Hilger & Watts 1964.

References for Chapter 6

DALLOS, P.: The Auditory Periphery. New York — London: Academic Press 1973.

EVANS, E. F., WILSON, J. P.: Psychophysics and Physiology of Hearing. London: Academic Press 1977.

HENDERSON, D., HAMERNIK, R. P., DARSHAN, S. D., MILLS, H. H. (eds.): Effects of Noise on Hearing. New York: Raven Press 1976.

KEIDEL, W. D., NEFF, W. D. (eds.): Handbook of Sensory Physiology. Berlin — Heidelberg — New York: Springer Verlag 1974, 1975, 1976, Vol. V/1, Vol. V/2, Vol. V/3.

MOORE, B. C. J.: An Introduction to the Psychology of Hearing. London: Academic Press 1982.

PICKLES, J. O.: An Introduction to the Physiology of Hearing. London: Academic Press 1982.

ROEDERER, J. G.: Introduction to the Physics and Psychophysics of Music, 2nd ed. Berlin — Heidelberg — New York: Springer 1975.

TOBIAS, J. V. (ed.): Foundations of Modern Auditory Theory. New York: Academic Press 1970, 1972, Vol. I, Vol. II.

WEBSTER, W. R. ATKIN, L. M.: Central auditory processing. In: GAZZANIGA, M. S., BLAKEMORE, C. (eds.) Handbook of Psychobiology. New York: Academic Press 1975.

References for Chapter 7

BRODAL, A., POMPEIANO, O. (eds.): Basic Aspects of Central Vestibular Mechanisms. Amsterdam: Elsevier Publishing 1972.
KORNHUBER, H. H. (ed.): Handbook of Sensory Physiology. Berlin: Springer-Verlag 1974, Vol. VI/1, VI/2.

References for Chapter 8 and 9

Series: Olfaction and Taste.
V DENTON, D. A. COGHLAN, J. P. (eds.): Olfaction and Taste.
New York — San Francisco — London: Academic Press 1975.
VI LE MAGNEN, J., MAC LEOD, P. (eds.): Olfaction and Taste.
London — Washington DC: Information Retrieval 1977.
VII VAN DER STARRE, H. (ed.): Olfaction and Taste.
London — Washington DC: IRL Press 1980.
BEIDLER, L. M. (ed.): Taste. In: Handbook of Sensory Physiology. Berlin — Heidelberg — New York: Springer 1971, Vol. IV/1.
BEIDLER, L. M. (ed.): Olfaction. In: Handbook of Sensory Physiology. Berlin — Heidelberg — New York: Springer 1971, Vol. IV/2.
BREIPOHL, W. (ed.): Olfaction and Endocrine Regulation. London: IRL Press 1982.
CAIN, W. S. (ed.): Odors: Evaluation, Utilization, and Control. Ann. N. Y., Sci. **237,** 1–439 (1974).
KARE, M. R., MALLER, O. (eds.): The Chemical Senses and Nutrition. New York — San Francisco — London: Academic Press 1977.
NORRIS, M. D. (ed): Perception of Behavioral Chemicals. Amsterdam — New York — Oxford: Elsevier/North Holland 1981.
SHEPHERD, G. M.: The Olfactory Bulb as a Simple Cortical System: Experimental Analysis and Functional Implications. In: SCHMITT, F. O. (ed.): The Neurosciences; Second Study Program. New York: Rockefeller University Press 1970, pp. 539–552.
SHEPHERD, G. M.: Synaptic Organization of the Mammalian Olfactory Bulb. Physiol. Rev. **52,** 864–917 (1972).
SHEPHERD, G. M.: The Synaptic Organization of the Brain. New York — London — Toronto: Oxford University Press 1974.

References for Chapter 10

ANDERSON, B.: Receptors subserving hunger and thirst. In: Handbook of Sensory Physiology, Vol. III/I (ed,. E. NEIL), p. 187. Berlin — Heidelberg — New York: Springer 1972.
ANDERSON, B.: Regulation of Water Intake. Physiol. Rev. **58,** 582, 1978.
CODE, C. F. (ed.): Handbook of Physiology. Section 6: Alimentary Canal, Vol. I: Control of Food and Water Intake. Washington: American Physiological Society 1967.
FITZSIMONS, J. T.: The Physiology of Thirst and Sodium Appetite (Monographs of the Physiological Society, No. 35). Cambridge, England: Cambridge University Press 1979.
HAYWARD, J. N.: Functional and Morphological Aspects of Hypothalamic Neurons. Physiol. Rev. **57,** 574, 1977.
LEIBOWITZ, S. F.: Neurochemical systems of the hypothalamus. Control of feeding and drinking behavior and water-electrolyte excretion. In: P. J. MORGANE, J. PANKSEPP (eds.): Handbook of the Hypothalamus, Vol. 3, Part A, Behavioral Studies of the Hypothalamus. New York, Basel: Marcel Dekker 1980.
MAYER, J.: Regulation of Energy Intake and Body Weight: Glucosatatic Theory and Lipostatic Hypothesis. Ann. N. Y. Acad. Sci. **63,** 15, 1955.

Novin, D., Wyrwicka, W., Bray, G.A. (eds.): Hunger. Basic Mechanisms and Clinical Implications. New York: Raven Press 1976.

Peters, G., Fitzsimons, J.T., Peters-Haefeli, L.: Control Mechanisms of Drinking. Berlin — Heidelberg — New York: Springer 1975.

Pilgrim, F.H.: Human food attitudes and consumption. In: Handbook of Physiology. Sect. 6: Alimentary Canal, Vol. I: Control of Food and Water Intake (ed. C.F. Code), p. 139. Washington: American Physiological Society 1967.

Rolls, B.J., Wood, R.J., Rolls, E.T.: Thirst. The initiation, maintenance, and termination of drinking. In: I.M. Sprague and A.N. Epstein (eds.), Progress in Psychobiology and Physiological Psychology, Vol. 9. New York: Academic Press 1980.

Stunkard, A.J. (ed.): Obesity. Philadelphia: Saunders 1980.

Thompson, C.I.: Controls of Eating. Jamaica, New York: Spectrum 1980.

Wolf, A.V.: Thirst: Physiology of the Urge to Drink and Problems of Water Lack. Springfield/ Ill.: Ch. C. Thomas 1958.

12 Answer Key

Chapter 1

Q1.1: Modality (sense), qualities

Q 1.2: a) M; b) I; c) Q; d) M; e) M; f) Q; g) Q; h) I; i) M

Q 1.3: c

Q 1.4: A learned or acquired reflex in which a particular stimulus regularly elicits a particular activity

Q 1.5: a, d

Q 1.6: b, d

Q 1.7: a, b

Q 1.8: Time, space, quality, intensity (quantity) (in any order)

Q 1.9: a, c, d

Q 1.10: 5

Q 1.11: c

Q 1.12: e

Chapter 2

Q 2.1: c, b, a, d, f, e

Q 2.2: b

Q 2.3: c, e

Q 2.4: c

Q 2.5: c, d

Q 2.6: e

Q 2.7: a

Q 2.8: f

Q 2.9: Senses of position, movement, force

Q 2.10: b, c, e

Q 2.11: e

Q 2.12: b, e, f, g, i

Q 2.13: e, f

Q 2.14: d

Q 2.15: a, b, d

Q 2.16: b, e

Q 2.17: a

Q 2.18: c

Q 2.19: d

Q 2.20: a

Q 2.21: d

Chapter 3

Q 3.1: Mechano-, thermo-, chemo-, and photoreceptors

Q 3.2: b, c

Q 3.3: a, c, d

Q 3.4: c

Q 3.5: b, d

Q 3.6: b, e

Q 3.7: d

Q 3.8: The seven main regions are: spinal cord, medulla oblongata, pons, midbrain, diencephalon, telencephalon, and cerebellum. Medulla, pons, and midbrain together are called the brain stem.

Q 3.9: a, d

Q 3.10: b, c, d

Q 3.11: The difference threshold of a neuron is the smallest change in a stimulus parameter that produces a measurable change in its discharge rate.

Q 3.12:   b, c, d
Q 3.13:   As in Fig. 3–10
Q 3.14:   b, c, d
Q 3.15:   c
Q 3.16:   b, c
Q 3.17:   d
Q 3.18:   b
Q 3.19:   a, c
Q 3.20:   c
Q 3.21:   a, c
Q 3.22:   d

Chapter 4

Q 4.1:   b
Q 4.2:   d
Q 4.3:   Sensory, affective, auto-
          nomic and motor compo-
          nents
Q 4.4:   Depression
Q 4.5:   c
Q 4.6:   a
Q 4.7:   d
Q 4.8:   c
Q 4.9:   d, e
Q 4.10:   e
Q 4.11:   a
Q 4.12:   b
Q 4.13:   b
Q 4.14:   e
Q 4.15:   I: b, c, d, e, II: a, f
Q 4.16:   a
Q 4.17:   b
Q 4.18:   d
Q 4.19:   b
Q 4.20:   c

Chapter 5

Q 5.1:   c
Q 5.2:   Read, near-sighted, con-
          cave
Q 5.3:   b, c, d, f
Q 5.4:   1f + g, 2d, 3b, 4e, 5c, 6h
Q 5.5:   b, d

Q 5.6:   d
Q 5.7:   a, b, c, d, e, f
Q 5.8:   1.25 (minutes of arc)$^{-1}$
Q 5.9:   a, d, e
Q 5.10:   b
Q 5.11:   c
Q 5.13:   b, f
Q 5.14:   a, d, f
Q 5.15:   Activation, inhibition, in-
          hibition, activation, an-
          tagonistic, smaller
Q 5.16:   a, c, e
Q 6.17:   b, c
Q 5.18:   a
Q 5.19:   c, e
Q 5.20:   c, d
Q 5.21:   b

Chapter 6

Q 6.1:   b, a, d, c
Q 6.2:   d
Q 6.3:   c
Q 6.4:   a, c
Q 6.5:   a, c, f
Q 6.6:   b
Q 6.7:   b
Q 6.8:   c
Q 6.9:   c
Q 6.10:   b
Q 6.11:   b
Q 6.12:   c
Q 6.13:   b
Q 6.14:   a
Q 6.15:   a, d, f, g
Q 6.16:   a

Chapter 7

Q 7.1:   a, b, d, e, f
Q 7.2:   b
Q 7.3:   a, b, c
Q 7.4:   c
Q 7.5:   a, b, c, d

Chapter 8

Q 8.1:	c
Q 8.2:	Facial and glossopharyngeal nerves; nucleus of the solitary tract, ventral thalamus, postcentral gyrus
Q 8.3:	1d, 2c, 3b, 4a, 5d, 6b, 7d
Q 8.4:	c
Q 8.5:	1a, 2d
Q 8.6:	d
Q 8.7:	a, b
Q 8.8:	b, c, e

Chapter 9

Q 9.1:	A: b, B: d
Q 9.2:	a, c, d
Q 9.3:	For example: flowery, etheric, musky, camphorous, sweaty, rotten, pungent
Q 9.4:	b
Q 9.5:	c
Q 9.6:	b
Q 9.7:	b
Q 9.8:	b, c, d

Chapter 10

Q 10.1:	b
Q 10.2:	c
Q 10.3:	a, d
Q 10.4:	b, e
Q 10.5:	b
Q 10.6:	a, b, c
Q 10.7:	Short-term control: a, b, d; long-term control: a, c
Q 10.9:	Preabsorptive satiety: b, c, d, f; postabsorptive satiety; a, c, e, f

13 Subject Index

abducens nerve   78
acceleration detector   40–42
accessory nerve   78
accommodation, eye   149
acetylsalicylic acid   137, 138
achromatic series, color vision   163
acid, analgesic   138
acidification, pain   134
acoustical impedance matching   212
acuity, luminance effect   160
–, visual   145, 158–160
adaptation, cone component   161
–, dark   11–13, 174
–, hearing   222
–, light/dark   174
–, mechanoreceptor   37
–, odor stimulus   27
–, olfaction   252
–, pain   128, 129
–, receptor   69, 71
–, retina   158
–, rod component   161
–, sensation   27
–, taste   242
–, thermoreception   54, 61
–, thirst   262
–, vision   161, 178, 179
–, visual   197
–, warm stimulus   27
ADH, thirst   263
afferent inhibition   65
afterimage, visual   158
ageusia   242
agnosia, visual   102, 189
alcohol, visceral sensation   66
algesic substance   134–140
amacrine   176
amacrine cell   153
ampulla, vestibular organ   226
analgesia   134
–, SPA   141
–, stimulation produced   141
analgesic, acetylsalicylic acid   137, 138

–, acid   138
–, aspirin   137, 138
–, morphia   138
–, morphine   138
–, morphium   138
–, narcotic   138, 139
–, non-narcotic   137, 138
anesthesia dolorosa   135
– –, dorsal root transection   141
–, cocaine   139
–, ethyl chloride   139
–, infiltration   139, 140
–, lidocaine   139
–, local   134, 139, 140
–, mepivacaine   139
–, procaine   139
–, therapeutic local   140
angina pectoris   119, 126
animal, consciousness   13
–, identity   13
–, subjectivity   13
annular ligament, ear   201
anorexia nervosa   270
anosmia   250, 255
anterolateral funiculus   91
antidepressant, pain treatment   139
antidiuretic hormone, thirst   263
anvil, middle ear   200
anxiety, pain   120
aorta, pressure receptor   64
appendicitis   119
–, pain   133
appetite   269
ARAS   94
artery, central retina   148
articular receptor   49, s. a. receptor
artificial kidney   259
aspirin   137, 138
association area, cerebral cortex   101, 102
astigmatism, Placido's disk   151
–, vision   151
asymbolia, pain   135
atrium, stretch receptor   260

Fundamentals of
Neurophysiology

Editor: **R. F. Schmidt**
With contributions by J. Dudel, W. Jänig, R. F. Schmidt,
M. Zimmermann

Translated from the German by M. A. Biederman-
Thorson

3rd revised edition. 1985. 139 figures. IX, 346 pages
(Springer Study Edition). ISBN 3-540-96147-X

This is the third edition of Professor Schmidt's popular
book which presents both the essential concepts relevant
to an introductory understanding of neurophysiology and
the most important results of recent neuroscientific
research.
All of the chapters have been updated, including major
revisions to the sections on the autonomic nervous
system and the integrative function of the central nervous
system. Key features of the third edition include:
– new presentation of smooth muscle fiber physiology
– increased emphasis on postsynaptic adrenergic receptors
– coverage of brain metabolism and blood flow
– insights into recent results of research on split-brain
  and aphasic patients.
No prior knowledge of anatomy or physiology is
assumed, and each term is defined and explained as it is
introduced. A collection of early rendered illustrations
enhance the instructional quality of the work. Since its
publication in 1975 nearly 50.000 copies of this work
have been sold worldwide.

G. Thews, P. Vaupel

Autonomic Functions in
Human Physiology

Springer-Verlag
Berlin Heidelberg
New York Tokyo

Translated from the German by M. A. Biederman-
Thorson
1984. 171 figures. IX, 384 pages. ISBN 3-540-13217-1

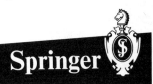

Springer

Human Physiology

Editors: **R. F. Schmidt, G. Thews**

Translated from the German by
M. A. Biederman-Thorson

1983. 569 figures (most in color).
XXI, 725 pages. ISBN 3-540-11669-9

From the reviews:
"**Human Physiology** is a good English translation of Schmidt and Thew's textbook which
has appeared in numerous German editions.
Although there is already an impressive
number of English and American textbooks
for the large medical market, this one could
eventually become a bestseller. The presentation is excellent. The figures are of a uniformly
high standard (mostly they are schematic, in
black, grey, white and red, but with original
records included as required), genuinely help
understanding and are well integrated with the
text. The chapters on neuroscience and the
accounts of the cardiovascular and respiratory
systems are in my opinion superior to those in
comparable medical physiology textbooks.
This will be good enough for some potential
purchasers and **Human Physiology** will be seen
by many dental and medical students as a
good first choice of textbook on the subject."

Nature

Springer-Verlag
Berlin Heidelberg
New York Tokyo

Springer